Recent Advances in Renal Physiology and Pharmacology

Proceedings of the Fifteenth Annual A. N. Richards Symposium, held at Jefferson Medical College in Philadelphia, Pennsylvania, 14-15 May 1973

Sponsored by The Physiological Society of Philadelphia

Recent Advances in Renal Physiology and Pharmacology

Edited by
Laurence G. Wesson, M.D.
Jefferson Medical College

and

George M. Fanelli, Jr., Ph.D.
Merck Institute for Therapeutic Research

MTP
Medical and Technical Publishing Co. Ltd.
Lancaster

Published by
MTP
MEDICAL AND TECHNICAL PUBLISHING CO. LTD.
St. Leonards House
Lancaster, England

First Published by
UNIVERSITY PARK PRESS
Chamber of Commerce Building
Baltimore, Maryland 21202

Printed in the United States of America

ISBN 085200116-9

Contents

VASCULAR AND TUBULAR ASPECTS OF RENAL FUNCTION

RENIN-ANGIOTENSIN SYSTEM

DIURETICS

CLINICAL ASPECTS OF RENAL FUNCTION

Foreword

This volume, containing contributions to the proceedings of the Fifteenth Alfred Newton Richards Symposium, is the first published collection in the Symposium's brief history. Sponsored by The Physiological Society of Philadelphia, an organization which Dr. Richards strongly supported, the symposia are an expansion of the Richards Memorial Lecture Series. This series, presented annually since 1959, is represented in the present symposium by Dr. Gerhard Giebisch's lecture.

Appropriately, kidney function is the subject of this volume. Dr. Richards developed a keen interest in the study of the kidney and made monumental contributions to this field. Stimulated by the technical achievements of Robert Chambers, Dr. Richards and his associates created the subscience of micropuncture investigation of kidney function. The prominence of micropuncture technology is seen in this symposium.

This symposium, *Recent Advances in Renal Physiology and Pharmacology,* illuminates the advances of a broad spectrum comprising molecular structure, clinical applications of knowledge, homeostatic mechanisms, and the molecular biology of transport systems. Although the subject areas are familiar, the many technological advances and conceptual reversals to canonical renal physiology attest to the continuing vigor of this science as a significant area for research.

This symposium was made possible by generous contributions from Abbott Laboratories, Ayerst Laboratories, Hoechst Pharmaceuticals, Lakeside Laboratories, Lederle Laboratories, McNeil Laboratories, Merck Sharp and Dohme Research Laboratories, Penwalt Corporation, A. H. Robins Co., W. H. Rorer, Inc., Sandoz Pharmaceuticals, G. D. Searle and Co., Smith Kline Corp., Sterling-Winthrop Research Institute, The Upjohn Co., The Wellcome Research Laboratories, and Wyeth Laboratories. The editors and The Physiological Society of Philadelphia acknowledge with sincere thanks these contributions.

Laurence G. Wesson
George M. Fanelli, Jr.

Participants in the Symposium

A. Clifford Barger, M.D.
Dept. of Physiology
Harvard Medical School
Boston, Mass. 02115

Karl H. Beyer, Jr., M.D., Ph.D.
Merck Institute for Therapeutic Research
West Point, Pa. 19486

Emile L. Boulpaep, M.D.
Dept. of Physiology
Yale University School of Medicine
New Haven, Conn. 06510

Maurice B. Burg, M.D.
Laboratory of Kidney and Electrolyte Metabolism
National Heart and Lung Institute
National Institutes of Health
Bethesda, Md. 20014

Mortimer M. Civan, M.D.
Dept. of Physiology
University of Pennsylvania School of Medicine
Philadelphia, Pa. 19104

Leo B. Czyzewski, Ph.D.
Hoffmann-La Roche Inc.
Nutley, N.J. 07110

S.L. Engel, Ph.D.
Squibb Institute for Medical Research
Princeton, N.J. 08540

George M. Fanelli, Jr., Ph.D.
Merck Institute for Therapeutic Research
West Point, Pa. 19486

Gerhard Giebisch, M.D.
Dept. of Physiology
Yale University School of Medicine
New Haven, Conn. 06510

Martin Goldberg, M.D.
Dept. of Medicine
University of Pennsylvania School of Medicine
Philadelphia, Pa. 19104

Robert Z. Gussin, Ph.D.
Lederle Laboratories
Division of American Cyanamid Co.
Pearl River, N.Y. 10965

Patrick H. Hernandez, Ph.D.
Sterling-Winthrop Research Institute
Rensselaer, N.Y. 12144

Lorenz M. Hofmann, Ph.D.
G.D. Searle and Co.
Chicago, Ill. 60680

Arnost Kleinzeller, M.D., Ph.D., D.Sc.
Dept. of Physiology
University of Pennsylvania School of Medicine
Philadelphia, Pa. 19104

Garland R. Marshall, Ph.D.
Dept. of Physiology and Biophysics
Washington University School of Medicine
St. Louis, Mo. 63130

Gilbert H. Mudge, M.D.
Dept. of Pharmacology and Toxicology
Dartmouth Medical School
Hanover, N.H. 03755

Philip Needleman, Ph.D.
Dept. of Pharmacology
Washington University
School of Medicine
St. Louis, Mo. 63130

Barbara R. Rennick, M.D.
Dept. of Pharmacology and Therapeutics
State University of New York
Medical School
Buffalo, N.Y. 14214

Richard L. Riley, Ph.D.
Dept. of Physiology and Biophysics
Hahnemann Medical College
Philadelphia, Pa. 19102

Bertram Sacktor, Ph.D.
Gerontological Research Center
National Institute of Child Health and Human Development
Baltimore, Md. 21224

Robert W. Schrier, M.D.
Dept. of Medicine
University of Colorado Medical Center
Denver, Col. 80220

Alexander Scriabine, M.D.
Merck Institute for Therapeutic Research
West Point, Pa. 19486

Thomas H. Steele, M.D.
Dept. of Medicine
University of Wisconsin Center for the Health Sciences
Madison, Wisc. 53706

Charles S. Sweet, Ph.D.
Merck Institute for Therapeutic Research
West Point, Pa. 19486

Samuel O. Thier, M.D.
Dept. of Medicine
University of Pennsylvania
School of Medicine
Philadelphia, Pa. 19104

Heinz Valtin, M.D.
Dept. of Physiology
Dartmouth Medical School
Hanover, N.H. 03755

Irwin M. Weiner, M.D.
Dept. of Pharmacology
State University of New York
Upstate Medical Center
Syracuse, N.Y. 13210

Laurence G. Wesson, M.D.
Dept. of Medicine
Jefferson Medical College
Philadelphia, Pa. 19107

Virgil D. Wiebelhaus, Ph.D.
Smith, Kline, and French Laboratories
Division of Smith Kline Corporation
Philadelphia, Pa. 19101

Gerald R. Zins, Ph.D.
The Upjohn Company
Kalamazoo, Mich. 49001

Pathways of Sugar Transport in Renal Cells

Arnost Kleinzeller
Department of Physiology
University of Pennsylvania School of Medicine
Philadelphia, Pennsylvania

Evidence concerning pathways of sugar transport in renal cells was examined.

1. Phosphorylation of D-galactose, 2-deoxy-D-glucose, and 2-deoxy-D-galactose takes place within the cells and is not part of the transport step. Methyl glycosides are not phosphorylated.
2. The pathways of active sugar accumulation in slices of rabbit kidney cortex were studied on the basis of their electrolyte requirements and inhibition by selective reagents and competing sugars: (a) the Na-independent transport of 2-deoxy-D-hexoses differs from the Na-dependent transport by its lack of stimulation by K^+ and by its reduced sensitivity to phloridzin. D-galactose is simultaneously transported by both Na-dependent and Na-independent pathways; (b) the pattern of competition of sugars for transport sites allows thus far discrimination between two systems: the carrier shared by D-glucose and D-galactose requires hydroxyls on C_2 (in the position found in D-glucose), C_3, and C_6, and a free C_1-OH is not essential, while the D-galactose - 2-deoxy-D-galactose pathway requires a free C_1-OH as well as C_4-OH (in the position of D-galactose) and C_6-OH.
3. At the antiluminal face of flounder kidney tubules, at least three carriers with differing specificities were characterized: a pathway for α-methyl-D-glucoside; a D-glucose and 2-deoxy-D-glucose pathway; a D-galactose - 2-deoxy-D-galactose transport system. No conclusive evidence for active sugar transport at the antiluminal face was found.
4. In the flounder (and probably also the rat) kidney tubule α-methyl-D-glucoside is reabsorbed by an active step at the luminal cell face, followed by a carrier-mediated passive outflow at the antiluminal cell face.
5. Multiple transport pathways for sugars with overlapping specificities and (in part) different cellular localizations are postulated.

The concept of one pathway for the reabsorption of various sugars in the renal tubule stems from two sources. First, observations of Homer Smith and J. A. Shannon and their students (see Smith, 1951) showed that the tubular reabsorption of sugars such as galactose or xylose was inhibited by elevated glucose concentrations, suggesting the sharing of a common transport mechanism in the renal tubule. Second, the active cellular accumulation of some free sugars by intestinal (Crane, 1960; Csáky and Thale, 1960) and renal (Krane and Crane, 1959) epithelial cells led to the suggestion (Csáky and Fernald, 1961) of identical (or very similar) transport mechanisms in both tissues, illustrated by the following scheme (Fig. 1). Here, the active transport step is localized at the luminal brush border, producing a cellular accumulation of the free sugar. The defined structural requirements for active sugar transport by intestinal cells (Crane, 1960) implied one carrier of a rather wide specificity for various sugars. The sugars accumulated in the cells against their concentration gradient were then assumed to pass the antiluminal (serosal) face of the cells in accordance with their chemical gradient, possibly by a carrier-mediated process (e.g. facilitated diffusion). The observation that in renal cells *in vitro* the cellular accumulation of sugars such as D-galactose was Na-dependent (Kleinzeller and Kotyk, 1961), as previously demonstrated for intestinal sugar transport (Csáky and Thale, 1960), strengthened the analogy of transport mechanisms for sugars in both tissues and contributed to the view that one carrier with a rather wide specificity mediated the active transport of various sugars.

Experimental approaches available for an investigation of whether one or several pathways are involved in the transport of a solute in any cell are rather limited. If one pathway of active sugar transport were involved, one would expect identical electrolyte requirements as well as identical patterns of inhibition by reagents selective for the sugar transport system (such as phloridzin) or by other sugar species competing for the shared carrier. In renal cells, in addition to problems of cellular polarity (shared by all epithelial

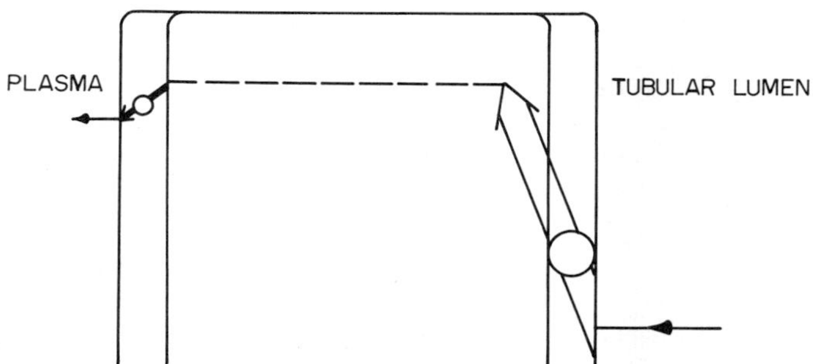

Fig. 1. Simple scheme of transepithelial active sugar transport: White arrow, active transport step; black arrow, carrier-mediated transport (e.g., facilitated diffusion).

cells), the experimental problems are compounded by the complex architecture of the tissue.

Before summarizing present evidence in favor of a multiplicity of transport pathways for sugars in renal tubular cells, it appears appropriate to re-examine the possible relationship between transport and metabolism of some sugars in renal cells.

TRANSPORT AND PHOSPHORYLATION OF SUGARS IN RENAL CELLS

Several years ago we observed major differences in values of free tissue sugars in slices of rabbit kidney cortex when employing different analytical procedures. In the procedure used hitherto in our and other laboratories the analyzed tissue was placed in a solution of $ZnSO_4$ and homogenized. Subsequently, proteins and sugar phosphates were precipitated by the addition of $Ba(OH)_2$. Values obtained for free sugars by this classical Somogyi (1945) procedure were considerably higher for many sugars, such as D-galactose or 2-deoxy-D-glucose, than those found when the tissue was deproteinized with trichloroacetic acid (TCA) and the TCA-free extract fractionated on a Dowex-1 ion exchange column (Kleinzeller, McAvoy, and Griffin, 1973). However, identical values for free tissue sugar were obtained by both methods if, prior to the $ZnSO_4$ + $Ba(OH)_2$ procedure, the tissue enzymes were first inactivated. In the absence of inactivation, the longer the tissue was at room temperature in contact with $ZnSO_4$, the higher values of free sugar were found in the Somogyi supernatant. Thus, as opposed to a widely held belief, a Zn-activated phosphatase catalyses the hydrolysis of sugar phosphates to free sugar. No indication of phosphorylation of α-methyl-D-glucoside (or methyl glycosides of other D-hexoses) was observed, as previously noted by Segal *et al.* (1973) concerning α-methyl-D-glucoside.

The following evidence suggests that the phosphorylation of model sugars such as D-galactose, 2-deoxy-D-glucose, and 2-deoxy-D-galactose takes place within the cells and does not constitute part of the transport step (Kleinzeller *et al.*, 1973). Figure 2 clearly shows that with increasing external pH, the near-steady-state distribution of total (i.e., free plus phosphorylated) tissue galactose in the cells increased while free tissue galactose remained constant. On the other hand, with increasing pH both free and total tissue 2-deoxy-D-galactose decreased. Using tissue homogenates, the same pH dependence could be demonstrated for the phosphorylation of both sugars, i.e., the phosphorylation of galactose increased whereas that of 2-deoxy-D-galactose decreased. Thus, the phosphorylation step is not restricted to preparations with intact cell membranes.

Second, efflux experiments showed that, during the outflow of free D-galactose from the cells, the tissue pool of D-galactose-1-phosphate also decreased with the same rate constants, suggesting that a steady state exists within the cells between free and phosphorylated D-galactose, the dephos-

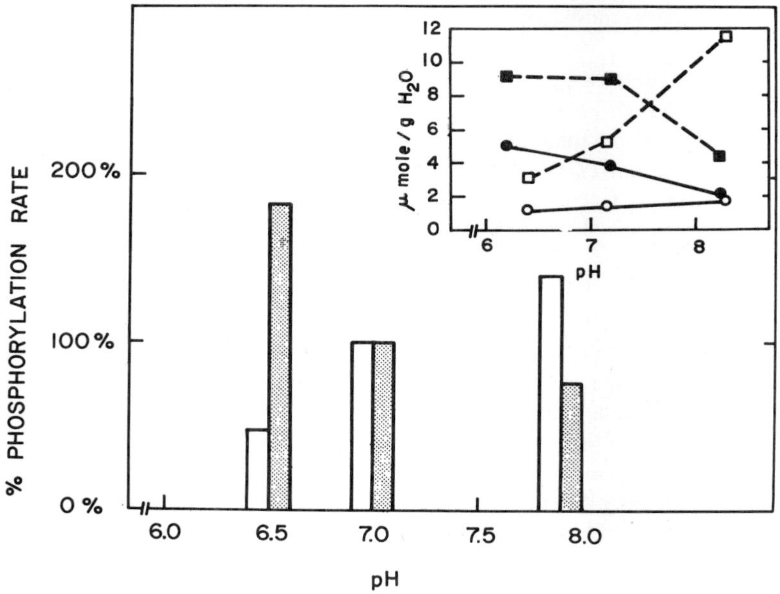

Fig. 2. Effect of pH on the uptake and phosphorylation of D-galactose and 2-deoxy-D-galactose in renal cortex tissue. Insert: Effect of pH on the sugar uptake by slices. Tissue was incubated aerobically (O_2) at 25°C for 60 min in Na-salines at varying pH. Substrates, 1 mM. Each point is the mean of three analyses: ○, □, D-galactose; ●, ■, 2-deoxy-D-galactose; ○, ●, free tissue sugar; □, ■, total (free plus phosphorylated) tissue sugar. Bar graph: Percentage rate of sugar phosphorylation in kidney cortex homogenate (pH 7.0 = 100%). White bars, D-galactose; shaded bars, 2-deoxy-D-galactose.

phorylation of galactose phosphate being the rate-limiting step for the efflux of the free sugar. Using slices of rabbit kidney cortex, the efflux of 2-deoxy-D-glucose or 2-deoxy-D-galactose was not associated with a decrease of the respective phosphates, confirming an observation of Elsas and Macdonell (1972) concerning the former sugar.

Finally, using galactose-1-phosphate as a model, the activation of the dephosphorylation step by Zn^{2+} was demonstrated in homogenates of kidney tissue.

These data are therefore compatible with the following scheme of events. Here the free external sugar (S_o) is transported across the cell membrane (M) by a carrier-mediated process, the active influx of the studied model sugars being energized directly (by ATP) or indirectly (via an electrolyte gradient) by the cell metabolism. Within the cell the free sugar (S_i) is phosphorylated (SP) by a kinase. The reverse process, i.e., hydrolysis of the cellular sugar phosphate, is brought about by a Zn^{2+}-activated phosphatase. In this scheme, K with the appropriate subscript represents the respective rate constants.

EVIDENCE FOR A MULTIPLICITY OF TRANSPORT PATHWAYS

The Electrolyte Requirement

Many of the actively transported sugars were shown (Kleinzeller, Kolínská, and Beneš, 1967; Kleinzeller, 1970b) to require external Na^+ for their cellular accumulation, and K^+ was found to stimulate the active sugar transport. On the other hand, the transport of 2-deoxy-D-sugars was independent of Na^+ and did not require external K^+ (Kleinzeller, 1970b). A considerable portion of D-galactose is also accumulated by renal tubular cells by a Na^+-independent mechanism (Kleinzeller, 1970b) as shown in Fig. 3. These results suggested the possibility of different direct energy sources for the active transport of both groups of sugars. Whereas the Na-dependent transport of sugars such as α-methyl-D-glucoside might be brought about by a mechanism of the Na-gradient type (Almendares and Kleinzeller, 1971), it had to be postulated that the Na-independent active transport of 2-deoxy-hexoses and some other sugars is directly coupled to cellular metabolism, since no evidence was found for other solute gradients capable of driving the up-hill transport of these sugars.

The pH dependence of the active transport of some model sugars (Kleinzeller *et al.*, 1970) suggested a further complication. It had been shown earlier (Fig. 2) that increasing pH had opposite effects on the uptake of sugars such

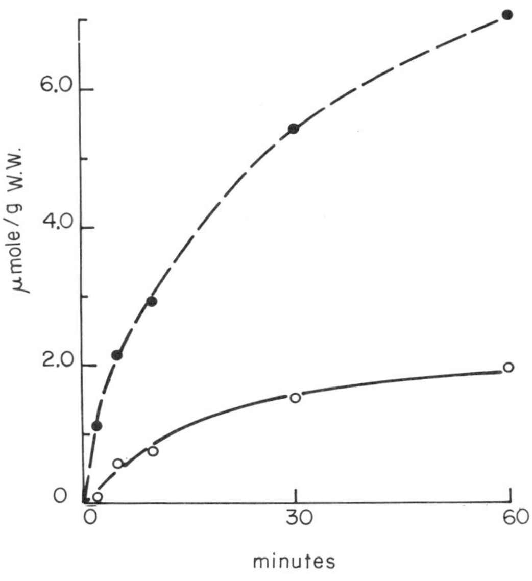

Fig. 3. Uptake of D-galactose by renal cortex slices. Tissue incubated aerobically (O_2) at 25°C for 60 min in Na-free saline (LiCl replacing NaCl) in the presence of 1 mM D-galactose. ○, free tissue sugar; ●, tissue galactose-1 phosphate.

Table 1. Effect of phloridzin and phloretin on sugar accumulation in slices of rabbit kidney cortex

Sugar	Saline	Phloridzin K_i (mM)	Phloretin K_i (mM)
α-Methyl-D-glucoside	Na^+	0.007	0.2
2-Deoxy-D-glucose	Na^+	0.6	0.2
2-Deoxy-D-galactose	Na^+	0.9	0.5
D-Galactose	Na^+	0.06	0.3
D-Galactose	Li^+	0.7	0.4

The tissue was incubated aerobically (O_2) in salines at 25°C for 20 min with 0.5 and 1 mM of the sugars and varying concentrations of the inhibitor. Values of K_i were computed using the Hunter-Downs plot.

as D-galactose and 2-deoxy-D-glucose, as opposed to 2-deoxy-D-galactose. Thus, the possibility of differing pathways for the Na-independent transport of 2-deoxy-glucose and 2-deoxy-galactose had to be considered.

Effect of Inhibitors

The inhibitory action of phloridzin and its aglycon, phloretin, on the active sugar accumulation in slices of rabbit kidney cortex allowed discrimination between two transport pathways (Kleinzeller, 1972). Based on measurements of the inhibition constants (Table 1), the Na-dependent transport pathway for α-methyl-D-glucoside is about 30 times more sensitive to phloridzin than to phloretin. On the other hand, the K_i for the phloridzin inhibition of the Na-independent transport of 2-deoxy-hexoses is two to three times higher than that for phloretin. A comparison of the K_i for the inhibition of D-galactose transport by phloridzin and phloretin in the presence and absence of Na^+ was of particular interest (unpublished data). In the presence of Na^+, the K_i for the phloridzin inhibition was intermediate between that for α-methyl-D-glucoside and the 2-deoxy-D-sugars. In the absence of Na^+, the values of K_i for both inhibitors were of the same order as those found for the inhibition of the 2-deoxy-hexoses. It follows that, in the presence of Na^+, D-galactose is transported simultaneously by both Na-dependent and Na-independent pathways.

Competition of Sugars for Transport Sites

Kinetic data obtained using slices of kidney cortex indicated some discrepancies between the values of transport K_m for a given sugar and the K_i for its competitive inhibitory effect on the transport of another sugar species; such discrepancies would not be expected if one carrier were involved in the transport of both sugars. Therefore, multiple transport pathways with some overlapping specificities have been suggested (Kleinzeller, 1970a). A similar conclusion was independently drawn on the basis of competition of sugars for transport pathways in renal tubules *in vivo* (Silverman, Aganon, and Chinard, 1970). A more detailed investigation of the patterns of specificity of sugar transport in slices of rabbit kidney cortex is now yielding new information (Kleinzeller *et al.*, unpublished). Using [^{3}H] 2-deoxy-D-galactose, no competitive inhibition of the transport of this sugar by 2-deoxy-D-glucose was observed, although the cellular accumulation of 2-deoxy-D-glucose was inhibited by its galactose anomer. This observation provided further indication, in addition to that arising from differing patterns of pH effects on the transport of these two sugars, in favor of different pathways for the Na-independent transport of these two 2-deoxy-D-hexoses.

An active, Na-dependent accumulation of β-methyl-D-galactoside by renal cells was found. Figure 4 shows that the cellular accumulation of this sugar is competitively inhibited by the methyl glycosides of D-glucose, D-galactose, and L-arabinose (pentose homolog of D-galactose), as well as by the hexoses D-glucose and D-galactose. Since the reverse is also true, i.e., β-methyl-D-galactoside inhibits the transport of the above sugars, a single carrier is shared for their transport. Furthermore, it follows that a free hydroxyl on C_1 and its steric position is not essential for the interaction of these sugars with the carrier. On the other hand, α-methyl-D-mannoside and α-methyl-2-deoxy-D-

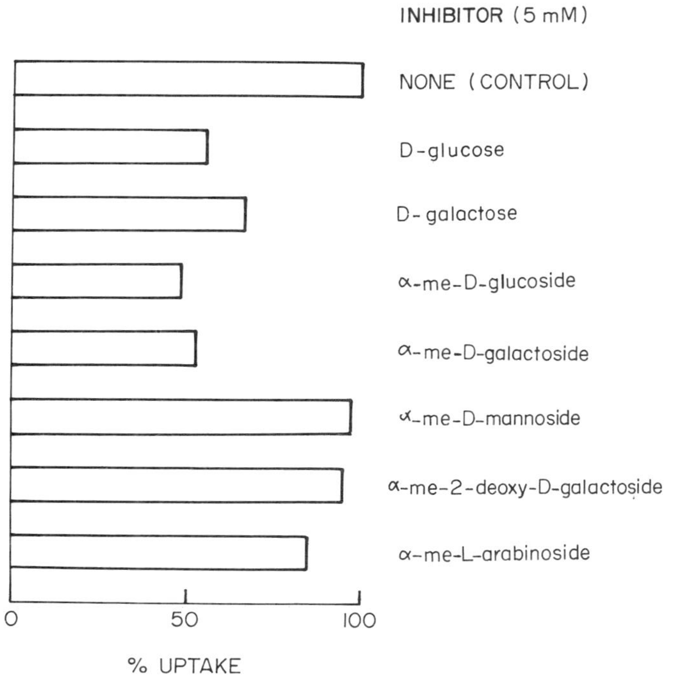

Fig. 4. Competitive inhibition of β-methyl-D-galactoside accumulation in kidney cortex slices. Tissue incubated aerobically (O_2) at 25°C for 60 min in the presence of 1 mM substrate, without (control, 100%) or with 5 mM other sugars (percentage of uptake of control). Each result represents the mean of at least five analyses. Mean accumulation ratio for β-methyl-D-galactoside is 3.0.

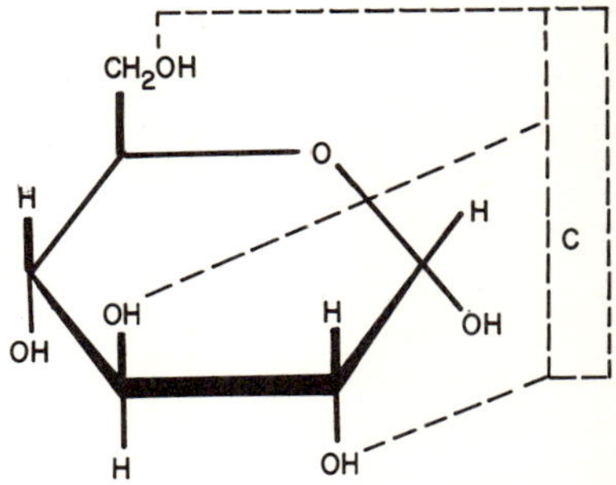

Fig. 5. Structural requirements for the D-glucose - D-galactose transport pathway in renal cortex cells. C, Carrier.

galactoside did not inhibit the accumulation of β-methyl-D-galactoside. Thus, the presence of a hydroxyl on C_2 in the position found in D-glucose (or galactose) is essential for the sugar-carrier interaction. Furthermore, 3-O-methyl-D-glucose, as well as 6-deoxy-D-glucose and its α-methyl derivative were not actively transported by renal cells. Therefore, free hydroxyls on C_3 and C_6 also appear to be part of the structural requirements for this carrier (see Fig. 5).

Figure 6 shows the results of a similar study using 2-deoxy-D-galactose as substrate. It will be noticed that the active cellular accumulation of this sugar was not inhibited by the methyl-glycosides of various sugars. Moreover, methylation of the hydroxyl of 2-deoxy-D-galactose on C_1 prevented the active accumulation of this sugar. We have shown previously that D-galactose was a potent inhibitor of the active accumulation of 2-deoxy-galactose,

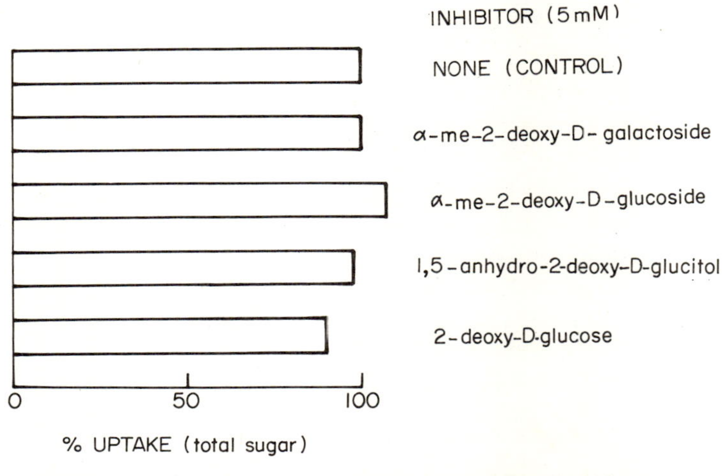

Fig. 6. Competitive inhibition of 2-deoxy-D-galactose uptake in kidney cortex slices. Conditions for incubation and presentation of data as in Fig. 4.

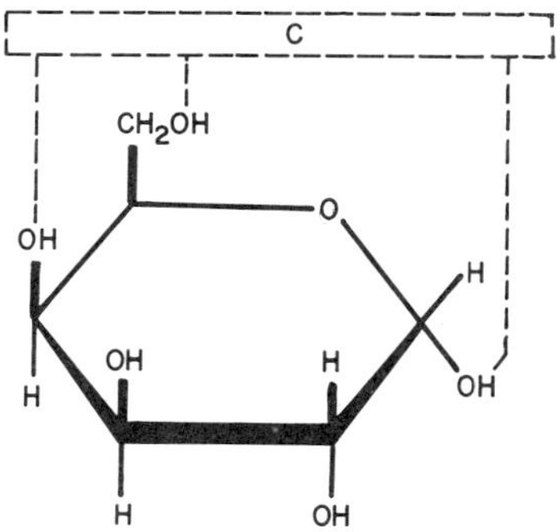

Fig. 7. Structural requirements for the D-galactose - 2-deoxy-D-galactose transport pathway in kidney cortex cells. C, Carrier

whereas D-glucose was ineffective. The structural requirements for the active transport of 2-deoxy-D-galactose thus include a free hydroxyl on C_1 and a hydroxyl on C_4 in the position found in D-galactose. Moreover, since 6-deoxy-galactose (D- and L-) is not actively transported by renal cells (Kleinzeller *et al.*, 1967; Kleinzeller *et al.*, unpublished) C_6-OH also appears to be required for the carrier-sugar interaction. In view of the above data it is not surprising that saccharides without C_1-OH (i.e., 1,5-anhydro-D-glucitol and its 2-deoxy-derivative) were ineffective as inhibitors of the active transport of 2-deoxy-D-galactose. These structural requirements are summarized in Fig. 7.

The above data, and also similar observations concerning the D-glucose derivatives, confirm and extend the conclusion (Kleinzeller *et al.*, 1970) as to a multiplicity and overlapping specificity of transport pathways for sugars in renal cells. In spite of the crucial positions of C_1 and C_6, evidence presented above indicates that phosphorylation on these preferred positions does not constitute a step in the actual transport process.

THE LOCALIZATION OF SUGAR TRANSPORT PROCESSES IN RENAL CELLS

The elegant investigation of Silverman *et al.* (1970) provided evidence for at least two transport pathways for sugars at the luminal face of renal cells with some overlapping specificities, and one pathway for sugar entry at the antiluminal cellular face. We undertook to investigate the specificity of sugar transport at the antiluminal face of flounder renal tubules. The teased tubule of the flounder kidney is particularly suited for such study, since it closes up at its ends and thus offers only the antiluminal face for the entry of solutes. Using this preparation, three distinct carrier-mediated pathways of sugar transport have been defined on the basis of the pattern of competitive inhibition studies (Kleinzeller and McAvoy, 1973): (1) the pathway of α-methyl-D-glucoside, with little affinity for D-glucose or D-galactose; (2) the pathway commonly shared by 2-deoxy-D-glucose and D-glucose; (3) the pathway shared by D-galactose and 2-deoxy-D-galactose. Only in the case of 2-deoxy-D-glucose were indications obtained for an uphill transport system at the antiluminal face. Clearance studies (Kleinzeller, McAvoy, and Pritchard, 1972) showed that α-methyl-D-glucoside is rapidly reabsorbed in the flounder kidney tubule and that during this process a marked cellular accumulation of the sugar in the renal tubular cells took place. The scheme shown in Fig. 1 therefore describes the transport of this sugar in renal cells of the flounder. Work in progress (Kleinzeller and Kormi, unpublished) has now demonstrated a rapid and practically complete reabsorption of α-methyl-glucoside in the rat, again associated with a marked cellular accumulation of this sugar. However, data presented at this conference by Dr. Thier (Ausiello, Segal, and Thier, 1972) require a cautionary note. In the absence of direct information concerning the transport system for this sugar at the antiluminal face of the renal tubular cell of the rat, such a result may only be taken as an indication that the scheme in Fig. 1 is also applicable here. Certainly, the fact that the brush border of renal tubular cells is capable of interacting with α-methyl-glucoside (Sacktor, personal communication) suggests that the active transport step for this sugar is localized at the luminal face of the renal tubular cells.

The sum total of data presented here provides clear evidence for a multiplicity of transport pathways of sugars in renal cells. Only painstaking studies of their respective structural requirements and localization (at the cellular level as well as in the nephron) may provide the rationale for a better understanding of the molecular mechanisms involved in the transport of sugars in renal cells.

ACKNOWLEDGMENTS

The reported investigation was supported by U. S. Public Health Service Grant No. 5 RO1 AM 12619, which is gratefully acknowledged.

REFERENCES

Almendares, J.A., and A. Kleinzeller. 1971. The ouabain inhibition of sugar transport in kidney cortex cells. Archs. Biochem. Biophys. 145: 511–519.

Ausiello, D.A., S. Segal, and S.O. Thier. 1972. Cellular accumulation of L-lysine in rat kidney cortex in vivo. Am. J. Physiol. 222: 1473–1478.

Crane, R.K. 1960. Intestinal absorption of sugars. Physiol. Rev. 40: 789–825.

Csáky, T.Z., and G.W. Fernald. 1961. Localization of the "sugar pump" in the intestinal epithelium. Nature (Lond.), 191: 709–710.

Csáky, T.Z., and M. Thale. 1960. Effect of ionic environment on the intestinal sugar transport. J. Physiol. 151: 59–65.

Elsas, L.J., and R.C. Macdonell, Jr. 1972. Hexose transport and phosphorylation by hamster kidney cortex slices and everted jejunal rings. Biochim. Biophys. Acta 255: 948–959.

Kleinzeller, A. 1970 a. The specificity of the active sugar transport in kidney cortex cells. Biochim. Biophys. Acta 211: 264–276.

Kleinzeller, A. 1970 b. Active sugar transport in renal cortex cells: The electrolyte requirement. Biochim. Biophys. Acta 211: 277–292.

Kleinzeller, A. 1972. The Na-independent transport of sugar in renal tubular cells. *In* E. Heinz (ed.), Na-linked transport of organic solutes, Springer Verlag, Berlin, pp. 109–115.

Kleinzeller, A., D.A. Ausiello, J.A. Almendares, and A.H. Davis. 1970. The effect of pH on sugar transport and ion distribution in kidney cortex cells. Biochim. Biophys. Acta 211: 293–307.

Kleinzeller, A., J. Kolínská, and I. Beneš. 1967. Transport of monosaccharides in kidney cortex cells. Biochem. J. 104: 852–860.

Kleinzeller, A., and A. Kotyk. 1961. Cations and transport of galactose in kidney cortex slices. Biochim. Biophys. Acta 54: 367–369.

Kleinzeller, A., and E.M. McAvoy. 1973. Sugar transport across the peritubular face of renal cells of the flounder. J. Gen. Physiol. 62: 169–184.

Kleinzeller, A., E.M. McAvoy, and P. Griffin. 1973. Transport and phosphorylation of sugars in renal cells. Fed. Proc. 32: 382 (abstr.).

Kleinzeller, A., E.M. McAvoy, and J. Pritchard. 1972. The renal handling of some sugars by the flounder. Bull. Mt. Desert Island Biol. Lab. 12: 64–66.

Krane, S.M., and R.K. Crane. 1959. The accumulation of D-galactose against a concentration gradient by slices of rabbit kidney cortex. J. Biol. Chem. 234: 211–216.

Segal, S., M. Genel, P. Holtzapple, and C. Rea. 1973. Transport of α-methyl-D-glucoside by human kidney cortex. Metabolism 22: 67–76.

Silverman, M., M.A. Aganon, and F.P. Chinard. 1970. Specificity of monosaccharide transport in dog kidney. Am. J. Physiol. 218: 743–750.

Smith, H.W. 1951. The Kidney. Oxford University Press, New York, pp. 101–104.

Somogyi, M. 1945. Determination of blood sugar. J. Biol. Chem. 160: 69–73.

The Interactions of D-Glucose with the Renal Brush Border

Bertram Sacktor, Russell W. Chesney, Michael E. Mitchell, and Peter S. Aronson

Gerontology Research Center
National Institute of Child Health and Human Development
National Institutes of Health
Baltimore City Hospitals
Baltimore, Maryland

The experiments described in this review show that D-glucose interacts in a highly specific manner with isolated renal proximal tubule luminal membranes. The transport of the sugar into membrane-bound vesicles was found. The membranal system was stereospecific, saturable, inhibited by phloridzin and D-glucose analogs, and selectively influenced by Na^+. These findings characterize, in part, the interactions of D-glucose with isolated brush-border membranes. The properties of the *in vitro* membrane system are compared with those of the transport of D-glucose in the intact animal. Each functional feature of sugar transport *in vivo* has its direct counterpart in the brush border system. This excellent correlation between the mechanisms of transport in the brush border membrane and in the intact organism strongly supports the view that the isolated membranes serve advantageously as a model system in studies of the molecular basis of transport in the renal tubule.

The early studies of Shannon and Fisher (1938) and Walker *et al.* (1941), and more recently those of Kleinzeller, Kolinska, and Benes (1967) and Tune and Burg (1971), have led to the concept that the resorption of D-glucose in the kidney is an uphill transport process, energy and Na^+ dependent, sensitive to phloridzin, and localized to the luminal cell membrane of the proximal tubular cell. The preparations used in these studies have ranged from the intact animal, to renal cortical slices, to segments of the isolated tubule. These physiological findings, although contributing significantly to an understanding of the overall sugar transport system in the kidney, do not provide direct information on the molecular mechanisms of the membrane transport.

With the development of procedures for the isolation and biochemical characterization of the renal brush border (Berger and Sacktor, 1970), highly purified preparations of the membrane are now available for an experimental inquiry into the biochemical mechanisms of sugar transport. In this presentation we shall describe some of our studies on the interactions of D-glucose with these isolated rabbit renal membranes, and relate the findings with this model system to what is known of the mechanism of transport in more physiological systems. The observations may also permit some conclusions to be drawn on the biochemical basis of glucose transport in renal tubules.

The renal brush borders used in these studies were isolated from New Zealand white male rabbits weighing 2–3 kg essentially by a modification (Berger and Sacktor, 1970) of the procedure of Thuneberg and Rostgaard (1968). A biochemical evaluation of the preparation, demonstrating the effectiveness of the separation of the luminal membrane from other subcellular components, was made previously (Berger and Sacktor, 1970), and is summarized in Table 1. ATP:NMN adenylyl transferase was used to indicate nuclear contamination. Cytochrome oxidase served as a marker for mitochondria. Lysosomes were indicated by β-glucuronidase, and glucose-6-phosphatase was the marker for microsomes. The specific activities of these enzymes in the final brush border fraction were significantly lower than those in the unfractionated homogenate. Additionally, considerably less than 1% of each of the four enzymes was found in the preparation. In clear contradistinction to the distribution of these enzymes, the disaccharidase, trehalase, showed specific activity increased 12-fold as compared with that of the original homogenate. Some preparations had increases in specific activity as great as 20-fold. The disaccharidase, maltase, had a distribution pattern almost identical with that of trehalase, and, like trehalase, showed a progressive increase in specific activity during the purification of the brush border, resulting in a specific activity approximately 14 times that in the homogenate. Other enzymatic activities found in these preparations of renal brush borders include alkaline phosphatase, a ouabain-sensitive (Na^+ + K^+) ATPase, an oligomycin-insensitive Mg^{2+} ATPase, and a Ca^{2+}-activated ATPase (Berger and Sacktor, 1970). The specific activities of these enzymes were increased 3- to 5-fold in the brush border preparations and activities were found in other subcellular fractions of the renal cortex. Thus, trehalase was considered the preferred enzyme marker for the proximal tubule luminal membrane, and the isolated brush border preparations used in these studies of the interactions of D-glucose with the membranes were randomly examined for trehalase activity.

In addition to evaluating biochemically the preparation of tubular luminal membranes, correlated morphological examinations by phase and electron microscopy were performed. As illustrated in Fig. 1, the preparation of isolated brush borders was homogeneous with only rare contamination with mitochondrial fragments. The microvilli were well preserved and appeared as

Table 1. Biochemical evaluation of the isolated brush border preparation

Enzyme	Specific activity		Percentage recovery[a]	
	Homogenate	Brush borders	All fractions	Brush borders
Trehalase	4.0	48.5	97	13
ATP:NMN adenylyl transferase	1.95	0	67	0
Cytochrome oxidase	0.78	0.04	50	0.2
β-Glucuronidase	0.80	0.15	90	0.6
Glucose-6-phosphatase	3.75	1.30	88	0.1

[a]The percentage recovery is based on the activity in the homogenate, set at 100%. From Berger and Sacktor, 1970.

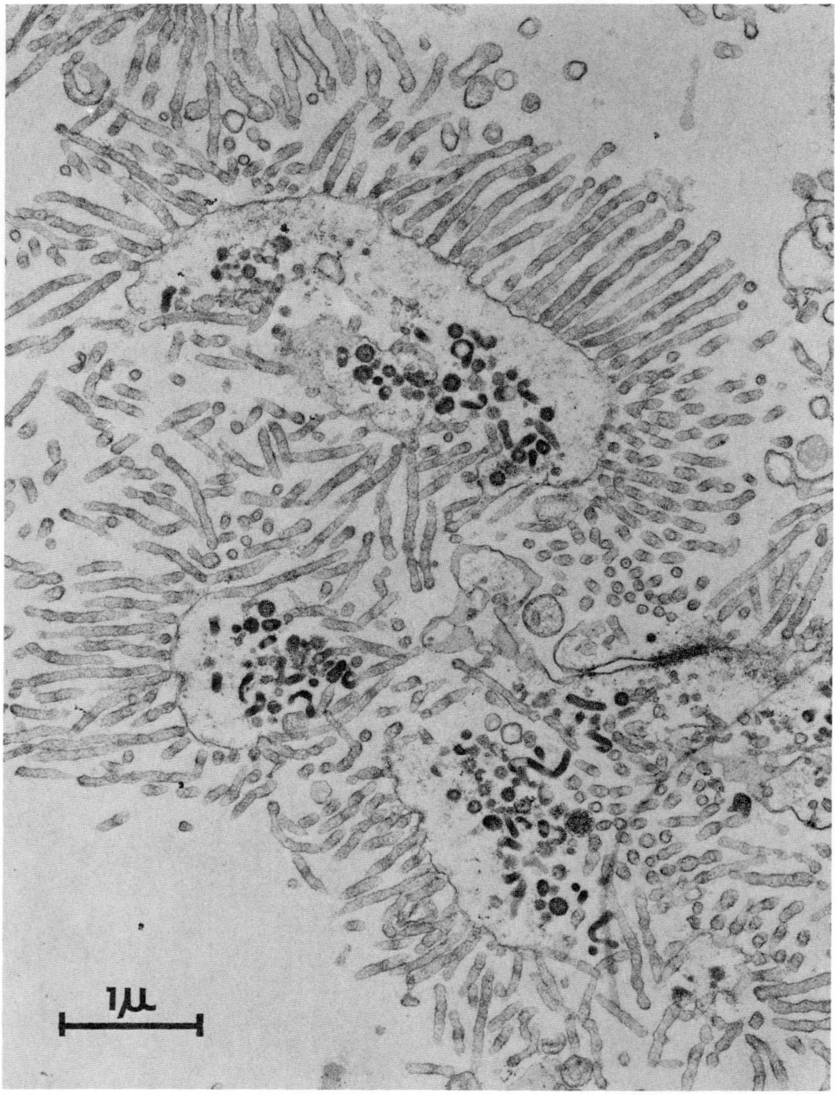

Fig. 1. Electron micrograph of the isolated brush border membranes from rabbit renal cortex. Line, 1 μm. × 23,650.

finger-like projections. Often the entire apical membrane vesiculated with the microvilli extending outward. Occasionally, tight junction structures were seen attached to the brush borders, suggesting the shearing together of the apical membranes of adjacent tubular cells. Higher magnification of the micrographs revealed fibrillar-like figures within and running the length of the microvillus.

Except when otherwise noted, incubations of the membranes with labeled sugar were carried out in Krebs-Ringer bicarbonate buffer, pH 7.4, at 37°C for 1 min, as described in detail elsewhere (Chesney, Sacktor, and Rowen, 1973). The reactions were terminated by rapid dilution and pouring the incubation mixture through Millipore filters. The filters were thoroughly washed, dissolved in scintillation fluid, and counted. All results were corrected for nonspecific binding, as described previously (Chesney, Sacktor, and Rowen, 1973).

In examining the relationship between the D-glucose concentration in the medium and the D-glucose interaction with the membranes, the concentration of the sugar was varied about six orders of magnitude, from 0.1 μM to 100 mM. As shown in Fig. 2, deviation from a linear relationship, hence suggestion of saturability, was evident with concentrations of D-galactose exceeding 5mM. Saturation was incomplete, however, in that a plateau was not reached at concentrations as high as 100 mM. At concentrations below 2mM, D-glucose uptake was dependent in a linear fashion on D-glucose concentration (Aronson and Sacktor, 1973).

The interaction of D-glucose with the luminal membrane was found to be stereospecific. As illustrated in Fig. 3, the uptake of 1 mM D-glucose by the membranes was about four times that of 1 mM L-glucose under these experimental conditions. Moreover, phloridzin significantly inhibited the uptake of D-glucose, whereas the uptake of L-glucose by the membranes was

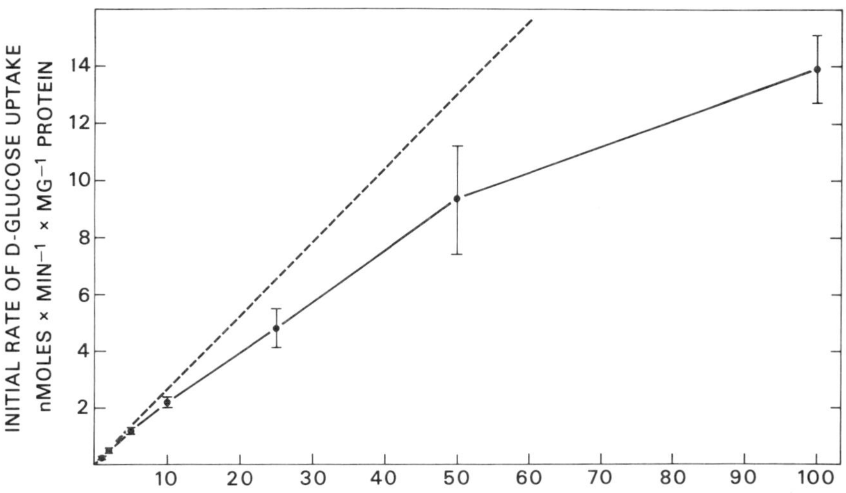

Fig. 2. The dependence of the rate of uptake of D-glucose by renal brush border membranes on the concentration of D-glucose. Mannitol was added so that the sum of the mannitol and D-glucose concentration was always 100 mM; hence, all incubation mixtures were equiosmotic. The dashed line indicates a hypothetical linear relationship between concentration of sugar and initial rate of uptake. (From Aronson and Sacktor, 1973)

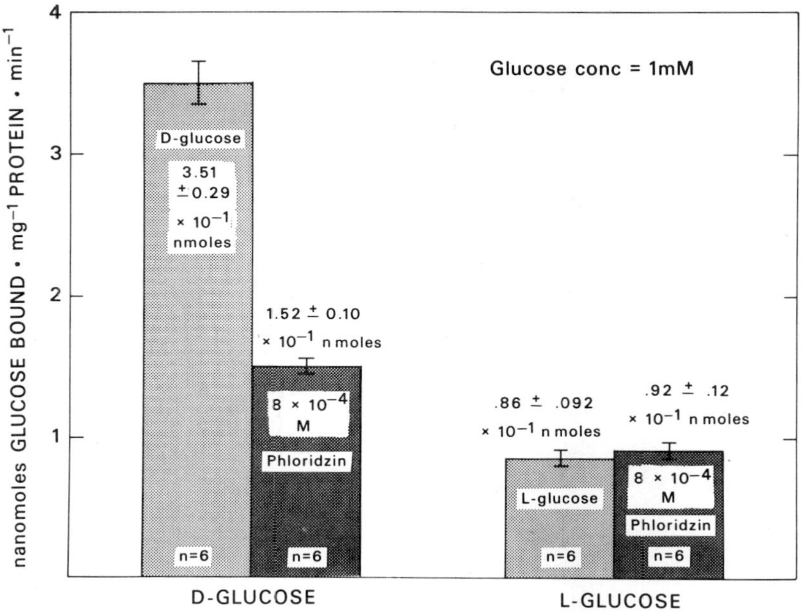

Fig. 3. Comparison of the effect of phloridzin on the interactions of D- and L-glucose with brush border membranes.

insensitive to phloridzin. Other notable differences between the interactions of D- and L-glucose with the brush border membranes were described by Chesney, Sacktor, and Rowen (1973). These included the findings that, when D- and L-glucose were incubated together, the total sugar uptake was the sum of the D-glucose uptake alone plus the L-glucose uptake alone, indicating no effect of one isomer on the interaction of the other. Additionally, D-galactose, an inhibitor of D-glucose uptake, had no effect on the uptake of L-glucose. These findings strongly indicated that the two stereoisomers did not share the same carrier transport system on the proximal tubule luminal membrane.

Phloridzin, the classical inhibitor of active sugar transport in the kidney, was found to inhibit the uptake of D-glucose by the renal brush border membrane (Chesney, Sacktor, and Rowen, 1973). In the μM range of D-glucose, kinetics typical of competitive inhibition were observed, as shown in Fig. 4a. The apparent K_i was approximately 2×10^{-4} M. In the mM range of D-glucose, the kinetics of the inhibition were not consistent with competitive inhibition (Fig. 4b).

It had been reported that inhibition of sugar transport by phloridzin was effected in the absence of detectable levels of the glycoside in the tissues, indicating that the site of phloridzin action was at the membrane level (Stirling, 1967). Since phloridzin inhibited sugar transport competitively and without penetrating the membrane, it had been presumed that the binding site for phloridzin was identical with the receptor site for D-glucose (Frasch *et al.,* 1970). Thus, a study of the binding of phloridzin to the membrane might provide insight into the interaction of D-glucose with the membrane. Accordingly, the interaction of labeled phloridzin with isolated renal proximal tubule luminal membranes was investigated (Chesney, Sacktor, and Kleinzeller, 1974). The binding of phloridzin was greatly dependent on the concentration of the glycoside in the reaction medium. The presence of at least two receptor sites for phloridzin in the brush border membrane was clearly indicated from a Scatchard plot, as shown in Fig. 5. It was calculated that for the binding system that was saturated at low levels of phloridzin the $K_{\text{phloridzin}}$ was 8 μM and 8 $\times$ 10^{-2} nM could interact with 1 mg of membrane protein. At the other receptor site the $K_{\text{phloridzin}}$ was 2.5 mM and 1.25 nM interacted with 1 mg of brush border membrane. These results were in general agreement with the report by Frasch *et al.* (1970) of two binding systems for phloridzin in rat kidney preparations.

It was shown above that phloridzin was a potent inhibitor of the uptake of D-glucose. The converse was also found, namely, that D-glucose inhibited the binding of phloridzin to the brush border membranes (Chesney, Sacktor, and Kleinzeller, 1974). The action of D-glucose at the high-affinity class of phloridzin binding sites is described in Fig. 6. Kinetics typical of competitive inhibition were observed. The apparent K_i was approximately 1 mM. In other experiments it was found that 1 mM L-glucose had no influence on the high-affinity binding of phloridzin. On the other hand, D-galactose, like

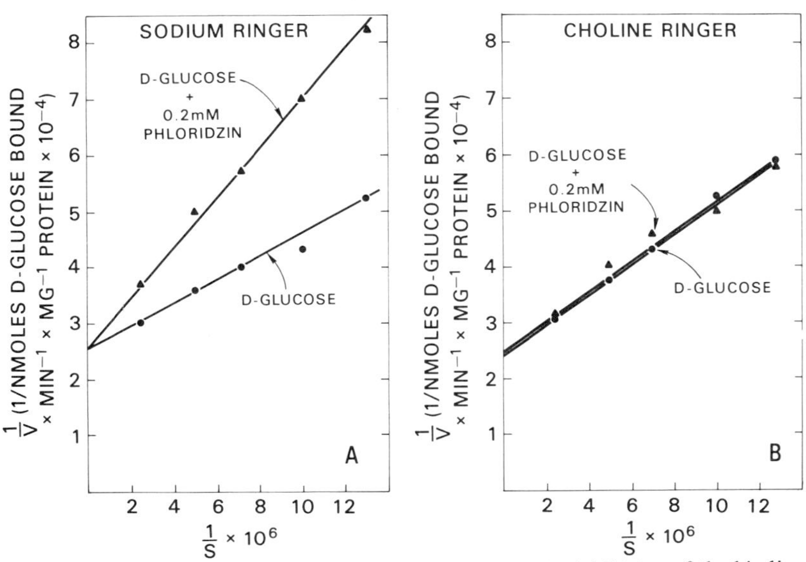

Fig. 4. Lineweaver-Burk plots describing the kinetics of the inhibition of the binding of D-glucose by phloridzin. (From Chesney, Sacktor, and Rowen, 1973.)

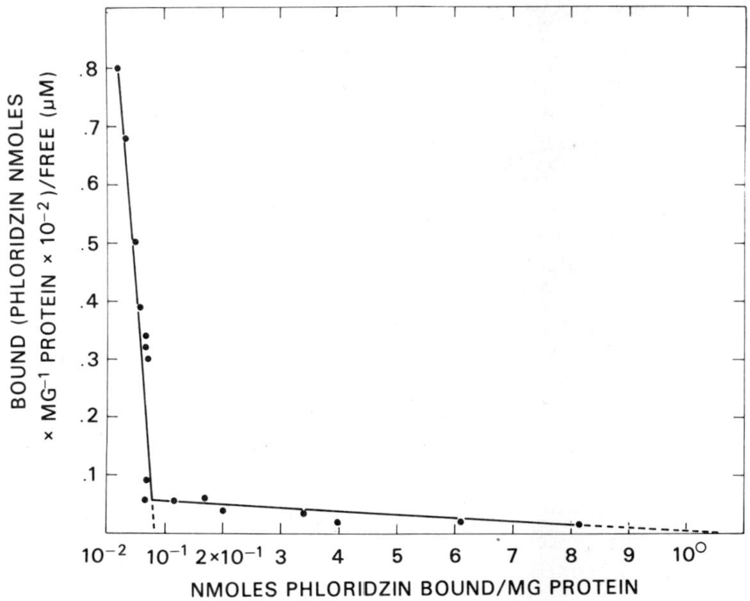

Fig. 5. A Scatchard plot characterizing the relationship between the concentration of phloridzin and its binding. (From Chesney, Sacktor, and Kleinzeller, 1974.)

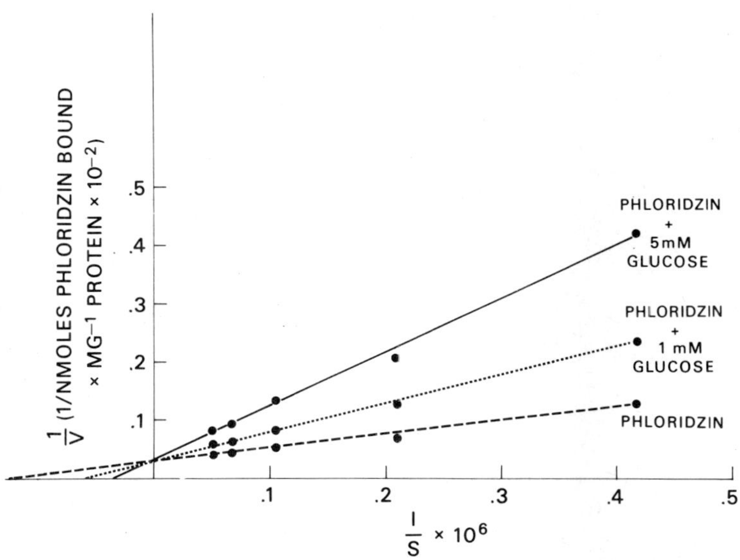

Fig. 6. Lineweaver-Burk plots describing the kinetics of the inhibition of the high-affinity phloridzin binding by D-glucose. (From Chesney, Sacktor, and Kleinzeller, 1974.)

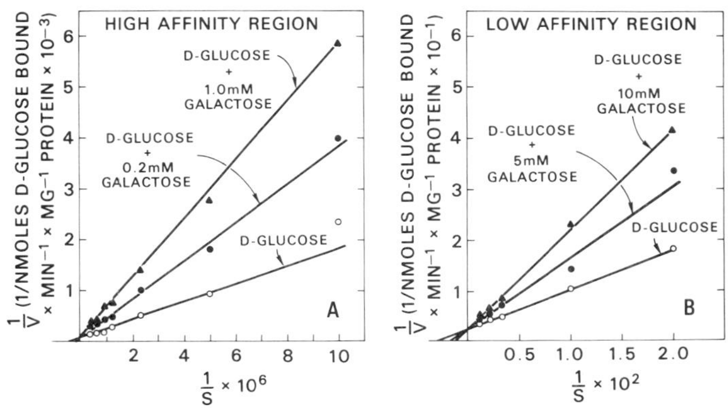

Fig. 7. Lineweaver-Burk plots describing the kinetics of the inhibition of the binding of D-glucose by D-galactose. (Chesney and Sacktor, 1973.)

D-glucose, inhibited the binding of phloridzin. When compared at a concentration of 10 mM, however, D-galactose was not as effective an inhibitor of phloridzin binding as was D-glucose (Chesney, Sacktor, and Kleinzeller, 1974).

Previous investigations had suggested that D-glucose and D-galactose were resorbed in the intact kidney by similar mechanisms (Pitts, 1968), and that the two sugars shared a common pathway (Krane and Crane, 1959; Curran, 1972). Thus, the interactions of these two sugars and other D-glucose analogs with isolated brush border membranes were examined (Chesney and Sacktor, 1973). Figure 7 describes the inhibition by D-galactose of the interactions of D-glucose with the proximal tubule luminal membrane. Kinetics typical of competitive inhibition were found. In the μM range (Fig. 7a) the apparent K_i value was estimated to be about 0.2 mM. In the D-glucose range of D-glucose uptake (Fig. 7b) the K_i value was approximately 8 mM. The mutual interactions of D-glucose and D-galactose with mM the brush border membrane were characterized additionally by experiments described in Fig. 8. The observation that D-galactose was taken up at a rate about 40% that of D-glucose should be noted. Moreover, when [^{3}H] D-galactose and [^{14}C] D-glucose were incubated simultaneously, the value for each labeled sugar was always less than the uptake of each of the species when incubated alone. D-galactose inhibited D-glucose uptake, and D-glucose inhibited D-galactose uptake. Therefore, these data supported the view that D-glucose and D-galactose had common or closely associated carrier sites on the renal brush border membrane.

The interaction of D-glucose with the luminal membranes was examined further by Aronson and Sacktor (1973), in part to resolve the question of whether this interaction represented solely the specific binding of the sugar to receptor sites on the membrane or reflected a preliminary

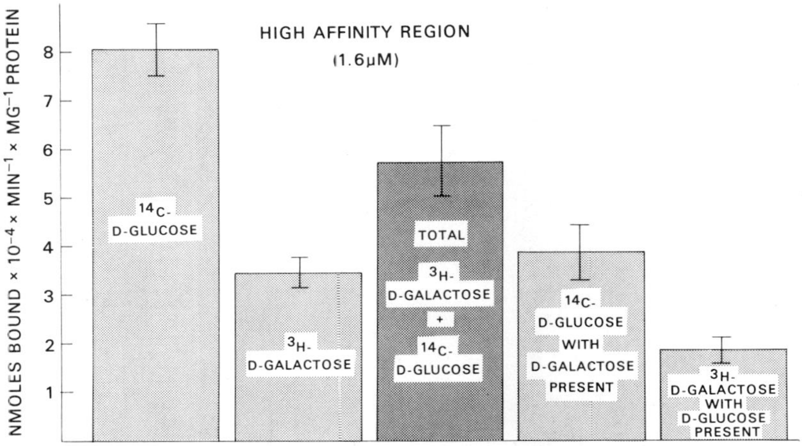

Fig. 8. The mutually competitive uptake of D-glucose and D-galactose.

association followed by the transport of D-glucose into membrane-bound vesicles. If the latter were true, then the isolated brush border membranes could be utilized additionally as a simple, but useful, model to examine many facets of the complex mechanism of sugar transport in the kidney.

As shown in Table 2, when brush border membranes were incubated with 1 mM D-glucose for 24 min at 20°C, at which time steady-state levels of uptake were approached, and then the incubation mixtures were diluted 1:10 in a sugar-free medium and reincubated for an additional 30 sec before the reactions were terminated by Millipore filtration, there was efflux of the previously retained D-glucose. At 20°C, about 35% of the D-glucose was released in the half-minute. Thus, the initial rate of efflux was comparable to the initial rate of influx. Moreover, the rate of efflux was temperature sensitive, as was shown previously for the rate of influx. Remarkably, phloridzin completely inhibited the efflux of D-glucose. If this interaction of

Table 2. Effect of temperature and phloridzin on initial rate of efflux of D-glucose

Experiment	Efflux in 30 sec (%)
Undiluted	0.338 nM/mg prot. (0)
Diluted 1:10,0°C	10 ± 2
Diluted 1:10,20°C	34 ± 2
Diluted 1:10,37°C	58 ± 1
Diluted 1:10,20°C in 1 mM phloridzin	0 ± 2

From Aronson and Sacktor, 1973.

Table 3. Effect of preincubation with sugars on initial rate of uptake of D-glucose

Preincubation (24 min) (mM)	Incubation (30 sec) (mM)	D-glucose uptake (%)
50 Mannitol	25 D-glucose 25 Mannitol	6.02 nM/min/mg prot (100)
50 L-glucose	25 D-glucose 25 L-glucose	107 ± 13
50 D-glucose	25 D-glucose 25 Mannitol	143 ± 11

From Aronson and Sacktor, 1973.

D-glucose with the brush border membrane was simple binding, phloridzin would be expected to displace glucose and augment efflux. These findings are, therefore, consistent with the hypothesis that D-glucose uptake by this system was freely reversible, and that during influx D-glucose was transported to the inside space of membrane vesicles and during efflux the sugar underwent transmembrane movement that was phloridzin sensitive.

Further confirmation that the interaction of D-glucose with the luminal membranes was carrier-mediated transport rather than simple binding came from studies on the effects of preloading the brush border membrane vesicles with sugars. As shown in Table 3, preloading the membranes with D-glucose significantly augmented the uptake of D-glucose relative to a control in which the membranes were preloaded with mannitol. The effect was stereospecific, since preloading with L-glucose gave results not significantly different from those with mannitol. These findings demonstrated that the isolated membranes exhibited the phenomenon of countertransport or facilitated exchange diffusion, a well-established characteristic of carrier-mediated transport systems.

The effects of Na^+ on the transport of D-glucose by the brush border membranes were also examined by Aronson and Sacktor (1973), and some of the findings are reported in Table 4. When the membrane vesicles were prepared in Na^+ or choline medium, thus presumably being loaded with that cation, and then incubated in a medium containing the same cation, there was little difference in rates of D-glucose uptake between the Na^+ and choline systems. Therefore, Na^+ *per se* was not required for the transport of D-glucose into the membrane vesicles, in agreement with the findings of Chesney, Sacktor, and Rowen (1973). However, if Na^+ was added externally to a membrane preparation isolated with choline at the instant of incubation, thereby causing a transient Na^+ gradient from outside to inside, the rate of D-glucose uptake was enhanced by 60%. A Li^+ gradient was ineffective. On

Table 4. Effect of sodium on the initial rate of uptake of 1 mM D-glucose

Incubation medium (mM)	Preparation medium (mM)	D-glucose uptake (%)
130 Sodium	130 Sodium	0.308 nM/min/mg prot (100)
130 Choline	130 Choline	88 ± 7
65 Choline 65 Sodium	130 Choline	140 ± 10
65 Choline 65 Sodium	130 Sodium	89 ± 3
65 Lithium 65 Choline	130 Choline	72 ± 2

From Aronson and Sacktor, 1973.

the other hand, if choline was added externally to a membrane preparation isolated with Na^+, thereby reversing the Na^+ gradient, the transport of D-glucose was inhibited. These findings indicated that, whereas the transport of D-glucose into brush border membrane vesicles did not require Na^+, the process was significantly facilitated by a Na^+ gradient.

The experiments described in this presentation showed that D-glucose interacted in a highly specific manner with isolated renal proximal tubule luminal membranes. The transport of the sugar into membrane-bound vesicles

Table 5. Properties of glucose transport systems *in vivo* and with model membranes

In vivo	Brush border membrane model
Active transport across proximal tubule luminal membrane	Carrier-mediated transport by membrane
T_m behavior mM range	Saturability mM range
Stereospecific	Stereospecific
Inhibited by phloridzin	Inhibited by phloridzin
Competitive with galactose and D-glucose analogs	Inhibited
Na^+ dependent	Dependence on Na^+ gradient

was found. The membranal system was stereospecific, saturable, inhibited by phloridzin and D-glucose analogs, and selectively influenced by Na^+. These findings characterized, in part, the interactions of D-glucose with isolated brush border membranes. In Table 5 the properties of the *in vitro* membrane systems are compared with those of the transport of D-glucose in the intact animal. Each functional feature of sugar transport *in vivo* had its direct counterpart in the brush border systems. This excellent correlation between the mechanisms of transport in the brush border membrane and in the intact organism strongly supports the view that the isolated membranes serve advantageously as a model system in studies of the molecular basis of transport in the renal tubule.

ACKNOWLEDGMENTS

The excellent technical assistance of Margaret A. Weston and Janice A. Barnes is acknowledged. Electron micrographs were skillfully prepared by Joanne P. Alsruhe.

REFERENCES

Aronson, P. S., and B. Sacktor. 1973. Glucose transport by isolated brush border membranes. To be published.

Berger, S. J., and B. Sacktor. 1970. Isolation and characterization of brush borders from rabbit kidney. J. Cell Biol. 47: 637–645.

Chesney, R. W., and B. Sacktor. 1973. Unpublished data.

Chesney, R. W., B. Sacktor, and A. Kleinzeller. 1974. The binding of phloridzin to the isolated luminal membrane of the renal proximal tubule and the interactions of phloridzin and D-glucose at the receptor sites on the brush border membrane. Biochim. Biophys. Acta 332: 263–277.

Chesney, R. W., B. Sacktor, and R. Rowen. 1973. The binding of D-glucose to the isolated luminal membrane of the renal proximal tubule. J. Biol. Chem. 248(6): 2182–2191.

Curran, P. F. 1972. Active transport of amino acids and sugars. Archs Intern. Med. 129: 258–269.

Frasch, W., P. P. Frohnert, F. Bode, K. Baumann, and R. Kinne. 1970. Competitive inhibition of phloridzin binding by D-glucose and the influence of sodium: a study on isolated brush border membrane of rat kidney. Pflügers Arch. Ges. Physiol. 320: 265–284.

Kleinzeller, A., J. Kolinska, and I. Benes. 1967. Transport of monosaccharides in kidney-cortex cells. Biochem. J. 104: 852–860.

Krane, S. M., and R. K. Crane, 1959. The accumulation of D-galactose against a concentration gradient by slices of rabbit kidney cortex. J. Biol. Chem. 234(2): 211–216.

Pitts, R. F. 1968. Physiology of the kidney and body fluids, 2nd ed., Yearbook Medical Publishers, Chicago.

Shannon, J. A., and S. Fisher. 1938. The renal tubular reabsorption of glucose in the normal dog. Am. J. Physiol. 122: 765–774.

Stirling, C. E. 1967. High resolution radioautography of phloridzin-3H in rings of hamster intestine. J. Cell Biol. 35: 605–618.

Thuneberg, L., and J. Rostgaard. 1968. Isolation of brush border fragments from homogenates of rat and rabbit kidney cortex. Exp. Cell Res. 51: 123–140.

Tune, B. M., and M. B. Burg. 1971. Glucose transport by proximal renal tubules. Am. J. Physiol. 221: 580–585.

Walker, A., P. Bott, J. Oliver, and M. MacDowell. 1941. The collection and analysis of fluid from single nephrons of the mammalian kidney. Am. J. Physiol. 134(3): 580–595.

Active Sodium Transport and the Sodium Pool

Mortimer M. Civan
Departments of Physiology and Medicine
University of Pennsylvania School of Medicine
Philadelphia, Pennsylvania

Active sodium transport across epithelia proceeds by sodium entry from the mucosal medium into the transporting cells and extrusion of sodium from these cells into the serosal medium. Measurement of the sodium transport pool is essential in order to characterize these two processes, and in order to relate the mechanisms of cell volume regulation to transepithelial transport. Study of the transport pool has been limited by technical and conceptual difficulties. It is now possible to isolate the transporting epithelial cells from one model system, the urinary bladder of the toad, and to measure their intracellular sodium content. Recent studies using nuclear magnetic resonance suggest that far less intracellular sodium may be bound than had been estimated from previous such studies. However, rigorous measurement of the active transport pool must await more precise quantification of subcellular binding and compartmentalization of sodium. Such investigations are currently in progress.

A variety of *in vitro* model systems have been applied to the study of active sodium transport across renal tubular cells. Of particular interest has been the urinary bladder of the toad (Leaf, 1965), partly because the transport properties of this convenient preparation can be largely ascribed to a single complete layer of epithelial cells (DiBona, Civan, and Leaf, 1969). There is evidence that under appropriate conditions the tissue can actively transport not only Na^+, but also Cl^- (Finn, Handler, and Orloff, 1967; Davies, Martin, and Sharp, 1968), and H_3O^+ (Frazier and Vanatta, 1971; Ludens and Fanestil, 1972), while both vasopressin and aldosterone exert marked effects upon the preparation (Leaf, 1965). Thus, toad bladder appears to be a functional analog of the distal nephron.

Primarily on the basis of intracellular electrical measurements (Frazier, 1962; Civan and Frazier, 1968), active sodium transport has been considered to proceed across toad bladder in two steps: sodium entry from the mucosal medium into the transporting cells, and sodium extrusion from the cell into the serosal medium. In order to characterize these steps more precisely and to relate changes in intracellular composition to changes in transepithelial transport, the concept of a transport pool for sodium is of considerable value (Frazier, Dempsey, and Leaf, 1962). The pool may be defined as that amount of sodium which has entered the epithelial cells from the bathing media and which is readily available for subsequent extrusion into the serosal medium by the sodium pump, a transfer mechanism dependent upon metabolic energy and capable of transporting sodium against an electrochemical gradient. Defined in these terms, the transport pool is not necessarily identical with the intracellular sodium content of the transporting cells.

ISOLATION OF TRANSPORTING CELLS

Early efforts (Crabbé, 1963; Frazier *et al.*, 1962; Janáček and Rybová, 1967; Janáček, Rybová, and Slavíková, 1971; Sharp and Leaf, 1964) to measure the sodium pool of the whole tissue led to conflicting reports, partly because these early measurements necessarily included contributions not only from the epithelial cells, but also from the underlying submucosal and serosal tissue. This experimental difficulty has been resolved with the development by Gatzy and Berndt (1968) of a technique to isolate sheets of intact epithelial cells from the surface of toad bladder. Their technique has since been modified by investigators in several laboratories (Macknight, Leaf, and Civan, 1970; Macknight, DiBona, Leaf, and Civan, 1971; Lipton and Edelman, 1971; Handler, Preston, and Orloff, 1972). Our approach has been to remove and blot the tissue at the conclusion of an experiment, and finally to simply scrape off the epithelial cells with a glass slide. This simple procedure permits analysis of an intact and relatively pure phase of epithelial cells. From observation under phase and electron microscopy, less than 2–3% of the volume of cell scrapings arise from submucosal contamination (Macknight, DiBona, Leaf, and Civan, 1971).

CORRECTION FOR SODIUM IN THE EXTRACELLULAR SPACE

Using this technique the size of the sodium pool is calculated from the sodium content of the isolated cells, from the extracellular sodium concentration of the bulk bathing media, and from a measure of the extracellular space of the cell scrapings. Of these measurements, only the choice of a suitable marker of the extracellular space is a likely source of serious experimental error. In principle, the ideal marker would penetrate the same space throughout which sodium is freely diffusible. Thus the molecule of choice would be the smallest marker which does not freely penetrate the intracellular space of the transporting cells. It has long been assumed that inulin is the most appropriate marker of the extracellular space of toad bladder. Recently, Drs. Anthony Macknight, Qais Al-Awqati, Alexander Leaf, and I re-examined this problem. The results have indicated that the smaller molecules SO_4, mannitol, and sucrose all penetrate the epithelial cells, and that inulin is indeed an appropriate extracellular marker.

Thus the technical problems of isolating the transporting cells and choosing the proper marker of the extracellular space have been resolved. However, another more fundamental problem must also be considered. In certain other epithelia (Kaye *et al.*, 1966; Tormey and Diamond, 1967; Diamond and Bossert, 1967), evidence has been presented suggesting that active transport results in the establishment of a standing gradient for ions throughout the intercellular space. Thus, the concentration of sodium ions in the lateral-basal spaces of the epithelium may be rather different from the sodium concentration of the bulk bathing media. In such an event the true sodium content in the extracellular space would exceed the correction factor calculated by multiplying the extracellular volume by the sodium concentration of the bulk bathing medium. If this error were large, the sodium pool would seem to be directly dependent upon the rate of active sodium transport. In order to investigate whether this problem might be a source of serious error, the following experiments were performed in collaboration with Drs. Macknight and Leaf.

Paired hemibladders were mounted in Lucite chambers. Initially, both mucosal and serosal surfaces were bathed with sodium Ringer's solution and continuously short circuited. Once the short-circuit current had stabilized, the chambers were drained, filled with the appropriate solutions, and the experimental procedure performed. At the conclusion of the experiment, the epithelial cells were removed from both experimental and control sides and analyzed.

When the mucosal medium bathing toad bladder is rendered sodium free, the short-circuit current falls markedly and the sodium content of the cells is significantly reduced (Macknight, Civan, and Leaf, unpublished). The short-circuit current may also be virtually abolished by adding 10 mM ouabain to the serosal bathing medium. Ouabain, which has been thought to be a relatively specific inhibitor of the sodium pump (Herrera, 1966), produced a marked increase in the sodium pool (Macknight, DiBona, Leaf, and Civan, 1971). Similarly, the short-circuit current was increased by two very different maneuvers. First, vasopressin was added to a final serosal concentration of 100 mU/ml. The hormone increases the short-circuit current largely or entirely by enhancing sodium entry into the tissue (Civan, Kedem, and Leaf, 1966; Civan and Frazier, 1968; Macknight *et al.*, 1970; Macknight, Leaf, and Civan, 1971; Handler, Preston, and Orloff, 1972; Yonath and Civan, 1971). The stimulation of short-circuit current was accompanied by an increase in the size of the sodium pool. On the other hand, stimulation of the sodium pump by aerating previously anoxic tissues was associated with an increase in short-circuit current, but with a fall in the size of the sodium pool (Macknight, DiBona, Leaf, and Civan, 1971).

It is clear that changes in the size of the sodium pool and changes in the magnitude of the short-circuit current may be entirely dissociated in our hands, in a manner logically consistent with other information we have concerning the mechanisms of action of these four maneuvers. It seems, therefore, that the techniques described provide a direct measure of the sodium pool.

COMPARTMENTALIZATION

Of even greater concern than the technical difficulties in measuring the total intracellular sodium content have been the conceptual and technical difficulties in determining the distribution and state both of the sodium and water within the cells. Thus it has been unclear just what fraction of the total sodium content constitutes the sodium pool.

Relatively few hard data are as yet available concerning subcellular compartmentalization in, for example, the nucleus and the mitochondria. It is known from the studies of Loewenstein and Kanno (1963) that the nuclear membrane of some cells has a high electrical resistance, and the results obtained by both Mirsky and his colleagues (Allfrey *et al.,* 1961) and Siebert and his group (Siebert and Langendorf, 1970) have more directly indicated that the sodium concentrations in the nucleoplasm and cytoplasm may be very different. In addition, it has long been known that isolated mitochondria can accumulate ions against concentration gradients (MacFarlane and Spencer, 1953; Bartley and Davies, 1954). Thus there are indications that compartmentalization of sodium is indeed present within the subcellular organelles. The amount and significance of such compartmentalization is currently under study in our laboratory.

BINDING

Far more attention has been devoted to the possibility of binding of sodium to macromolecules within the cell. A considerable body of kinetic data, electrophysiologic data obtained with cation-selective microelectrodes, and thermodynamic calculations may be considered to reflect differential binding sites and structured water within the cell. In general these results may be interpreted equally or more plausibly in terms of subcellular compartmentalization and in terms of the complex transport properties of the plasma membrane. More recently, however, a number of studies based on the techniques of nuclear magnetic resonance (NMR) have purported to demonstrate in a far more cogent fashion that the intracellular sodium is largely bound (Cope, 1965, 1967a,b, 1970a,b; Czeisler, Fritz, and Swift, 1970; Ling and Cope, 1969; Martinez, Silvidi, and Stokes, 1969; Rotunno, Kowalewski, and Cereijido, 1967; Reisin *et al.*, 1970).

At least three components are necessary to conduct an NMR experiment. A large steady magnetic field is established along the z-axis, a smaller radiofrequency magnetic field is established along the x-axis, and a receiver coil is oriented along the y-axis. In the absence of a sample with suitable magnetic properties no signal is perceived since the three axes are mutually perpendicular. However, when nuclei with suitable magnetic properties are introduced into the apparatus, a signal is generated. Nuclei whose mass and/or charge numbers are odd possess the property of nuclear spin. A magnetic moment is associated with this spin of a charged body. In the presence of a large steady magnetic field an excess of such nuclei are aligned with the field. When the frequency of the oscillating magnetic field approaches the resonance frequency of the sodium nuclei, magnetic energy is absorbed, inducing a transition to a higher energy state. The intensity of the energy absorbed considered as a function of the frequency of the applied field constitutes the NMR spectrum of the nuclide under study. In practice, it is usually more convenient to obtain the same information by keeping the frequency of the oscillating field constant and sweeping the magnitude of the steady magnetic field through the resonance position.

Biological tissue may be packed into a test tube and the ^{23}Na NMR spectrum determined. The tissue may then be ashed, the volume restored by addition of solvent, and the NMR signal re-examined. Cope (1967a) was the first to observe that the intensity of the ^{23}Na signal before ashing of several preparations was 30–40% of that after ashing, and concluded that the NMR data defined two populations of Na nuclei. One population, constituting 60–70% of the total, was considered to be bound, while a second population, constituting 30–40% of the total, was hypothesized to be free and thought to be solely responsible for the NMR-visible signal. Similar results have now been obtained for a wide variety of biological tissues by a number of investigators who have reached similar conclusions. Despite the unanimity of the conclusions drawn from the published NMR data, it seemed that the data might arise from other mechanisms. Dr. Shporer and I therefore studied the NMR properties of ^{23}Na within a model system, sodium linoleate in water (Shporer and Civan, 1972). These studies, in fact, suggested an alternative interpretation.

The experimental sample was composed of thoroughly mixed equimolar amounts of NaOH and linoleic acid. The control sample was constituted from an identical amount of NaOH mixed with sufficient glycerol to equalize the volume with that of the experimental sample and to provide a comparable line width by increasing the viscosity of the reference solution. The relative integrated intensity of the signal from the sodium linoleate was far smaller than that for the reference signal, although both test tubes contained identical numbers of Na nuclei in identical volumes. On the basis of five such measurements from each of two different experiments containing different samples of material, the central line constituted 39 and 34%, respectively, of the total integrated intensity. The derivative of the NMR spectrum was also recorded. In this more sensitive mode of signal detection two additional satellite signals were easily distinguished, one equally spaced on either side of the central spectral line from the Na linoleate, but not from the control sample (Fig. 1).

One might conclude that binding of 61–66% of the sodium nuclei broadened the ^{23}Na signal beyond detection and that all of the observable

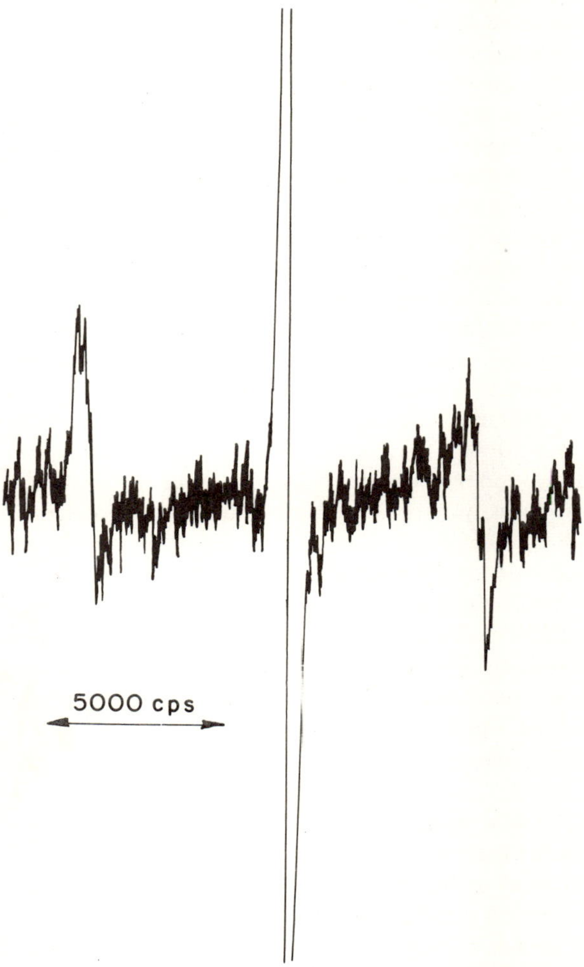

Fig. 1. Derivative of the ^{23}Na signal obtained from sodium linoleate in water (Shporer and Civan, 1972). Two satellite lines are easily distinguished, one on each side of the central signal. (Reprinted with the permission of the Rockefeller University Press.)

signal arose from the 34–39% of the Na nuclei which were free. Such an interpretation, however, would leave inexplicable the observation that satellite signals were clearly demonstrable, an observation in qualitative and quantitative agreement with the concept of a first-order quadrupolar interaction. Nuclides such as ^{23}Na and ^{39}K possess a spin quantum number of 3/2 and a quadrupole moment; therefore, in the presence of an asymmetrical electrical environment, the four possible energy levels will be modified by an electrical energy term. The three permitted energy transitions will then be characterized by different decrements in energy, such that two of the spectral lines will be equally displaced from the central signal (Abragam, 1961). Thus the observed central spectral line arises not from a selected population of the total sodium nuclei, but rather from a single energy transition characterizing all of the sodium nuclei from the soap. Similarly, the fractions of the ^{23}Na spectrum which are not visible in the absorption mode reflect not different populations of sodium nuclei, but rather different energy transitions characterizing all the sodium nuclei.

This interpretation is supported by an examination of the NMR spectrum of the ^{17}O of $H_2{}^{17}O$ in the same model system, sodium linoleate in water (Civan and Shporer, 1972). Since ^{17}O has a spin number of 5/2, a first-order quadrupolar effect for this nuclide should lead to the appearance of four satellite signals, two on each side of the central signal (Abragam, 1961). The expected satellite signals were, in fact, observed using the derivative mode of analysis (Fig. 2).

The basis for the quadrupolar effects in this system cannot be specified from our data. Binding of sodium ions would be only one possible way in which a quadrupolar effect could be produced. The significance of the data lies not in that some fraction of the sodium ions might or might not have been bound, but rather that calculation of the visible fraction of the NMR spectrum for ^{23}Na does not, in itself, permit estimation of the putative binding. Irrespective of the precise fraction, if any, of sodium bound, the approach which had been applied to biological tissue would inevitably lead to an estimate of 60% of the sodium apparently bound. Similar data have since been obtained with unoriented liquid crystals of lecithin-Na-cholate in water (Lindblom, 1971), oriented liquid crystals of Na-decyl sulfate-decyl alcohol-Na_2SO_4 in water (Chen and Reeves, 1972), and oriented DNA samples (Edzes, Rupprecht, and Berendsen, 1972).

It was, of course, uncertain whether the data obtained with biological tissue also reflected a nuclear quadrupolar effect on the ^{23}Na spectrum. Dr. Shporer and I did not observe satellite signals in the frog striated muscle samples we examined. However, because of both technical and theoretical considerations, such a negative result is not helpful in determining whether the NMR data obtained with biological tissue arise from the existence of two distinct populations of Na nuclei with binding of the larger fraction rendering its signal invisible, or from a quadrupolar effect obscuring 60% of the spectral intensity of all the Na nuclei. On the other hand, a review of the published

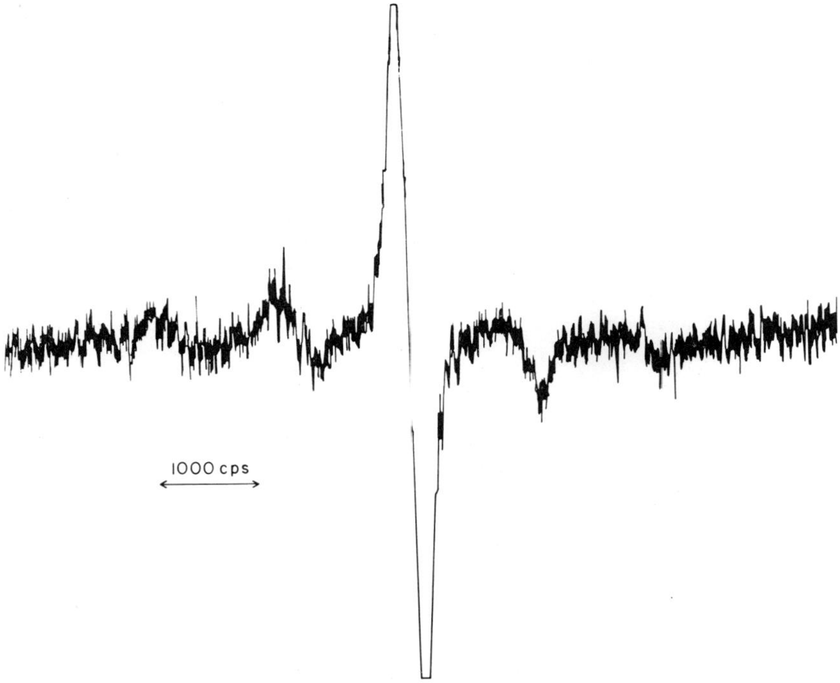

Fig. 2. Derivative of the ^{17}O signal of $H_2\ ^{17}O$ obtained from sodium linoleate in water (Civan and Shporer, 1972). Four satellite signals are clearly distinguished, two on either side of the central signal. (Reprinted with the permission of the Rockefeller University Press.)

data did suggest that a nuclear quadrupolar effect is the more likely mechanism (Shporer and Civan, 1972). The nonvisible fraction of the ^{23}Na spectrum obtained from almost all of the great variety of tissues examined has been close to 60% of the anticipated value, despite the very different compositions of these tissues (Table 1). Such a finding must be considered fortuitous within the framework of two distinct populations of sodium nuclei, but is directly predicted from the concept of a nuclear quadrupolar effect.

Our alternative interpretation of the biological data has received strong support from the studies of striated muscle by Berendsen and Edzes (1973). Although two components of the spin-spin relaxation time were observed, as had been noted previously, only a single spin-lattice relaxation time could be detected. On the basis of these newer data, it seems clear that the NMR data thus far published do not permit ready calculation of the amount of sodium presumed bound within the cell.

I might add that Dr. Shporer and I have been conducting further studies of the ^{23}Na spectrum of frog striated muscle in an effort to quantify the

Table 1. Reported apparent percentage binding of ^{23}Na in biological tissues estimated from NMR studies of ^{23}Na

Tissue	Apparent binding (%)	Reference
Frog muscle	63–72	Cope, 1967a
	58–65	Ling and Cope, 1969
	37	Martinez *et al.*, 1969
	55–63	Czeisler *et al.*, 1970
Rat muscle	65–72	Cope, 1967a
	62	Cope, 1970a
Homogenated frog muscle	65–74	Cope, 1967a
Rabbit muscle actomyosin	48	Cope, 1967a
Frog skin	57–64	Rotunno *et al.*, 1967
	44	Reisin *et al.*, 1970
Rat testicle	24	Reisin *et al.*, 1970
Rabbit kidney	58–70	Cope, 1967a
Rat kidney	67	Cope, 1970a
Rabbit brain	60–70	Cope, 1967a
Rat brain	67	Cope, 1970a
Rabbit myelinated nerve	56	Cope, 1970b
Frog liver	66	Martinez *et al.*, 1969

Shporer and Civan, 1972. Reprinted with permission of the Rockefeller University Press.

amount of the putative binding, assuming that the sodium nuclei do undergo a first-order quadrupolar interaction within frog striated muscle. In these recent studies it has become necessary to define more precisely just what is meant by 'binding.' If, in phenomenologic terms, we consider the bound state to be characterized by severely restricted molecular movement of sodium with respect to its environment, then our preliminary data suggest that only some 1% of the total intracellular sodium is actually bound.

SUMMARY

I should like to stress that the relationship of transepithelial transport to the composition of the intracellular fluids has yet to be rigorously defined. In this regard, precise measurement of the sodium transport pool would be of enormous value. The technical problems in isolating the transporting cells and measuring their intracellular chemical contents have been largely resolved, using at least one suitable model system for renal tubular transport. However, it is still uncertain what fraction of the total sodium content constitutes the sodium pool. The formidable technical and conceptual problems arising from possible subcellular compartmentalization and binding are currently under study.

ACKNOWLEDGMENTS

It is a pleasure to acknowledge the kind permission of the Rockefeller University Press to reproduce Table 1, Fig. 1 (Shporer and Civan, 1972), and Fig. 2 (Civan and Shporer, 1972).

This study was supported in part by a Grant-in-Aid (71-847) from the American Heart Association and Research Grant GB-40040X from the National Science Foundation. The author is an Established Investigator of the American Heart Association.

REFERENCES

Abragam, A. 1961. The Principles of Nuclear Magnetism. Clarendon Press, Oxford.

Allfrey, V.G., R. Meudt, J.W. Hopkins, and A.E. Mirsky. 1961. Sodium-dependent "transport" reactions in the cell nucleus and their role in protein and nucleic acid synthesis. Proc. Natl. Acad. Sci. 47: 907–932.

Bartley, W., and R.E. Davies. 1954. Active transport of ions by sub-cellular particles. Biochem. J. 57: 37–49.

Berendsen, H.J.C., and H.T. Edzes. 1973. The observation and general interpretation of sodium magnetic resonance in biological material. Ann. N.Y. Acad. Sci. 204: 459–480.

Chen, D.M., and L.W. Reeves. 1972. Sodium magnetic resonance in lyotropic nematic phases and the implications for observation in living systems. J. Am. Chem. Soc. 94: 4384–4386.

Civan, M.M., and H.S. Frazier. 1968. The site of the stimulating action of vasopressin on sodium transport in toad bladder. J. Gen. Physiol. 51: 589–605.

Civan, M.M., O. Kedem, and A. Leaf. 1966. Effect of vasopressin on toad bladder under conditions of zero net sodium transport. Am. J. Physiol. 211: 569–575.

Civan, M.M., and M. Shporer. 1972. ^{17}O NMR spectrum of $H_2\,^{17}O$ in frog striated muscle. Biophys. J. 12: 404–413.

Cope, F.W. 1965. Nuclear magnetic resonance evidence for complexing of sodium ions in muscle. Proc. Natl. Acad. Sci. 54: 225–227.

Cope, F.W. 1967a. NMR evidence for complexing of Na^+ in muscle, kidney and brain, and by actinomysin. The relation of cellular complexing of Na^+ to water structure and to transport kinetics. J. Gen. Physiol. 50: 1353–1375.

Cope, F.W. 1967b. A non-equilibrium thermodynamic theory of leakage of complexed Na^+ from muscle, with NMR evidence that the non-complexed fraction of muscle Na^+ is intra-vacuolar rather than extra-cellular. Bull. Math. Biophys. 29: 691–704.

Cope, F.W. 1970a. Spin-echo nuclear magnetic resonance evidence for complexing of sodium ion in muscle, brain and kidney. Biophys. J. 10: 843–858.

Cope, F.W. 1970b. Complexing of sodium ions in myelinated nerve by nuclear magnetic resonance. Physiol. Chem. Phys. 2: 545–550.
Crabbé, J. 1963. Site of action of aldosterone on the bladder of the toad. Nature (Lond.) 200: 787–788.
Czeisler, J.L., O.G. Fritz, Jr., and T.J. Swift. 1970. Direct evidence from nuclear magnetic resonance studies for bound sodium in frog skeletal muscle. Biophys. J. 10: 260–268.
Davies, H.E.F., D.G. Martin, and G.W.G. Sharp. 1968. Differences in the physiological characteristics of bladders from different geographical sources. Biochim. Biophys. Acta 150: 315–318.
Diamond, J.M., and W.G. Bossert. 1967. Standing-gradient osmotic flow: A mechanism for coupling of water and solute transport in epithelia. J. Gen. Physiol. 50: 2061–2083.
DiBona, D.R., M.M. Civan, and A. Leaf. 1969. The anatomic site of the transepithelial permeability barriers of toad bladder. J. Cell Biol. 40: 1–7.
Edzes, H.T., A. Rupprecht, and H.J.C. Berendsen. 1972. Observation of quadrupolar NMR signals of ^{7}Li and ^{23}Na in hydrated oriented DNA. Biochem. Biophys. Res. Commun. 46: 790–794.
Finn, A.L., J.S. Handler, and J. Orloff. 1967. Active chloride transport in the isolated toad bladder. Am. J. Physiol. 213: 179–184.
Frazier, H.S. 1962. The electrical potential profile of the isolated toad bladder. J. Gen. Physiol. 45: 515–528.
Frazier, H.S., E.F. Dempsey, and A. Leaf. 1962. Movement of sodium across the mucosal surface of the isolated toad bladder and its modification by vasopressin. J. Gen. Physiol. 45: 529–543.
Frazier, L.W., and J.C. Vanatta. 1971. Excretion of H^+ and NH_4^+ by the urinary bladder of the acidotic toad and the effect of short-circuit current on the excretion. Biochim. Biophys. Acta 241: 20–29.
Gatzy, J.T., and W.O. Berndt. 1968. Isolated epithelial cells of the toad bladder. Their preparation, oxygen consumption and electrolyte content. J. Gen. Physiol. 51: 770–784.
Handler, J.S., A.S. Preston, and J. Orloff. 1972. Effect of ADH, aldosterone, ouabain, and amiloride on toad bladder epithelial cells. Am. J. Physiol. 222: 1071–1074.
Herrera, F.C. 1966. Action of ouabain on sodium transport in the toad urinary bladder. Am. J. Physiol. 210: 980–986.
Janáček, K., and R. Rybová. 1967. Stimulation of the sodium pump in frog bladder by oxytocin. Nature (Lond.) 215: 992–993.
Janáček, K., R. Rybová, and M. Slavíková. 1971. Independent stimulation of sodium entry and sodium extrusion in frog urinary bladder by aldosterone. Pflügers Arch. Ges. Physiol. 326: 316–323.
Kaye, G.I., H.O. Wheeler, R.T. Whitlock, and N. Lane. 1966. Fluid transport in the rabbit gall bladder: a combined physiological and electron microscopic study. J. Cell Biol. 30: 237–268.
Leaf, A. 1965. Transepithelial transport and its hormonal control in toad bladder. Ergeb. Physiol. 56: 215–263.
Lindblom, G. 1971. Ion binding in liquid crystals studied by NMR. III. ^{23}Na quadrupolar effects in a model membrane system. Acta Chem. Scand. 25: 2767–2768.
Ling, G.N., and F.W. Cope. 1969. Potassium ion: Is the bulk of intracellular K^+ adsorbed? Science (Wash.) 163: 1335–1336.
Lipton, P., and I.S. Edelman. 1971. Effects of aldosterone and vasopressin on electrolytes of toad bladder epithelial cells. Am. J. Physiol. 221: 733–741.

Loewenstein, W.R., and Y. Kanno. 1963. The electrical conductance and potential across the membrane of some cell nuclei. J. Cell Biol. 16: 421–425.

Ludens, J. H., and D. D. Fanestil. 1972. Acidification of urine by the isolated urinary bladder of the toad. Amer. J. Physiol. 223: 1338–1344.

MacFarlane, M.G., and A.G. Spencer. 1953. Changes in the water, sodium and potassium content of rat-liver mitochondria during metabolism. Biochem. J. 54: 569–575.

Macknight, A.D.C., D.R. DiBona, A. Leaf, and M.M. Civan. 1971. Measurements of the composition of epithelial cells from the toad urinary bladder. J. Membrane Biol. 6: 108–126.

Macknight, A.D.C., A. Leaf, and M.M. Civan. 1970. Vasopressin: evidence for the cellular site of the induced permeability change. Biophys. Biochim. Acta 222: 560–563.

Macknight, A.D.C., A. Leaf, and M.M. Civan. 1971. Effects of vasopressin on the water and ionic composition of toad bladder epithelial cells. J. Membrane Biol. 6: 127–137.

Martinez, D., A.A. Silvidi, and R.M. Stokes. 1969. Nuclear magnetic resonance studies of sodium ions in isolated frog muscle and liver. Biophys. J. 9: 1256–1260.

Reisin, I.L., C.A. Rotunno, L. Corchs, V. Kowalewski, and M. Cereijido. 1970. The state of sodium in epithelial tissues as studied by nuclear magnetic resonance. Physiol. Chem. Phys. 2: 171–179.

Rotunno, C.A., V. Kowalewski, and M. Cereijido. 1967. Nuclear spin resonance evidence for complexing of sodium in frog skin. Biochim. Biophys. Acta 135: 170–173.

Sharp, G.W.G., and A. Leaf. 1964. Biological action of aldosterone *in vitro*. Nature (Lond.) 202: 1185–1188.

Shporer, M., and M.M. Civan. 1972. NMR of ^{23}Na linoleate-water: basis for an alternative interpretation of ^{23}Na spectra within cells. Biophys. J. 12: 114–122.

Siebert, G., and H. Langendorf. 1970. Ionenhaushalt im Zellkern. Naturwissenschaften 57: 119–124.

Tormey, J. McD., and J.M. Diamond. 1967. The ultrastructural route of fluid transport in rabbit gall bladder. J. Gen. Physiol. 50: 2031–2060.

Yonath, J., and M.M. Civan. 1971. Determination of the driving force of the Na^+-pump in toad bladder by means of vasopressin. J. Membrane Biol. 5: 366–385.

Amino Acid Transport in the Renal Tubule Cell

Samuel O. Thier
Department of Medicine
Hospital of the University of Pennsylvania
Philadelphia, Pennsylvania

The interpretation of studies of amino acid transport in the kidney based upon a model in which amino acids are filtered and reabsorbed has generated confusion. The confusion stems in large part from apparently contradictory results obtained in clearance studies when compared with studies in kidney cortex slices. A prime example of discrepant results from *in vitro* and *in vivo* studies is in the aminoaciduria, cystinuria. In cystinuria clearance studies have supported the view that cystine and the dibasic amino acids share and compete for the same reabsorptive mechanism. Studies in kidney cortex slices have failed to show competition between cystine and the dibasic amino acids, and further have failed to show a defect for cystine transport *in vitro* in the cystinuric subject. Studies of amino acid uptake by tubular cells *in vivo* were performed. Correlation of these *in vivo* uptake studies with route of amino acid delivery (luminal or antiluminal) and with simultaneous clearance studies suggest a more complex amino acid transport model in the kidney. It is postulated that amino acids are filtered, reabsorbed, and secreted. Cellular accumulation reflects uptake largely from the antiluminal surface of the tubular cell and is altered significantly by competition between amino acids for efflux. Support for this model is found in microinjection studies and double-indicator dilution studies.

The mechanisms by which the renal tubular cell transports amino acids are presently the focus of renewed investigative interest. The confusion resulting from apparently conflicting observations *in vivo* and *in vitro* has begun to be resolved. New concepts of renal amino acid transport capable of reconciling the conflicting data are emerging and one such concept will be the subject of this discussion.

Throughout this discussion it will be critical to recall principles which should have been, but were not always, evident to investigators of renal amino acid transport. Clearance studies give information only about *net* reabsorption or secretion and do not necessarily reflect events occurring specifically at the brush border. Studies of cellular accumulation *in vitro* are not necessarily examining the processes involved in transepithelial transport, nor can accumulation in tissue slices or isolated cells be assumed to represent entry via brush border *versus* lateral or basal cell membrane.

The basic concepts of amino acid transport generated from clearance studies and studies in kidney cortex slices will be reviewed briefly. Apparent inconsistencies between these major *in vivo* and *in vitro* techniques will be noted and, using observations based on the disease cystinuria, a concept of amino acid transport involving both reabsorption and secretion will be developed. Support for this concept also comes from microinjection and double-indicator dilution techniques.

CLEARANCE STUDIES

The renal handling of amino acids is a relatively young field of study. Kirk (1936) studied the clearance of amino acids and concluded that they were filtered and reabsorbed, urinary concentrations being lower than plasma concentrations. Despite the 'black-box' approach implicit in clearance studies a number of critical concepts of amino acid transport arose from these studies. To summarize briefly, renal clearance studies under physiological conditions revealed that (1) amino acids are actively reabsorbed by processes which are saturable at least for some amino acids (Pitts, 1943), (2) preference is shown for L over D amino acids (Crampton and Smyth, 1953) and (3) it is possible to distinguish neutral, from dibasic, from dicarboxylic, from imino acids (Webber, 1962, 1963; Webber, Brown, and Pitts, 1961; Scriver, Efron, and Schafer, 1964). These processes seem less well developed in the newborn, and amino acid clearance is increased in the newborn and decreases with age (Brodehl and Gellissen, 1968). Urinary pH affects the clearance of amino acids, clearance increasing with increasing urinary pH (Braun, Zschaler, and Weiss, 1967), and clearance was also increased by sugars (Fox, Thier, Rosenberg, and Segal, 1964a).

Extension of clearance studies to pathological states participated in the development of the concept that there were genetically determined stereospecific transport mechanisms at the luminal surface of tubular cells. In a disease of transport affecting one of these mechanisms the structurally similar amino acids sharing the mechanism would be expected to be cleared at increased rates. For example, in the disease cystinuria the dibasic amino acids lysine, arginine, and ornithine, and the structurally similar cystine, are cleared at markedly increased rates. It was assumed that these amino acids shared a common transport pathway for which they would compete (Dent, Heathcote, and Joron, 1954; Dent, Senior, and Walshe, 1954). Infusing one member of this group of amino acids did in fact increase the clearance of the others and supported the basic concept (Robson and Rose, 1957). Occasional reports appeared of cystine clearance exceeding inulin clearance (Frimpter *et al.*, 1962; Crawhall *et al.*, 1967) and of the appearance of a previously non-excreted substance such as the mixed disulfide cysteine-homocysteine (Frimpter, 1963), but were not reconciled with the basic concepts. The advantage of the clearance studies was that they dealt with the structurally intact kidney. The disadvantage was that cellular mechanisms could not be defined.

Transport of amino acids in renal tubular cells has been studied most extensively in slices of kidney cortex. Studies in proximal tubular fragments and cells have also been performed and in general have agreed with data from slices.

KIDNEY SLICE STUDIES

In kidney cortex slices the processes involved in amino acid accumulation were frequently considered interchangeably with processes involved in tubular reabsorption *in vivo*. Slice accumulation was found to be an energy-dependent process. Uptake occurs against a chemical gradient by saturable processes which achieve a steady state in 60–90 min (Rosenberg, Blair, and Segal, 1961). Accumulation is in part or totally dependent on medium sodium concentration (Fox, Thier, Rosenberg, and Segal, 1964b). An optimum potassium concentration in the medium of approximately 8 mEq/L has been defined with uptake falling off as potassium concentration is raised or lowered (Fox, Thier, Rosenberg, and Segal, 1964b). Sugars inhibit uptake of amino acids (Thier *et al.*, 1964). These observations in slices are consistent with the concept that the cellular processes are reflecting tubular reabsorption as measured in clearance studies; that is, increased clearance correlates with decreased cellular accumulation. There are, however, a few discrepancies. For example, uptake of amino acids in slices from newborns is higher than in adult tissue as measured by distribution ratios (concentration of intracellular fluid to concentration of medium) (Baerlocher, Scriver, and Mohyuddin, 1970; Segal, Rea, and Smith, 1971); this occurs despite increased clearance of amino acids in newborns. Kinetic analysis in slices from newborns indicates that the increased distribution ratios are due to reduced efflux (Webber, 1968), raising the possibility of a peritubular membrane efflux step. This step would potentially be more complex than diffusion. In addition, increasing pH in the incubation medium increases cellular accumulation in direct contrast to its effect on clearance (Segal and Crawhall, 1968; Segal *et al.*, 1967). However, the most disconcerting difference between *in vivo* and *in vitro* studies came from the studies of cystinuria. Rosenberg, Downing, and Segal (1962) demonstrated that in rat kidney cortex slices the dibasic amino acids lysine, arginine, and ornithine appeared to compete for the same uptake mechanism. Cystine, which according to clearance studies should have

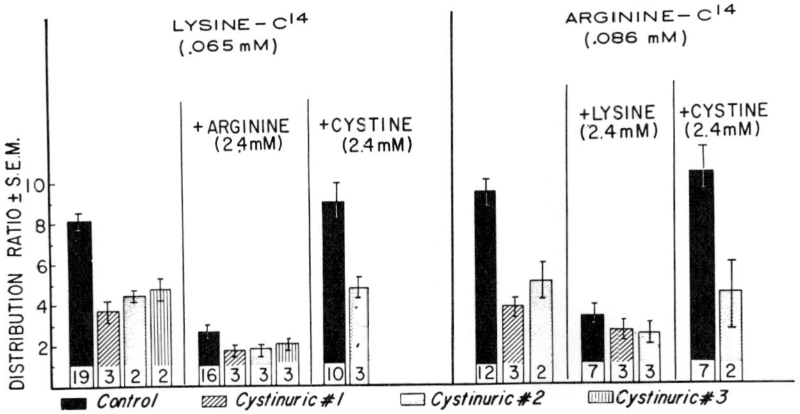

Fig. 1. Distribution ratios for kidney tissue of C^{14} lysine and C^{14} arginine after 30 min incubation without inhibitor and in the presence of arginine and cystine as inhibitors of lysine and lysine and cystine as inhibitors of arginine. The distribution ratio is defined as the ratio of the labeled amino acid concentration in the tissue to that of the incubation medium. (From Bartter, Lotz, Thier, Rosenberg, and Potts, 1965.)

shared this mechanism, neither inhibited nor was inhibited by dibasic amino acids. In subsequent study of renal cortical tissue from cystinuric and non-cystinuric patients obtained at the time of surgery, we obtained similar results (Fox, Thier, Rosenberg, Kiser, and Segal, 1964) (Fig. 1). In tissue from cystinuric subjects the accumulation of lysine and arginine was reduced. Arginine and ornithine inhibited lysine uptake, and lysine inhibited arginine uptake; the inhibition appeared to be competitive. Surprisingly, cystine did not inhibit either lysine or arginine accumulation. Obviously lysine and arginine might have a sufficiently greater affinity for the transport mechanism

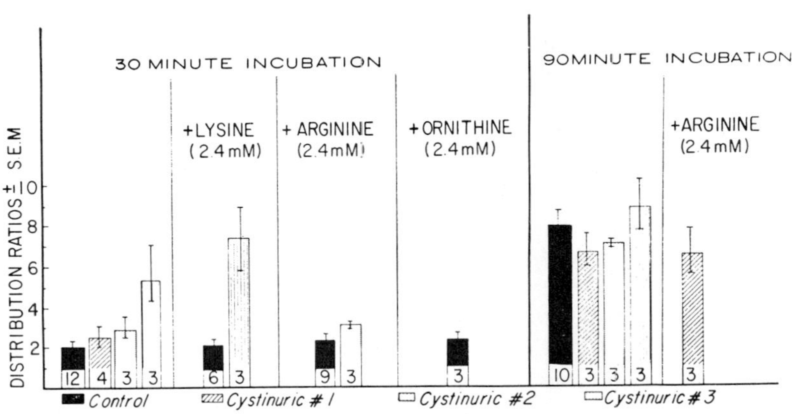

Fig. 2. Distribution ratios for kidney tissue from normal subjects incubated with [^{35}S] cystine (0.01 mM) alone or in the presence of lysine, arginine, or ornithine (From Bartter, Lotz, Thier, Rosenberg, and Potts, 1965.)

than cystine, resulting in an inability of cystine to displace them at achievable concentrations. If that were the case, cystine accumulation might be expected to be reduced by lysine or arginine. In fact, cystine uptake in cystinuric tissue was normal and was unaffected by lysine or arginine (Fig. 2). These findings in kidney slices were particularly disturbing, since in gut from the same patients defective cystine transport was demonstrable and interaction between cystine and dibasic amino acids occurred (Thier *et al.*, 1965). The question then was what was the slice measuring and what relationship did it have to tubular reabsorption *in vivo*. Wedeen and Thier (1971), studying cellular accumulation of para-aminohippuric acid (PAH) and alpha-aminoisobutysic acid (AIB) autoradiographically, noted that AIB accumulation was maximal in the straight segments of the proximal tubule. Since stopflow and more sophisticated microperfusion studies localized amino acid reabsorption to the proximal convolution, the autoradiographic studies suggested that uptake might be unrelated to transepithelial tubular reabosrption. It was subsequently noted by Wedeen that in kidney cortex slices sucrose and inulin distribute throughout the extracellular fluid but do not have access to proximal tubular lumina. In comparable slices AIB is concentrated in proximal tubule cells presumably without entering the lumen (Wedeen and Weiner, 1973). In order to examine luminal and cellular processes a series of collaborative studies were undertaken (Ausiello, Segal, and Thier, 1972; Greth, Thier, and Segal, 1973).

MATERIALS AND METHODS

Lysine was studied initially, but since it may bind to many cell components, including the cell membrane, its exact localization within the slice may be questioned. Cystine, on the other hand, is transported into the cell as cystine, and then rapidly metabolized to cysteine and reduced glutathione. Measurement of the metabolites of radioactive cystine assures that cell entry has occurred. In fact, the results of the cystine studies were exactly comparable to those obtained with lysine, but in the interest of brevity only the cystine data will be presented.

Cystine labeled with ^{35}S was injected into the tail vein of rats. At appropriate times the rats were sacrificed by stunning and decapitation. Blood was collected in heparinized dishes and the plasma was separated for counting and chromatography. Kidneys were removed and slices of cortex were made for analysis of intracellular radioactivity. Both kidney homogenates and plasma were reacted with N-ethylmaleimide (NEM) and analyzed on cellulose thin-layer chromatograms for cystine metabolites.

RESULTS

Figure 3 shows the disappearance of plasma radioactivity. A two-exponential decay is noted. The rapid decay is believed to represent entry into cells, while

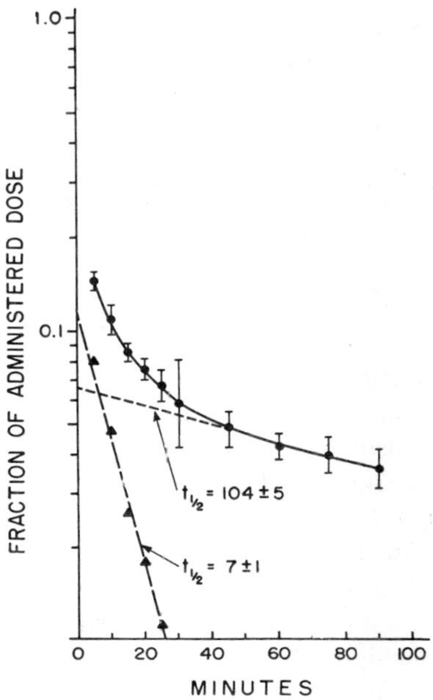

Fig. 3. The rate of disappearance of plasma radioactivity after injection of 28.8 μCi of L-[^{35}S]cystine. The log of the fraction of the administered dose in plasma and extracellular fluid is plotted *versus* time after injection. Each point is the average ± s.e. of six determinations. (From Greth, Thier, and Segal, 1973.)

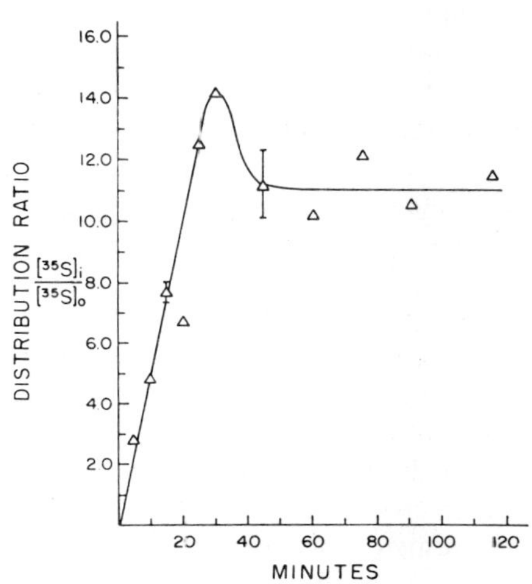

Fig. 4. The distribution ratio (cpm/ml of intracellular fluid divided by cpm/ml of plasma) plotted as a function of time after injection of 1.14 μCi of L-[^{35}S]cystine. Points with error bars represent average ± s.e. of 36 slices from three rats. Other points represent average of 12 slices from individual rats. (From Greth, Thier, and Segal, 1973.)

the slower decay probably represents cystine turnover. The plot of the distribution ratio of total intracellular ^{35}S to plasma ^{35}S as a function of time is presented in Fig. 4. The distribution ratio reaches a peak in 30 min and maintains a plateau out to 120 min. Figure 5 indicates that separation of cystine metabolites on thin-layer chromatograms reveals that the majority of ^{35}S is in cysteine and reduced glutathione. There is also an as yet unidentified metabolite (taurine, cysteic acid, or cysteinesulphinic acid). Even at 75 min all plasma radioactivity remains in cystine. If the total distribution ratio at each time point is multiplied by the percentage of radioactivity in each metabolite, the curves seen in Fig. 6 are obtained. The curve for cysteine mirrors the curve of the total ^{35}S distribution ratio. The combined radioactivity of reduced glutathione and the unidentified metabolite also roughly parallel the curve for total radioactivity.

Next, lysine at a concentration over 800 times greater than cystine was injected with the ^{35}S cystine. According to the classic view of the cystine-lysine interaction, cystine accumulation in the cell should be reduced. According to the view developed in slice studies there might be no change in cellular accumulation of cystine. In fact the presence of lysine increased the cellular accumulation of cystine (Fig. 7). In order to confirm that the increased distribution ratio measured by radioactivity reflects chemical concen-

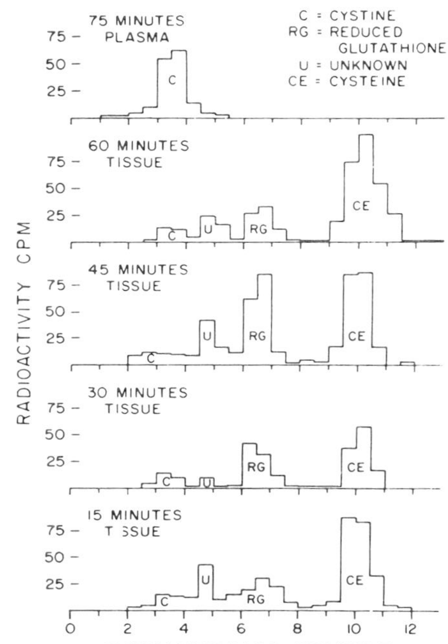

Fig. 5. Representative thin-layer chromatograms at various times after injection of L-[^{35}S] cystine. (From Greth, Thier, and Segal, 1973.)

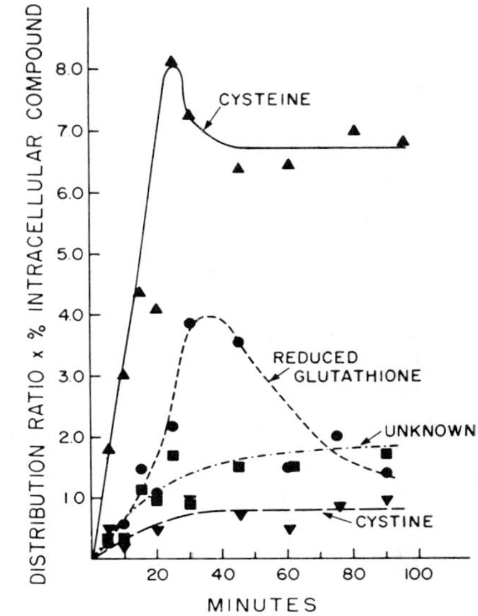

Fig. 6. The ratio of intracellular radioactivity for a given metabolite of cystine to extracellular radioactivity due to L-[^{35}S]cystine for various times after injection of 1.14 μCi L-[^{35}S] cystine. (From Greth, Thier, and Segal, 1973.)

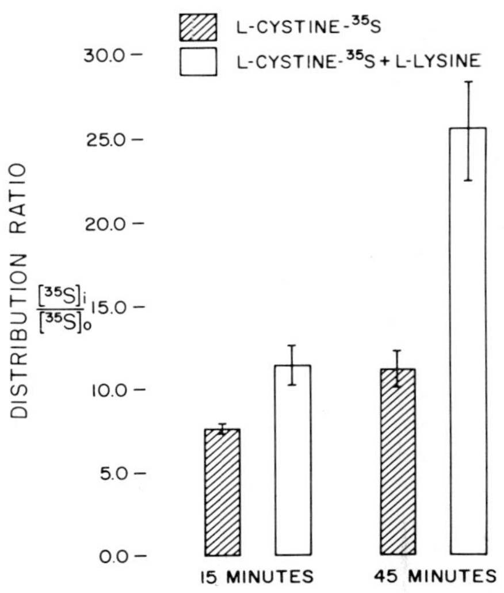

Fig. 7. Effect of L-lysine infusion on kidney uptake of L-[^{35}S]cystine at 15 and 45 minutes after infusion. (From Greth, Thier, and Segal, 1973.)

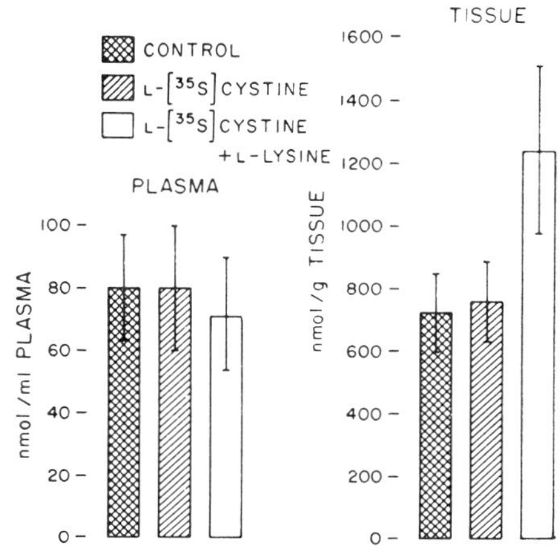

Fig. 8. The effect of an injection of L-cystine or L-cystine plus L-lysine on total cyst(e)ine levels in rat plasma and kidney tissue. Total cyst(e)ine was determined using the spectrophotometric method of Gaitonde. Each value is the average ± s.e. determined from four rats. (From Greth, Thier, and Segal, 1973.)

tration changes, tissues and plasma were reacted with dithiotreitol and total cystine plus cysteine measured. Figure 8 reveals that chemical measurements confirm the data generated by measurements of radioactivity.

In order to look at events at the antiluminal surface *in vivo*, the ureter of one kidney was ligated 10 min or 1 hr before the injection of amino acid. The

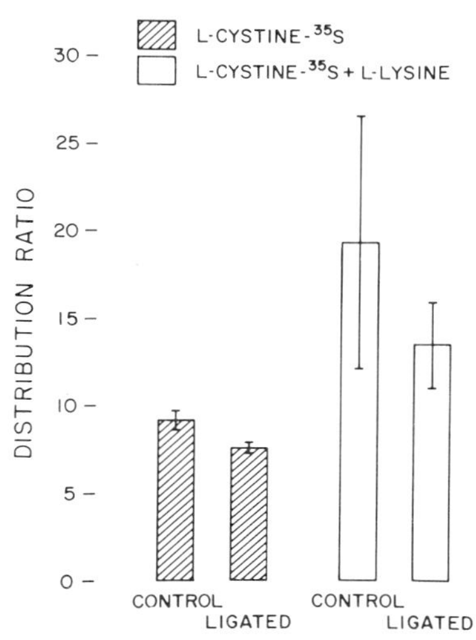

Fig. 9. Effect of ureter ligation on L-[^{35}S]cystine in presence and absence of L-lysine. (From Greth, Thier, and Segal, 1973.)

Table 1. Clearance of L-cystine and cellular accumulation of ^{35}S

Time period (min)	Fractional clearance ($C_{cystine}/C_{inulin}$ ±s.e.)	Distribution ratio ± s.d.	Urine lysine[a] (μM/ml)
Group 1			
0–15	4.02±0.52	7.7±0.3[b]	[c]
15–30	4.60±1.51		[c]
30–45	5.17±1.12	11.8±1.5	[c]
		11.2±1.3[b]	
Group 2			
0–15	24.0±0.7	11.5±2.3[b]	6.15
15–30	5.2±1.3	21.0±2.1[b]	0.0465
30–45	5.0±1.1	19.5±2.2	0.0028
		25.6±1.6[b]	

For the clearance studies each group consists of three rats. Group 1 represents control rats where labeled cystine was injected at zero time. Rats in group 2 were injected with L-lysine in addition.

[a]Representative urine lysine concentrations are given for a single rat in each time period.

[b]These values are intended for comparison and were determined on a comparable group of rats not in the clearance studies. Each value is the average ±s.d. for 48 tissue slices from four rats. The other values are obtained from kidneys removed at the end of the clearance studies.

[c]Unmeasurably low, less than 0.001 μM/ml.

(From Greth, Thier, and Segal, 1973.)

animals were sacrificed 10 min or 45 min after injection. The varying time sequences were used to assess the role of reabsorption-replacement after ureteral ligation. In fact the results at all times were comparable, and indicate that cellular accumulation was preserved in the presence of ureter ligation (Fig. 9). Presumably cystine is being delivered to and accumulated from the antiluminal surface of the tubular cell. The effect of lysine on cystine accumulation is also preserved in the presence of ureter ligation.

Thus cellular accumulation of cystine and the effect of lysine on this accumulation occur with minimal contribution of luminal surface processes. In order to examine the interaction of cystine and lysine at the luminal surface of the tubular cell, standard clearance studies were conducted. Cystine clearance was measured before and after lysine injection. In addition, cellular accumulation was measured at appropriate times during clearance studies. The results (Table 1) indicate that lysine does indeed inhibit cystine reabsorption from the tubular lumen. However, despite increased clearance of cystine, cellular accumulation of cystine increased.

DISCUSSION

Using microperfusion techniques and looking specifically at luminal events, Silbernagl and Deetjen (1972) have confirmed that cystine and lysine interact at the luminal surface. Schwartzman, Blair, and Segal (1966) noted that in slices preloaded with lysine distribution ratios for cystine were increased and were increased even more for cysteine. They demonstrated that cysteine and the dibasic amino acids competed for efflux.

A model for further study is postulated in which amino acids are filtered, reabsorbed, and secreted. The reabsorptive process has its stereospecific mechanism in the brush border. This mechanism is similar to or identical with the mechanism, which is shared by cystine and the dibasic amino acid, which is defective in cystinuria as studied by clearance measurements. The transport pathways for cellular accumulation and/or secretion are located on the antiluminal surface. At this surface the dibasic amino acid transport system is independent of the cystine transport system. These systems are not affected in cystinuria. (In fact, in all tissues studied in cystinurics other than kidney and gut no defect is demonstrable.) Slice studies view predominantly the antiluminal surface uptake and therefore fail to reveal either the full defect in cystinuria or the interaction between cystine and the dibasic amino acids. Finally, once in the cell cystine is metabolized to cysteine which then competes with the dibasic amino acids for efflux. Thus, infusion of dibasic amino acids will increase cysteine in the cell (increasing the distribution ratio for ^{35}S in our studies), while at the same time inhibiting cystine reabsorption via the brush border.

This scheme is speculative, but it does fit the majority of the data and provides a model to be tested by experiment. Support for a role for antiluminal transport comes from the microinjection studies of Bergeron and the double-indicator dilution studies of Foulkes (1971). Bergeron and Vadeboncoeur (1971) have demonstrated significant antiluminal to luminal flux of amino acid, and Foulkes has demonstrated energy-dependent amino acid transport across the antiluminal membrane of the tubular cell.

The bidirectional amino acid transport model should be examined to see if the discrepancy between *in vivo* and *in vitro* studies with regard to pH effects and the amino aciduria of the newborn can be resolved. In addition, the concepts can be tested further utilizing isolated perfused tubules, microperfusion techniques, double-indicator dilution techniques, and models such as canine cystinuria in which clearance of cystine may strikingly exceed clearance of inulin and allow study of secretion (Bovee *et al.*, 1973).

ACKNOWLEDGMENT

This work was supported by research grant AM 10894 from the National Institutes of Health, and a grant from the John A. Hartford Foundation.

REFERENCES

Ausiello, D. A., S. Segal, and S. O. Thier. 1972. Cellular accumulation of L-lysine in rat kidney cortex *in vivo*. Am. J. Physiol. 222(6): 1473–1478.

Baerlocher, K. E., C. R. Scriver, and F. Mohyuddin. 1970. Ontogeny of iminoglycine transport in mammalian kidney. Proc. Natl. Acad. Sci. 65: 1009.

Bartter, F. C., M. Lotz, S. Thier, L. E. Rosenberg, and J. J. Potts, Jr. 1965. Cystinuria. Combined clinical staff conference at the National Institutes of Health. Annals Int. Med. 62: 796.

Bergeron, M., and M. Vadeboncoeur. 1971. Antiluminal transport of L-arginine and L-leucine following microinjections in peritubular capillaries of the rat. Nephron 8: 355.

Bovee, K. C., S. O. Thier, C. Rea, and S. Segal. 1974. The renal clearance of amino acids in canine cystinuria. Metabolism. 23: 51.

Braun, W., W. Zschaler, and C. H. R. Weiss. 1967. Der einflussvon anderungen des urin-pH auf die ausscheidung von aminosauren an der isoliert perfundierten rattenniere. Naunyn-Schmiedebergs Arch. Pharmak. Exp. Path. 256: 397.

Brodehl, J., and K. Gellissen. 1968. Endogenous renal transport of free amino acids in infancy and childhood. Pediatrics 42: 395.

Crampton, R. F., and D. H. Smyth. 1953. The excretion of the enantiomorphs of amino acids. J. Physiol. 122: 1.

Crawhall, J. C., E. F. Scowen, C. J. Thompson, and R. W. E. Watts. 1967. The renal clearance of amino acids in cystinuria. J. Clin. Invest. 46: 1162.

Dent, C. E., J. G. Heathcote, and G. E. Joron. 1954. The pathogenesis of cystinuria. I. Chromatographic and microbiological studies of the metabolism of sulphur-containing amino acids. J. Clin. Invest. 33: 1210.

Dent, C.E., B. Senior, and J.M. Walshe. 1954. The pathogenesis of cystinuria. II. Polarographic studies of the metabolism of sulphur-containing amino acids. J. Clin. Invest. 33: 1216.

Foulkes, E. C. 1971. Effects of heavy metals on renal aspartate transport and the nature of solute movement in kidney cortex slices. Biochim. Biophys. Acta 241: 815.

Fox, M., S. Thier, L. E. Rosenberg, W. Kiser, and S. Segal. 1964. Evidence against a single renal transport defect in cystinuria. New Eng. J. Med. 270: 556.

Fox, M., S. Thier, L. Rosenberg, and S. Segal. 1964a. Impaired renal tubular function induced by sugar infusion in man. J. Clin. Endoc. Metabol. 24(12): 1318.

Fox, M., S. Thier, L. E. Rosenberg, and S. Segal. 1964b. Ionic requirements for amino acid transport in the rat kidney cortex slices. I. Influence of extracellular ions. Biochim. Biophys. Acta 79: 167.

Frimpter, G. W. 1963. Cystinuria: metabolism of the disulfide of cysteine and homocysteine. J. Clin. Invest. 42: 1956.

Frimpter, G. W., M. Horwith, E. Furth, R. E. Fellows, and D. D. Thompson. 1962. Inulin and endogenous amino acid renal clearances in cystinuria: evidence for tubular secretion. J. Clin. Invest. 41: 281.

Greth, W. E., S. O. Thier, and S. Segal. 1973. Cellular accumulation of L-cystine in rat kidney cortex *in vivo*. J. Clin. Invest. 52(2): 454.

Kirk, E. 1936. Studies on the amino acid clearance. Acta Med. Scand. 89(5): 450.

Pitts, R. F. 1943. A renal reabsorptive mechanism in the dog common to glycine and creatine. Am. J. Physiol. 140: 156.

Robson, E. G., and G. A. Rose. 1957. The effect of intravenous lysine on the renal clearances of cystine, arginine and ornithine in normal subjects, in patients with cystinuria and Fanconi syndrome and in their relatives. Clin. Sci. 16: 75.

Rosenberg, L., A. Blair, and S. Segal. 1961. The transport of amino acids by rat kidney cortex slices. Biochim. Biophys. Acta 54: 479.
Rosenberg, L., S. Downing, and S. Segal. 1962. Competitive inhibition of dibasic amino acid transport in rat kidney. J. Biol. Chem. 237: 2265.
Schwartzman, L., A. Blair, and S. Segal. 1966. A common renal transport system for lysine, ornithine, arginine and cysteine. Biochem. Biophys. Res. Comm. 23: 220.
Scriver, C. R., M. L. Efron, and I. A. Schafer. 1964. Renal tubular transport of proline, hydroxyproline, and glycine in health and in familial hyperprolinemia. J. Clin. Invest. 43: 374.
Segal, S., and J. C. Crawhall. 1968. The characteristics of cysteine and cystine transport in the rat kidney. Proc. Natl. Acad. Sci. 59: 231.
Segal, S., C. Rea, and I. Smith. 1971. Separate transport systems for sugars amino acid uptake in rat kidney cortex slice. Biochim. Biophys. Acta 93: 106.
Segal, S., L. Schwartzman, A. Blair, and D. Bertoli. 1967. Dibasic amino acid transport in rat kidney cortex slices. Biochim. Biophys. Acta 135: 127.
Silbernagl, S., and P. Deetjen. 1972. The tubular reabsorption of L-cystine and L-cysteine. A common transport system with L-arginine or not? Pflügers Arch. Ges. Physiol. 337: 277.
Thier, S., M. Fox, L. E. Rosenberg, and S. Segal. 1964. Hexose inhibition of amino acid uptake in rat kidney cortex slice. Biochim. Biophys. Acta 93: 106.
Thier, S. O., S. Segal, M. Fox, A. Blair, and L. E. Rosenberg. 1965. Cystinuria: Defective intestinal transport of dibasic amino acids and cystine. J. Clin. Invest. 44: 442.
Webber, W. A. 1962. Interactions of neutral and acidic amino acids in renal tubular transport. Am. J. Physiol. 202: 577.
Webber, W. A. 1963. Characteristics of acidic amino acid transport in mammalian kidney. Can. J. Biochem. Physiol. 41: 131.
Webber, W. A. 1968. A comparison of the efflux rates of AIB from kidney cortex slices of mature and newborn rats. Can. J. Physiol. Pharmac. 46: 765.
Webber, W. A., J. L. Brown, and R. F. Pitts. 1961. Interactions of amino acids in renal tubular transport. Am. J. Physiol. 200: 380.
Wedeen, R. P., and S. O. Thier. 1971. Intrarenal distribution of nonmetabolized amino acids *in vivo*. Am. J. Physiol. 220: 507.
Wedeen, R. P., and B. Weiner. 1973. The distribution of *p*-aminohippuric acid in rat kidney slices. I. Tubular localization. Kidney Internatl. 3: 205.

Bidirectional Transport: Urate and Other Organic Anions

I. M. Weiner and G. M. Fanelli, Jr.
Department of Pharmacology
State University of New York
Upstate Medical Center
Syracuse, New York and
Merck Institute for Therapeutic Research
West Point, Pennsylvania

In 1933 J. Bordley III and A. N. Richards demonstrated in snakes and frogs that the concentrations of urate in glomerular filtrate and plasma were the same. The situation in mammals was for a time less clear because there were conflicting reports regarding the filterability of urate. Much of the difficulty may be attributable to the fact that the binding of urate to plasma proteins is temperature dependent (Sheikh and Møller, 1968). It is now generally accepted that at 37°C urate is freely filterable. In 1950 Berliner and his colleagues published their classic study of urate excretion in man (Berliner *et al.*, 1950). They provided evidence for the complete ultrafilterability of urate from plasma, that filtered urate was largely reabsorbed, and, in experiments involving intravenous urate loading, they demonstrated what appeared to be a transport maximum for urate reabsorption. A transport maximum for a particular compound implies that its transport is specifically mediated, and thus this finding provided a probable mechanism of action for uricosuric drugs, i.e., they are inhibitors of the transport system mediating urate reabsorption.

The full complexity of the urate excretory system was not appreciated until the late A. B. Gutman and his colleague T. F. Yü deduced that urate disposition in man involved tubular secretion as well as filtration and reabsorption (Gutman and Yü, 1961). Their salient findings were that salicylate in small doses and certain other substances caused decreases in the clearance of urate, suggesting that in addition to filtration and reabsorption there was a specifically mediated secretory flux for urate which was susceptible to inhibition. Proof of this 'three-component' hypothesis came from their demonstration of net urate secretion in human subjects, albeit under very stringent conditions (Gutman, Yü, and Berger, 1959). To pharmacologists, the great appeal of this three-component hypothesis is that it has the potential for explaining a great variety of drug effects on urate excretion, especially those complicated phenomena that result from the introduction of more than one drug into the system.

For most of this paper we shall relate a few of the older findings in man and lower mammals with some recent work, mainly in nonhuman primates, to develop a somewhat speculative elaboration of the three-component hypothesis which seems to be consistent with available information. If there is any use to such an exercise, it is to define the questions in such a way as to encourage attempts to disprove the tentative answers.

MOST OF URATE REABSORPTION OCCURS IN THE PROXIMAL TUBULE

All published applications of the stop-flow technique in mammals that normally reabsorb urate have identified the proximal tubule as the reabsorptive site (Fanelli, Bohn, and Stafford, 1970; Kessler, Hierholzer, and Gurd, 1959; Mudge *et al.*, 1968; Beechwood, Berndt, and Mudge, 1964; Yü *et al.*, 1960; Mudge, McAlary and Berndt, 1968). Figure 1 summarizes the results of a free-flow micropuncture study on urate disposition in the New World monkey *Cebus albifrons*. Three-quarters of the filtered urate is reabsorbed in the proximal segments of these surface nephrons. It should also be noted that the fraction of filtered urate is smaller in final urine than in the distal tubule. This may be the result of additional reabsorption in the collecting system or a consequence of greater fractional reabsorption in the proximal tubules of deeper nephrons not accessible to micropuncture. In either event it is clear that the proximal process is quantitatively most important.[1]

URICOSURIC DRUGS ACT BY DEPRESSING PROXIMAL REABSORPTION OF URATE

In the original stop-flow study on urate transport Kessler *et al.* (1959) demonstrated a blunting of the proximal concentration dip for urate as a consequence of probenecid administration. Table 1 gives data from the previously mentioned micropuncture study in *Cebus* and demonstrates again a mainly proximal site of uricosuric action. The drug in this case is an analog of probenecid which has qualitatively similar actions (Blanchard *et al.*, 1972). The best evidence that these effects are the result of inhibition of reabsorption and not stimulation of coextensive secretion comes from the microinjection study of Kramp, Lassiter, and Gottschalk (1971). They injected [^{14}C]

[1]The rat is exceptional in this respect. Although the net direction of urate transport is reabsorptive in this species, micropuncture experiments demonstrated net urate secretion in proximal tubules (Greger, Lang, and Deetjen, 1971; Lang, Greger, and Deetjen, 1972).

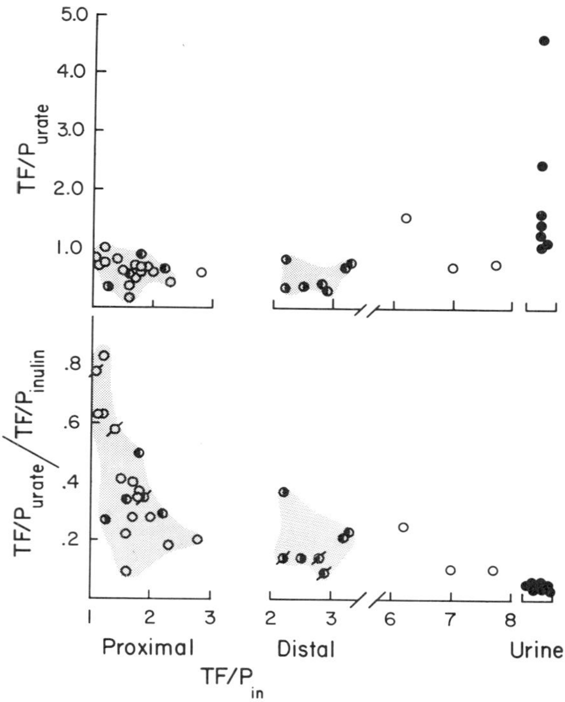

Fig. 1. Micropuncture analysis of urate excretion in *Cebus albifrons.* (From Roch-Ramel and Weiner, 1973.)

urate into various tubular segments of rats and estimated reabsorption from recovery of label in voided urine. Their results with three different inhibitors are given in part in Table 2. The fractional recovery of microinjected urate was enhanced by each of the substances tested, i.e., reabsorption was depressed.

Table 1. Fraction of filterated urate in nephron segments and urine

Condition	Proximal[a]	Distal	Urine
Control	0.40[b] (±0.04)	0.18 (±0.03)	0.05 (±0.005)
2-Nitroprobenecid	0.62 (±0.06)	0.51 (±0.03)	0.48 (±0.04)

[a]Does not take into account progressive decline with tubular length.
[b]Mean (±s.e.).
From Roch-Ramel and Weiner, 1973.

Table 2. Recovery of [^{14}C]urate in urine after injection into early proximal tubules of rats

Condition	Recovery (%)
Control	74 (±3)[a]
Probenecid	84 (±5)
Pyrazinoate	86 (±2)
p-Aminohippurate	85 (±5)

[a]Mean (± s.d.).
From Kramp *et al.*, 1971.

DRUGS THAT DEPRESS URATE REABSORPTION DO SO FROM THE LUMINAL ASPECT OF THE TUBULE

Yü and Gutman's (1959) demonstration in man that alkalosis enhanced the uricosuric activity of salicylate was the first and is still the best evidence that the tubular fluid concentration of drug is the critical parameter in uricosuric action. They demonstrated that alkalosis *per se* had minimal effects on urate clearance, but in the presence of salicylate, alkalosis, or more precisely alkaline urine, enhanced the excretion of salicylate in concert with the enhancement of its uricosuric action; that is, by suppressing the passive reabsorption of salicylate, more of the drug remained in the tubule to 'compete' for the active reabsorptive mechanism.

Figure 2 shows the same phenomena reproduced in *Cebus apella* monkeys. The lower panel shows the change in urate clearance ratio as a function of the concentration of salicylate in plasma. Of particular interest is the range of plasma concentrations between 200 and 750 μg/ml. It is apparent that some animals responded with a diminished urate clearance, the 'paradoxical' effect, while others demonstrated a uricosuric response. The two groups of animals were distinguished by their acid-base status. The animals showing urate retention were receiving infusions containing saline and mannitol, while those giving a uricosuric response were receiving infusions of sodium bicarbonate. If the changes in urate clearance ratio are plotted against the excretion of salicylate expressed as μg excreted per ml of glomerular filtration rate (GFR) (upper panel) a much more regular response is seen. At excretory rates of salicylate above 200 μg/ml GFR the response is uniformly uricosuric. It might be mentioned that monkeys of this species are somewhat less responsive to uricosuric drugs than are humans or chimpanzees. It is impossible to obtain a uricosuric response to salicylate in the nonalkalotic animal; severe salicylate intoxication and death occur before enough drug for the desired response can be infused (Weiner and Fanelli, unpublished).

Additional evidence for an intraluminal site of uricosuric action comes from studies of series of closely related compounds. In both the series of compounds related to phenylbutazone (Gutman *et al.*, 1960) and the series related to probenecid (Blanchard *et al.*, 1972) uricosuric potency is related, within limits, to rates of drug excretion.

URIC ACID IS SECRETED IN THE PROXIMAL TUBULE

In those mammals which show net tubular secretion of urate, stop-flow experiments demonstrate a proximal secretory peak (Yü *et al.*, 1960; Kessler *et al.*, 1959; Beechwood *et al.*, 1964; Mudge *et al.*, 1968). In the non-Dalma-

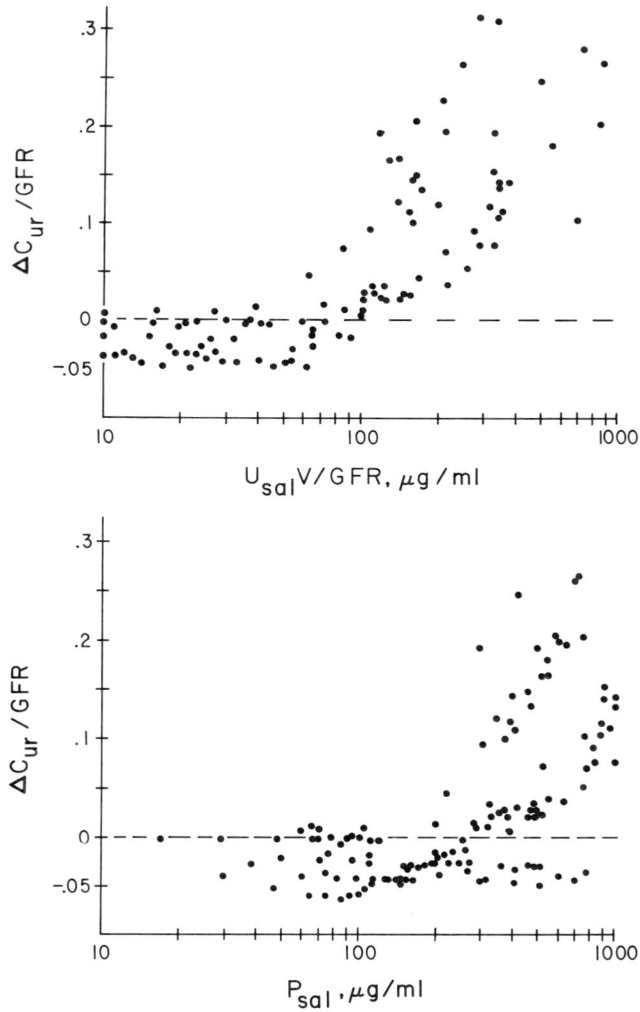

Fig. 2. The change in the ratio C_{urate}/GFR as a function of the concentration of salicylate in plasma (lower panel) and as a function of a parameter of salicylate excretion (upper panel). Each point is from a single clearance period.

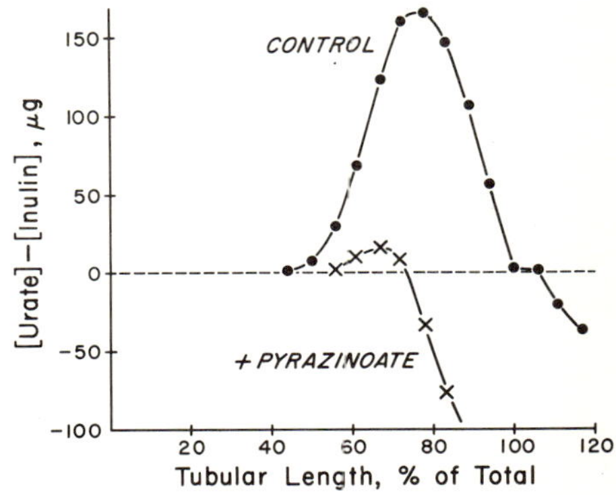

Fig. 3. The influence of pyrazinoate on the secretory movement of urate in the non-Dalmatian dog. (From Weiner and Tinker, 1972.)

tian dog, where net reabsorption of urate is a uniform finding, a proximal secretory flux for urate has been demonstrated, presumably coextensive with the reabosrptive region (Mudge *et al.*, 1968; Zins and Weiner, 1968). These experiments were done in animals subjected to massive osmotic diuresis. After occluding the ureter to minimize filtration, both urate and inulin were infused into the renal artery. The net transtubular influx of urate was taken to be equal to the difference between urate and inulin in the stop-flow samples collected after release of the ureteral occlusion. Figure 3 shows one such application of the technique; it demonstrates a large net influx of urate under control conditions. The influx was almost completely inhibited by the administration of pyrazinoate immediately before a second occlusion.

Apparently, demonstration of a proximal secretory flux has not been made in primates, although there is one study in man with an indirect technique which is consistent with proximal secretion (Podevin *et al.*, 1968).

THE SECRETORY FLUX FOR URATE (AND CONSEQUENTLY THE REABSORPTIVE FLUX) IS LARGE

This fact was fully anticipated by Mudge *et al.* (1968) when they deduced that the secretory and reabsorptive fluxes of urate were coextensive. The secretion of urate provides more urate for reabsorption and vice versa. In such a situation it is virtually impossible to deduce the magnitudes of the unidirectional fluxes from clearance experiments. However, experiments in chimpanzees have provided evidence that the secretory rate of urate is at least of the same order of magnitude as the rate of urate filtration, and from this it follows that the rate of reabsorption is at least almost twice as great as the rate of filtration. The experiments involved the most powerful uricosuric compound encountered thus far, the mercurial diuretic, mersalyl (Fanelli *et al.*, 1973).

Table 3. The effect of mersalyl on the clearance of urate in the chimpanzee

Condition	GFR (ml/min)	C_{urate}/GFR
Control[a]	96	0.094
Mersalyl[b]	100	1.78

[a]Mean of three consecutive clearance periods.
[b]Peak response after 2 mg Hg/kg.
From Fanelli *et al.*, 1973.

Table 3 depicts one such experiment. In this case urinary loss of volume due to the diuretic was replaced with saline, and GFR did not fall. After the diuretic was administered the contribution of net secretion was 78% of the filtered load. Since there is no assurance that the blockade of reabsorption was complete, or that the secretory process was entirely uninhibited by the diuretic, 78% of the filtered load is a minimal estimate of the secreted moiety.

Results of this type are not consistent with an older scheme for urate disposition in which an essentially unidirectional reabsorptive process exists in the proximal tubule and an independent secretory mechanism exists in the distal tubule. Were such a mechanism operative the maximum clearance ratio after complete blockade of the reabsorptive process would be 1 plus the control clearance ratio, or 1.094 in the experiment depicted. On the other hand, these results are entirely consistent with coextensive secretion and reabsorption.

A VARIETY OF COMPOUNDS, URICOSURIC OR NOT, INHIBIT THE SECRETORY FLUX

At the present time two techniques are especially useful in detecting a depression of urate secretion: (1) the modified stop-flow technique in the dog (Zins and Weiner, 1968) or a variant used by Nolan and Foulkes (1971); (2) the prevention of mercurial-induced net urate secretion in the chimpanzee. Table 4 is a list of compounds which have been shown to inhibit urate secretion by either or both of these techniques. Chlorothiazide and ethacrynic acid which gave positive results in the dog (Nolan and Foulkes, 1971) did not in the chimpanzee (Fanelli *et al.*, 1973), but this may reflect the fact that smaller doses of these compounds were used in the primate. In addition to those listed, other compounds, such as m-hydroxybenzoate (May and Weiner, 1971), also suppress urate excretion, but these have not been used in the test systems under consideration.

Of some interest is the fact that these inhibitions of urate secretion are dose related. Table 5 summarizes two experiments in chimpanzees demon-

Table 4. Organic compounds that inhibit secretion of urate

Compound	Species	References
PAH	Dog, chimpanzee	a, b, c
Chlorothiazide	Dog	a, b
Salicylate	Dog, chimpanzee	a, c
Probenecid	Dog, chimpanzee	b, c
Pyrazinoate	Dog, chimpanzee	b, c, d
Lactate	Dog	b
Ethacrynate	Dog	b
Furosemide	Dog	b
Bromcresol green	Chimpanzee	c
Diodrast	Chimpanzee	c
Phenol red	Chimpanzee	c

[a]Zins and Weiner, 1968.
[b]Nolan and Foulkes, 1971.
[c]Fanelli *et al.*, 1973.
[d]Weiner and Tinker, 1972.

strating this phenomenon. In the first experiment a small infusion of probenecid exerted a definite uricosuric response and did not block net urate secretion in response to mersalyl. In the second experiment a larger infusion of probenecid produced a somewhat greater uricosuric response, but in this instance the response to mersalyl was clearly blunted. The fact that probenecid produces a uricosuric effect at doses that do not seem seriously to compromise urate secretion probably accounts for the observation that a 'paradoxical' effect of probenecid is difficult to demonstrate (Yü and Gutman, 1955).

On the other hand, at least two compounds are quite effective in suppressing urate secretion at doses that are definitely not uricosuric. It will be shown later that pyrazinoic acid is a uricosuric agent, but at all but very high doses it causes urate retention. Pyrazinoate uniformly prevents mersalyl-

Table 5. The effects of two different levels of probenecid on the uricosuric response to mersalyl

Experiment	Condition	Loading dose (mg/kg)	Maintenance dose (mg/kg hr)	C_{urate}/GFR
1	Control			0.151
	Probenecid	0.25	0.30	0.321
	Mersalyl	1.5		1.42
2	Control			0.139
	Probenecid	12.5	15	0.534
	Mersalyl	1.9		0.626

From Fanelli *et al.*, 1973.

induced net secretion of urate in the chimpanzee (Fanelli *et al.*, 1973). Lactate is not uricosuric at any dose tested thus far; it also is a powerful inhibitor of the urate secretory flux (Nolan and Foulkes, 1971). The other compounds in Table 4 have been shown to possess uricosuric activity.

THE URATE SECRETORY MECHANISM IS PROBABLY DIFFERENT FROM THE P-AMINOHIPPURATE MECHANISM

As will be shown pyrazinoate is a very potent inhibitor of urate secretion, but is a very weak inhibitor of p-aminohippurate (PAH) secretion. Table 6 summarizes two experiments with chimpanzees. The first demonstrates almost complete suppression of urate excretion by pyrazinoate without any significant change in PAH clearance ratio. The second demonstrates inhibition of urate excretion without any depression of $T_{m_{PAH}}$. It might be argued that PAH has such high affinity for a common secretory mechanism that pyrazinoate cannot displace it; on the other hand urate would have weak affinity. It should be noted, however, that appreciable urate secretion persists in the face of high levels of PAH. In the second experiment in Table 6 pyrazinoate suppressed urate excretion presumably by inhibiting secretion that continued in the presence of PAH.

More cogent evidence to this point comes from experiments in which mersalyl-induced net secretion of urate was used as an indicator. Small doses of PAH did not prevent net secretion, but small doses of pyrazinoate did so (Fanelli *et al.*, 1973). Accordingly, pyrazinoate is a strong inhibitor of urate secretion and PAH is weaker, but as we have seen (Table 6) pyrazinoate is a very poor inhibitor of PAH secretion and it can be easily demonstrated that PAH inhibits pyrazinoate secretion (Weiner and Tinker, 1972; Fanelli and Weiner, 1973). Since the rank order of inhibitor potency varies depending on which transported substance is studied, it follows that at least two secretory mechanisms are operating. One, which is responsible for the bulk of urate secretion, is easily inhibited by pyrazinoate but only by massive doses of PAH. The other, which is responsible for most of the PAH secretion, and probably the excretion of many anionic drugs, is only weakly inhibited by

Table 6. Lack of effect of pyrazinoate on C_{PAH}/GFR and $T_{m_{PAH}}$

Experiment	P_{PZ}[a] (μg/ml)	GFR (ml/min)	C_{urate}/GFR	C_{PAH}/GFR	$T_{m_{PAH}}$ (mg/min)
1	0	105	0.071	5.5	
	125	113	0.011	5.6	
2	0	74	0.107		74
	115	71	0.027		79

The numbers are means from three or four clearance periods.
[a]Concentration of pyrazinoate in plasma.
From Fanelli and Weiner, 1973.

pyrazinoate. We believe that this hypothesis might be essential to the interpretation of drug effects on urate excretion and would encourage other attempts to validate or disprove it.

SOME COMPOUNDS THAT INFLUENCE URATE EXCRETION ARE THEMSELVES SECRETED AND REABSORBED BY ACTIVE TRANSPORT

At about the same time that the three-component hypothesis for the renal transport of urate was formulated, Kinter (1959) established the bidirectional active transport of PAH and Diodrast in the amphibian, *Necturus.* This phenomenon is now very well documented (Kinter, Leape, and Cohen, 1960; Tanner and Kinter, 1966; Tanner, 1967). Subsequently, bidirectional specific transport was demonstrated for a variety of anions in the mammalian kidney, including PAH (Cho and Cafruny, 1970). Two of these anions are of particular interest in relation to urate transport.

Meta-hydroxybenzoic acid is an isomer of salicylate. It differs from salicylate in that it is not lipid soluble and thus is not subject to extensive passive reabsorption. As shown in Fig. 4, based on experiments in *Cebus albifrons,* at low concentrations of this drug in plasma there is net secretion, while at higher concentrations there is net reabsorption of the drug. This reabsorptive process is relatively insensitive to changes in urine flow. Figure 5, based on stop-flow studies in the dog, demonstrates that both secretion and reabsorption are predominantly proximal tubular processes. This localization plus the lack of response to changes in urine flow suggest that reabsorption of this compound is specifically mediated. These results suggest further that closely related drugs, such as salicylate and probenecid, are likewise reabsorbed by the specific process and therefore inhibit urate reabsorption by

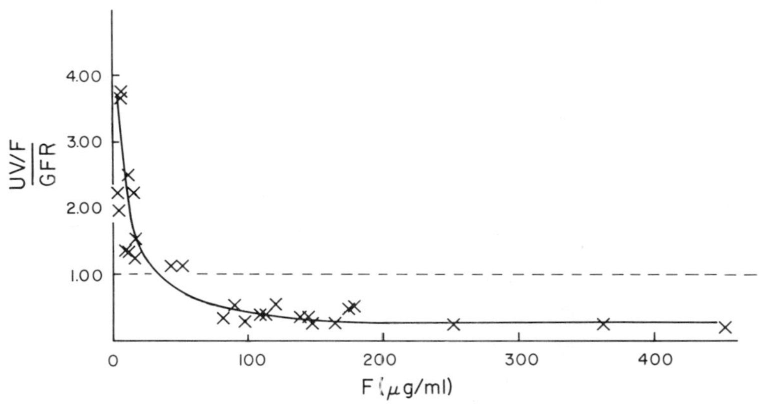

Fig. 4. The clearance ratio of m-hydroxybenzoate as a function of its concentration in plasma water (F). The experimental animals were monkeys, *Cebus albifrons.* (From May and Weiner, 1971.)

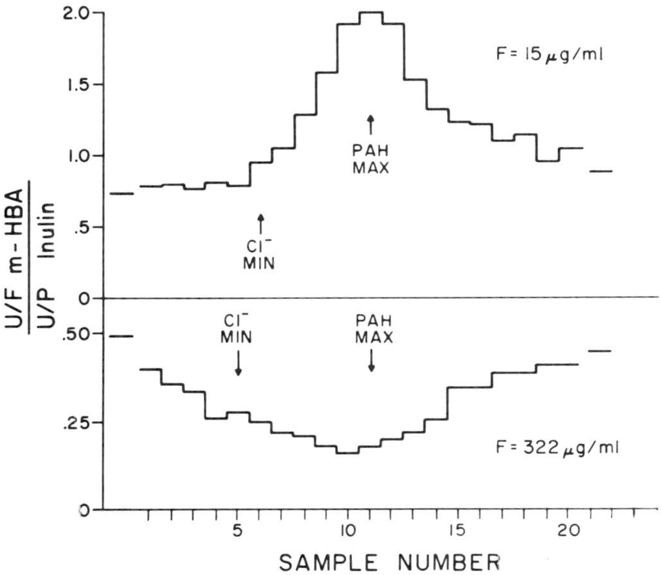

Fig. 5. Stop-flow analysis in a dog of the excretion of m-hydroxybenzoate at low (upper panel) and high (lower panel) concentrations in plasma water (F). Both experiments were performed with the same animal. PAH was also present in both phases of the experiment; its concentration in plasma was 3 μg/ml at the time of the first occlusion (upper panel) and 591 μg/ml in the second phase. PAH max indicates the sample with highest PAH concentration ratio, and Cl min the sample with the lowest chloride concentration. (From May and Weiner, 1970.)

competition. The difficulty with salicylate and probenecid is that they are also reabsorbed by passive transport, and therefore it is difficult to recognize their participation in an active reabsorptive process.

Pyrazinoic acid, the metabolite of pyrazinamide, which is responsible for effects on urate excretion, is also subjected to bidirectional transport. Table 7 summarizes an experiment in a chimpanzee which demonstrates that the clearance of pyrazinoate is greater than GFR (net secretion), but, after

Table 7. Effect of PAH on the clearance ratios of pyrazinoate and urate

Condition	GFR (ml/min)	P_{PZ} (μg/ml)	C_{PZ}/GFR	C_{urate}/GFR
Control	92			0.108
Pyrazinoate	98	64	1.6	0.012
PAH	101	77	0.59	0.021

Each number is the mean from three clearance periods.
From Fanelli and Weiner, 1973.

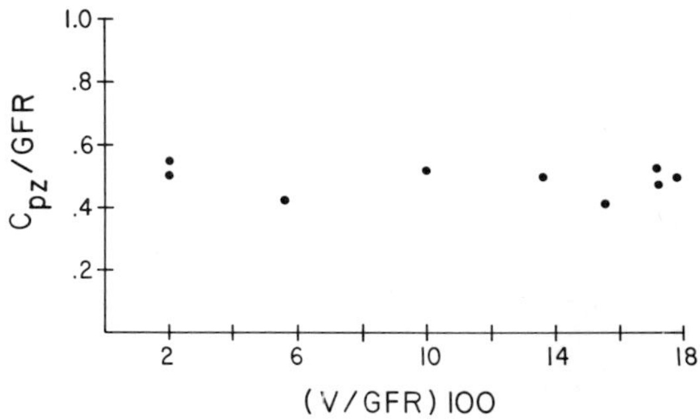

Fig. 6. The clearance ratio of pyrazinoate as a function of fractional water excretion. The data used to construct this figure are from Fanelli and Weiner (1973).

inhibition of secretion by PAH, there is net reabsorption of pyrazinoate. Other secreted anions, including Diodrast, sulfinpyrazone, and probenecid also inhibit pyrazinoate secretion and convert net tubular transport to reabsorption (Fanelli and Weiner, 1973). This reabsorptive process is almost entirely insensitive to changes in urine flow. This phenomenon is illustrated in Fig. 6. Before these data were obtained the animal was treated with probenecid to uncover net reabsorption; urine flow was varied by infusing the osmotic diuretic mannitol. These and other data led to the conclusion that

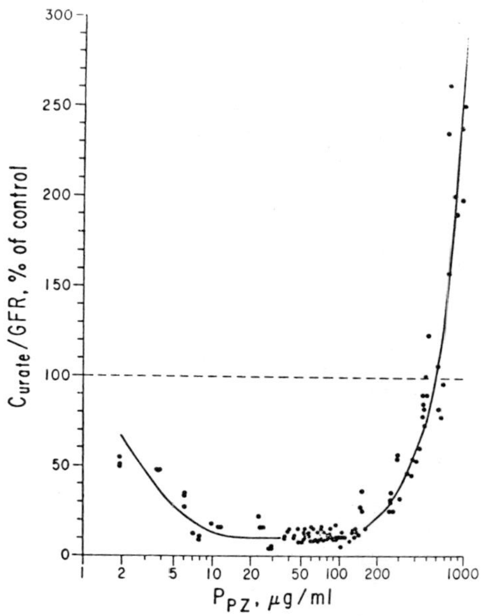

Fig. 7. The clearance ratio of urate as a function of the concentration of pyrazinoate in plasma. The urate data are expressed as percentages of control values. (From Fanelli and Weiner, 1973.)

pyrazinoate undergoes bidirectional transport in the proximal tubule (Weiner and Tinker, 1972; Fanelli and Weiner, 1973).

A DRUG SUBJECT TO BIDIRECTIONAL ACTIVE TRANSPORT MAY HAVE BIDIRECTIONAL EFFECTS ON URATE TRANSPORT

This phenomenon is illustrated with pyrazinoate in the chimpanzee (Fig. 7). At concentrations in plasma below 10 μg/ml there is a concentration-related inhibition of urate excretion which remains maximal until the plasma concentration of drug exceeds 200 μg/ml. At higher levels of drug urate clearance increases and at levels in excess of 600 μg/ml there is a definite uricosuric response.

CONCLUSIONS

Figure 8 summarizes the salient features of the preceding discussion. The essential features of the diagram are as follows.

1. Secretion of urate is not small relative to filtered load. In Fig. 8 secretion is arbitrarily set equal to filtered load, but it must be emphasized that unidirectional secretion has not been measured.
2. Reabsorption is larger than might be estimated from clearance experiments; both filtration and secretion contribute urate for reabsorption. In

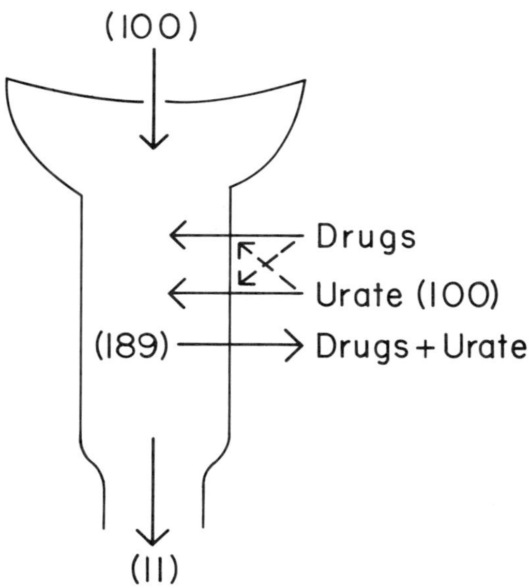

Fig. 8. A diagram summarizing the authors' views on the bidirectional transport of urate and some other organic anions.

Fig. 8 the magnitude of reabsorption is adjusted arbitrarily to give net excretion equal to 11% of filtered load.

3. In addition to the urate secretory mechanism, another arrow depicts the well-known organic anion secretory mechanism which is presumably responsible for most of drug secretion. The dotted arrows indicate that the two secretory mechanisms are not completely specific; i.e., a single substance may interact with both, albeit to different extents.
4. Both urate and drugs are reabsorbed by a single mechanism. There is no evidence for or against this postulate at the present time; the single mechanism is depicted for reasons of economy.

It should be noticed that this scheme provides two mechanisms by which one drug may inhibit the uricosuric activity of another. The inhibitory drug may either prevent uricosuric action by preventing secretion of the active agent and thereby minimizing its access to the site of action, or it may block urate secretion *per se.* For any single drug or combination of drugs the net effect on urate excretion will depend on the relative inhibitions of urate secretion and reabsorption. As has often been true for this field in recent decades, the central paper on the problem of drug interactions came from Dr. Gutman's laboratory (Yü, Dayton, and Gutman, 1963). It is of interest to extend the interpretation of the results reported therein in the light of this speculative construction (Fig. 8). Those authors found that when ordinarily uricosuric doses of salicylate and sulfinpyrazone were administered simultaneously, the responses to both drugs were virtually eliminated. The failure of salicylate to manifest its inhibition of urate reabsorption under these conditions was easily explained by the pharmacokinetic data. Sulfinpyrazone blocked the secretion of salicylate, thereby limiting its access to the site of uricosuric action. On the other hand, the excretion of sulfinpyrazone was not diminished by salicylate, i.e., its access to the site of uricosuric action was not embarrassed. However, in the situation of combined administration the balance of the effects of salicylate would be changed radically. The latter drug would still exert its characteristic inhibition of urate secretion, while its inhibition of reabsorption would be greatly diminished. This inhibition of urate secretion plus whatever inhibition of secretion would be contributed by sulfinpyrazone might so reduce the load of urate presented for reabsorption that the reabsorptive mechanism, albeit partially compromised by sulfinpyrazone, might nevertheless be able to reduce rejected (excreted) urate to normal levels. Obviously, the complexity of the phenomenon is great and a test of this speculation is not easily obtained.

ACKNOWLEDGMENTS

The work reported from I. M. Weiner's laboratory was for the most part supported by a grant from the National Heart and Lung Institute, HL-10595. The authors are indebted to Drs. J. E. Baer, K. H. Beyer, and C. A. Stone for their support of the work at the Merck Institute for Therapeutic Research. Numerous colleagues cited in the bibliography made much of the work possible. The authors note with sadness the recent death of A. B. Gutman whose contributions to this field provided a framework and powerful stimulus to our work.

REFERENCES

Beechwood, E. C., W. O. Berndt, and G. H. Mudge. 1964. Stop-flow analysis of tubular transport of uric acid in rabbits. Am. J. Physiol. 207: 1265–1272.

Berliner, R. W., J. G. Hilton, T. F. Yü, and T. J. Kennedy, Jr. 1950. The renal mechanisms for urate excretion in man. J. Clin. Invest. 29: 396–401.

Blanchard, K. C., D. Maroske, D. G. May, and I. M. Weiner. 1972. Uricosuric potency of 2-substituted analogs of probenecid. J. Pharmac. Exp. Ther. 180: 397–410.

Bordley, J., III, and A. N. Richards. 1933. Quantitative studies of the composition of glomerular urine. VIII. The concentration of uric acid in glomerular urine of snakes and frogs, determined by an ultramicroadaptation of Folin's method. J. Biol. Chem. 101: 193–221.

Cho, K. C., and E. J. Cafruny. 1970. Renal tubular reabsorption of p-aminohippurate acid (PAH) in the dog. J. Pharmac. Exp. Ther. 173: 1–12.

Fanelli, G. M., Jr., D. L. Bohn, S. S. Reilly, and I. M. Weiner. 1973. Effects of mercurial diuretics on renal transport of urate in the chimpanzee. Am. J. Physiol. 224: 985–992.

Fanelli, G. M., Jr., D. L. Bohn, and S. Stafford. 1970. Functional characteristics of renal urate transport in the *Cebus* monkey. Am. J. Physiol. 218: 627–636.

Fanelli, G. M., Jr., and I. M. Weiner. 1973. Pyrazinoate excretion in the chimpanzee; relation to urate disposition and the actions of uricosuric drugs. J. Clin. Invest. 52: 1946–1957.

Greger, R., F. Lang, and P. Deetjen. 1971. Handling of uric acid by the rat kidney. I. Microanalysis of uric acid in proximal tubular fluid. Eur. J. Physiol. 324: 279–287.

Gutman, A. B., P. G. Dayton, T. F. Yü, L. Berger, W. Chen, I. E. Sicam, and J. J. Burns. 1960. A study of the inverse relationship between pKa and rate of renal excretion of phenylbutazone analogs in man and dog. Am. J. Med. 29: 1017–1033.

Gutman, A. B., and T. F. Yü. 1961. A three component system for regulation of renal excretion of uric acid in man. Trans. Ass. Am. Physicians, Philadelphia 74: 353–364.

Gutman, A. B., T. F. Yü, and L. Berger. 1959. Tubular secretion of urate in man. J. Clin. Invest. 38: 1778–1781.

Kessler, R. H., K. Hierholzer, and R. S. Gurd. 1959. Localization of urate transport in the nephron of mongrel and Dalmatian dog kidney. Am. J. Physiol. 197: 601–603.

Kinter, W. B. 1959. Renal tubular transport of Diodrast-I^{131} and PAH in Necturus: evidence for simultaneous reabsorption and secretion. Am. J. Physiol. 196: 1141–1149.

Kinter, W. B., L. L. Leape, and J. J. Cohen. 1960. Autoradiographic study of Diodrast-I^{131} transport in *Necturus* kidney. Am. J. Physiol. 199: 931–941.

Kramp, R. A., W. E. Lassiter, and C. W. Gottschalk. 1971. Urate-2- ^{14}C transport in the rat nephron. J. Clin. Invest. 50: 35–48.
Lang, F., R. Greger, and P. Deetjen. 1972. Handling of uric acid by the rat kidney. II. Microperfusion studies on bidirectional transport of uric acid in the proximal tubule. Eur. J. Physiol. 335: 257–265.
May, D. G., and I. M. Weiner. 1970. Bidirectional active transport of m-hydroxybenzoate in proximal tubules of dogs. Am. J. Physiol. 218: 430–436.
May, D. G., and I. M. Weiner. 1971. The renal mechanisms for the excretion of m-hydroxybenzoic acid in *Cebus* monkeys: Relationship to urate transport. J. Pharmac. Exp. Ther. 176: 407–417.
Mudge, G. H., G. Cucchi, M. Platts, J. M. B. O'Connell, and W. O. Berndt. 1968. Renal excretion of uric acid in the dog. Am. J. Physiol. 215: 404–410.
Mudge, G. H., B. McAlary, and W. O. Berndt. 1968. Renal transport of uric acid in the guinea pig. Am. J. Physiol. 214: 875–879.
Nolan, R. P., and Foulkes, E. C. 1971. Studies on renal urate secretion in the dog. J. Pharmac. Exp. Ther. 179: 429–437.
Podevin, R., R. Andraillou, F. Paillard, J. Fontanella, and G. Richet. 1968. Etude chez l'homme de la cinétique d'apparition dans l'urine de l'acide urique 2-^{14}C. Nephron 5: 134–140.
Roch-Ramel, F., and I. M. Weiner. 1973. Excretion of urate by the kidneys of Cebus monkeys: A micropuncture study. Am. J. Physiol. 224: 1369–1374.
Sheikh, M. I., and J. V. Møller. 1968. Binding of urate to proteins of human and rabbit plasma. Biochim. Biophys. Acta 158: 456–458.
Tanner, G. A. 1967. Micropuncture study of PAH and Diodrast transport in Necturus kidney. Am. J. Physiol. 212: 1341–1346.
Tanner, G. A., and W. B. Kinter. 1966. Reabsorption and secretion of p-aminohippurate and Diodrast in Necturus kidney. Am. J. Physiol. 210: 221–231.
Weiner, I. M., and J. P. Tinker. 1972. Pharmacology of pyrazinamide. Metabolic and renal function studies related to the mechanism of drug induced urate retention. J. Pharmac. Exp. Ther. 180: 411–434.
Yü, T. F., L. Berger, S. Kupfer, and A. B. Gutman. 1960. Tubular secretion of urate in the dog. Am. J. Physiol. 199: 1199–1204.
Yü, T. F., P. G. Dayton, and A. B. Gutman. 1963. Mutual suppression of the uricosuric effects of sulfinpyrazone and salicylate. A study in the interactions between drugs. J. Clin. Invest. 42: 1330–1339.
Yü, T. F., and A. B. Gutman. 1955. Paradoxical retention of uric acid by uricosuric drugs in low dosage. Proc. Soc. Exp. Biol. Med. 90: 542–547.
Yü, T. F., and A. B. Gutman. 1959. Study of the paradoxical effects of salicylate in low, intermediate and high dosage on the renal mechanisms for excretion of urate in man. J. Clin. Invest. 38: 1298–1315.
Zins, G. R., and I. M. Weiner. 1968. Bidirectional urate transport limited to the proximal tubule in dogs. Am. J. Physiol. 215: 411–422.

Uricosuric Activity of Hydrocinnamic Acid Derivatives

P. H. Hernandez, J. H. Ackerman, A. Brousseau, and M. Zacek
Sterling-Winthrop Research Institute
Rensselaer, New York

The uricosuric activity of radiocontrast agents in man was first described when Bonsnes, Dill, and Dana (1944) reported that injections of Diodrast resulted in increased uric acid excretion. Mudge (1971) observed that standard doses of iopanoic acid used in oral cholecystography caused marked increases in uric acid excretion in the first 24-hr period. Postlethwaite and Kelly (1971) also reported that standard doses of iopanoic acid, calcium ipodate, iodipamide, and sodium diatrizoate produced a decrease in serum urate concentration, an increase in uric acid excretion, and an increase in the renal clearance of uric acid. The peak uricosuric activity for iopanoic acid was between 3 and 7 hr and the effect persisted for 5 or 6 days.

Almost without exception uricosuric agents are organic acids, highly lipid soluble, readily absorbed from the gastrointestinal tract, and excreted mainly as glucuronides (Gutman, 1966). Oral cholecystographic agents are iodinated compounds that have all or most of the characteristics described for uricosuric agents (McChesney and Banks, 1965).

The report by Postlethwaite and Kelly (1971) that the duration of the uricosuric activity of iopanoic acid in man lasted several days stimulated interest in the development of a new uricosuric agent that may have longer duration of action than probenecid. Since tyropanoic acid and iopanoic acid are iodinated derivatives of 3-amino hydrocinnamic acid (Fig. 1), a number of analogs of the latter were synthesized and tested for uricosuric activity in *Cebus albifrons* monkeys. The use of *Cebus* monkeys as a suitable model for the study of uric acid metabolism has been well established (Skeith and Healey, 1968; Fanelli, Bohn, and Stafford, 1970; Simkin, 1971). I. M. Weiner (personal communication) tested the effect of intravenous infusions of iopanoic acid, tyropanoic acid, and some of their analogs on uric acid excretion in *Cebus* monkeys and showed that tyropanoic acid and possibly the chlorinated analog of iopanoic acid had significant uricosuric activity in this species.

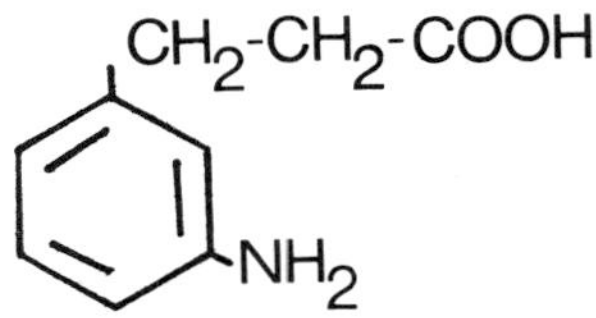

Fig. 1. Chemical structure of 3-amino hydrocinnamic acid.

The purpose of this study was to measure the uricosuric activity of several analogs of 3-amino hydrocinnamic acid after intravenous and oral administration to *Cebus albifrons* monkeys and to compare their potency with probenecid (Fig. 2).

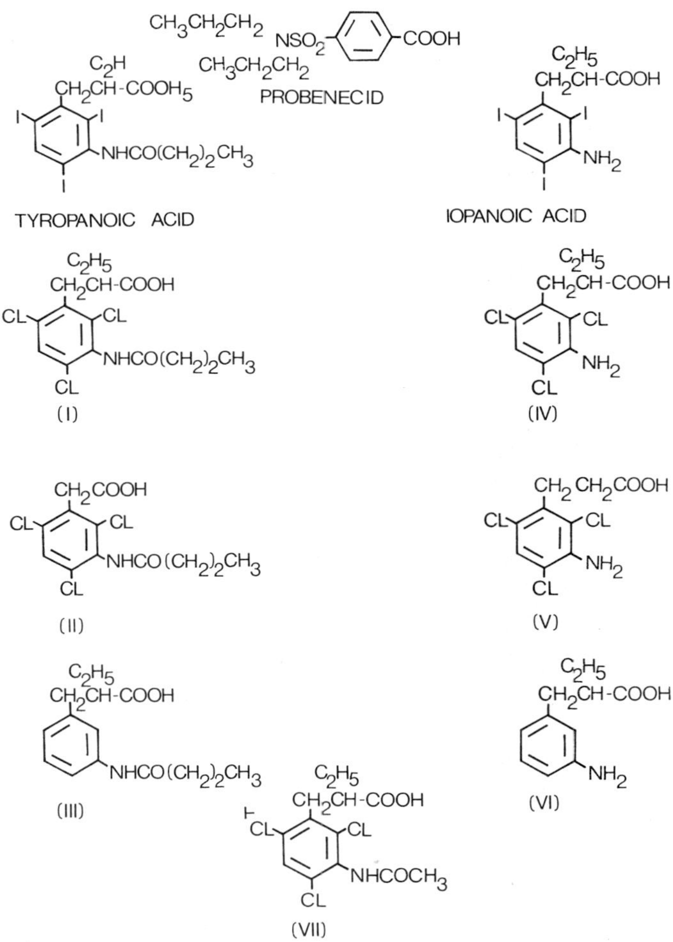

Fig. 2. Chemical structures of 3-amino hydrocinnamic acid analogs and probenecid.

METHODS

Female *Cebus albifrons* monkeys weighing 1.3–2.1 kg were fasted overnight and then anesthetized with pentobarbital sodium 30 mg/kg i.p. Two veins, usually a saphenous and a brachial, were cannulated with PE-50 tubing inserted through an 18-gauge thin-walled needle. One tube served for infusions and the other for blood sampling. The latter was kept filled with heparinized saline between samplings. A 5 Fr. polypropylene catheter was inserted into the bladder. Episiotomy was resorted to whenever necessary. Urine was allowed to drain continuously into collection cylinders and bladder emptying at the end of clearance periods was assisted by gently moving the catheter and occasionally applying suprapubic pressure.

Inulin clearance was used as a measure of glomerular filtration rate. A priming dose (50 mg/kg) was given intravenously followed by a constant infusion at 0.86 ml/min. The infusion contained mannitol 4%, inulin 0.2%, sodium chloride 0.9%, and was prepared with Sterile Water for Injection, U.S.P. Rectal temperature was monitored with a Tele-Thermometer and gooseneck lamps were used as a source of heat to help maintain body temperature.

After a sufficient length of time (a minimum of 1 hr) had elapsed to allow for equilibration the experiment was started. Two or three 10-min control clearance periods were carried out followed by eight 20-min periods after drug administration. Heparinized blood samples, 2.0–2.5 ml, were taken at the midpoint of most urine collection periods. At the conclusion of the experiment the packed red cells, separated from the plasma, were resuspended in sterile saline, filtered through gauze, and returned to the monkey.

For intravenous testing the compounds (0.1 mM/kg) were added to the constant infusion over 40 min. For oral testing the compounds (0.2 mM/kg) were dissolved in 4 ml of distilled water and sufficient NaOH to obtain a clear solution of the sodium salt and then administered orally via a 14 Fr. stomach tube. When the compounds were administered orally as the acids they were suspended in 1% gum tragacanth. The stomach tube was flushed with 3 ml of tap water.

A period of approximately three weeks was allowed between experiments for any one monkey.

The inulin content of plasma and urine samples was measured by the resorcinol method of Schreiner (1950). For plasma a 1:15 cadmium sulfate supernatant (Smith *et al.*, 1945) was prepared by mixing 0.25 ml of plasma, 2.5 ml of distilled water, 0.75 ml $CdSO_4$ solution (34.67 gm of $3CdSO_4^{=} \cdot 8H_2O$ plus 169 ml 1.0 N H_2SO_4 q.s. to 1000 ml with distilled water), and 0.25 ml of 1.0 N NaOH. The normalities of the NaOH and H_2SO_4 must be exactly equivalent. The tubes were allowed to stand for 10 min at room temperature and the supernatant was separated by centrifugation. Urine samples were diluted to 50 ml with distilled water and diluted again 1:25.

One-ml aliquots of the 1:15 cadmium sulfate plasma supernatants, appropriately diluted urine samples, inulin standards, and water (reagent blank) were reacted with 3.5 ml of a 2:7 mixture of alcoholic resorcinol (1 mg resorcinol per ml of 95% ethanol) and hydrochloric acid (224 ml of water added to 1000 ml of concentrated HC1). The samples were covered, placed in a water bath at 80°C for 25 min and then cooled in tap water for 3 min. Optical densities were read immediately in a Bausch and Lomb Spectronic 20 at 490 mμ.

Uric acid was determined by the modified carbonate-phosphotungstate method of Henry, Sobel, and Kim (1957). To 0.5 ml of plasma were added 4.0 ml of distilled water, 0.25 ml of 0.66 N H_2SO_4 and 0.25 ml of 10% sodium tungstate. After mixing, the tubes were centrifuged and the supernatants were decanted. Urine samples were diluted 1:3 with distilled water and used as such.

To 3 ml aliquots of the plasma sodium tungstate supernatant, appropriately diluted urine, uric acid standard, and water (reagent blank) were added 1 ml of 14% Na_2CO_3 and 1 ml of phosphotunstic acid. The samples were mixed, allowed to stand at room temperature for 20 min, and the optical densities were read at 660 mμ in a Bausch and Lomb Spectronic 20.

RESULTS AND DISCUSSION

The results of the intravenous study are summarized in Figs. 3 and 4 where each point represents the mean from four monkeys. Table 1 includes the standard errors and a comparison of the means with the corresponding

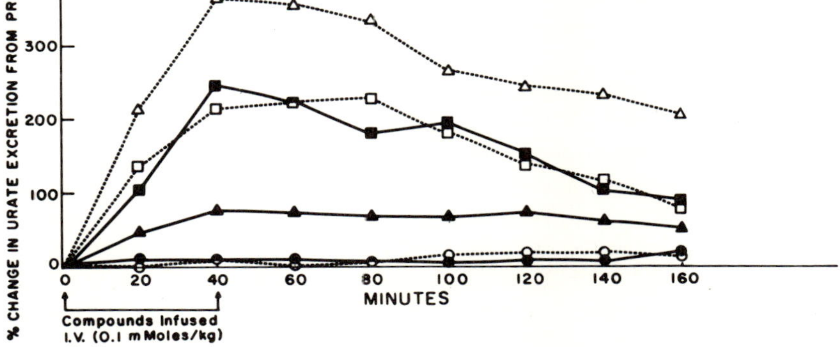

Fig. 3. Uricosuric activity of tyropanoic acid series in *Cebus albifrons* monkeys.

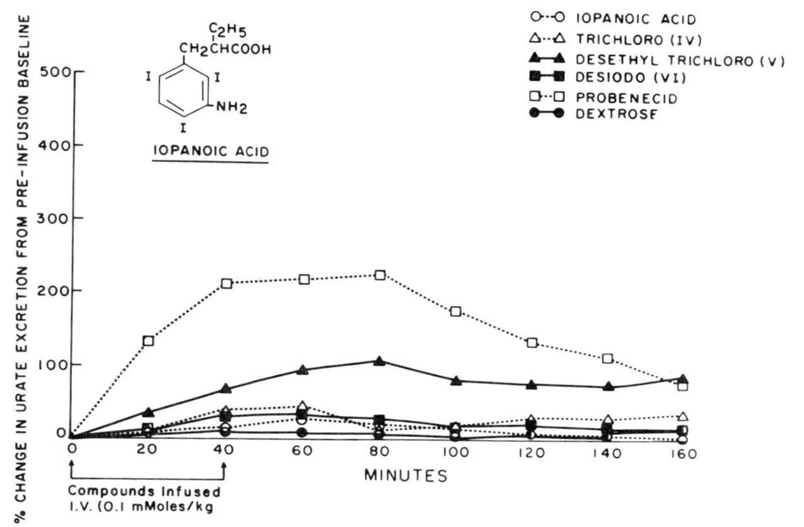

Fig. 4. Uricosuric activity of iopanoic acid series in *Cebus albifrons* monkeys.

dextrose control by Duncan's Multiple Range Test. Similar treatment of the data obtained from oral studies is shown in Fig. 5 and in Tables 2 and 3.

Since the glomerular filtration rate (GFR) (inulin clearance) was not altered by any of the compounds tested, an increase in the ratios C_{urate} (postmedication)/C_{urate} (premedication) represents a net increase in uric acid urinary excretion.

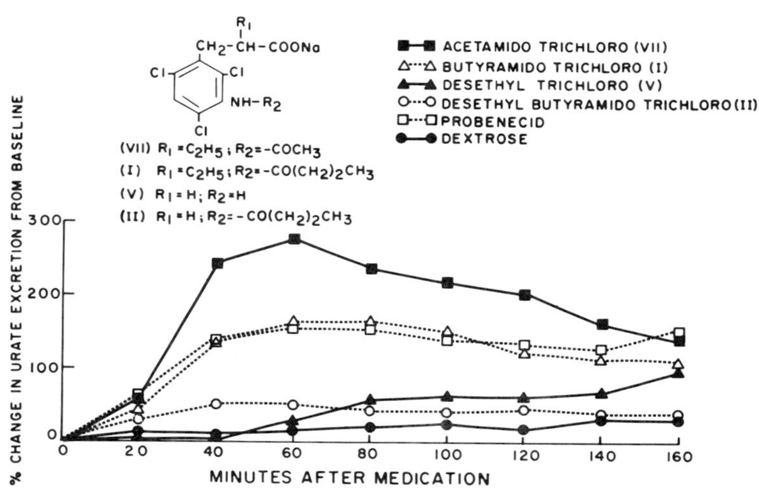

Fig. 5. Oral uricosuric activity in *Cebus albifrons* monkeys (0.2 mM/kg).

Table 1. Effect of several tyropanoic and iopanoic acid analogs on uric acid excretion in *Cebus albifrons* monkeys

	Postmedication clearance urate/GFR[a] / Premedication clearance urate/GFR							
	20 min	40 min	60 min	80 min	100 min	120 min	140 min	160 min
Tyropanoic acid	3.14[b] (0.24)	4.67[b] (0.27)	4.58[b] (0.22)	4.34[b] (0.24)	3.65[b] (0.18)	3.42[b] (0.03)	3.33[b] (0.13)	3.04[b] (0.18)
Butyramido trichloro (I)	2.04[b] (0.38)	3.47[b] (1.11)	3.21[b] (1.02)	2.80[b] (0.86)	2.96[b] (1.12)	2.51[b] (0.83)	2.06[b] (0.61)	1.90[b] (0.40)
Desethyl-butyramido trichloro (II)	1.47 (0.14)	1.78 (0.14)	1.73 (0.06)	1.68 (0.12)	1.68 (0.09)	1.74 (0.07)	1.62 (0.08)	1.51 (0.11)
Desiodo-butyramido (III)	0.96 (0.06)	1.10 (0.08)	1.04 (0.10)	1.06 (0.13)	1.14 (0.15)	1.18 (0.17)	1.17 (0.28)	1.15 (0.10)
Iopanoic acid	1.08 (0.11)	1.15 (0.04)	1.33 (0.04)	1.23 (0.08)	1.13 (0.04)	1.09 (0.11)	1.07 (0.10)	1.01 (0.13)
Trichloro (IV)	0.95 (0.08)	1.32 (0.08)	1.45 (0.12)	1.17 (0.08)	1.21 (0.04)	1.30 (0.04)	1.31 (0.08)	1.36 (0.20)
Desethyl trichloro (V)	1.35 (0.16)	1.70 (0.26)	1.92 (0.25)	2.08 (0.29)	1.81 (0.21)	1.78 (0.28)	1.76 (0.22)	1.86[b] (0.23)

Desiodo (VI)	1.10 (0.05)	1.34 (0.09)	1.33 (0.01)	1.27 (0.09)	1.23 (0.03)	1.21 (0.07)	1.18 (0.07)	1.17 (0.03)
Probenecid	2.37[b] (0.33)	3.15[b] (0.52)	3.24[b] (0.46)	3.28[b] (0.31)	2.80[b] (0.40)	2.38[b] (0.44)	2.17[b] (0.47)	1.80 (0.32)
Dextrose	1.11 (0.11)	1.11 (0.09)	1.11 (0.13)	1.08 (0.08)	1.05 (0.07)	1.07 (0.11)	1.08 (0.08)	1.18 (0.08)

All compounds infused i.v. (0.1 mM/kg/40 min).
[a]GFR (glomerular filtration rate) = clearance of inulin.
[b]$P < 0.05$; significantly different from corresponding dextrose mean (Duncan's Multiple Range Test). Means and standard errors (in parentheses) for $N = 5$.

Table 2. Effect of acetamido trichloro (VII), butyramido trichloro (I), and probenecid on uric acid excretion by *Cebus albifrons* monkeys after 0.2 mM/kg p.o. as sodium salts

	Postmedication clearance urate/GFR[a] / Premedication clearance urate/GFR							
	20 min	40 min	60 min	80 min	100 min	120 min	140 min	160 min
Acetamido trichloro (VII)	1.60 (0.29)	3.44[b] (0.63)	3.76[b] (0.31)	3.39[b] (0.18)	3.20[b] (0.26)	3.06[b] (0.19)	2.65[b] (0.23)	2.41[b] (0.29)
Butyramido trichloro (I)	1.42 (0.19)	2.39[b] (0.38)	2.66[b] (0.43)	2.65[b] (0.18)	2.54[b] (0.19)	2.23[b] (0.19)	2.15[b] (0.13)	2.10 (0.12)
Probenecid	1.66 (0.08)	2.38[b] (0.28)	2.57[b] (0.29)	2.55[b] (0.39)	2.44[b] (0.36)	2.37[b] (0.37)	2.33[b] (0.37)	2.54[b] (0.46)
Dextrose	1.13 (0.06)	1.12 (0.07)	1.19 (0.06)	1.23 (0.09)	1.28 (0.07)	1.20 (0.07)	1.30 (0.06)	1.34 (0.08)

[a]GFR (glomerular filtration rate) = clearance of inulin.
[b]$P < 0.05$; significantly different from corresponding dextrose mean (Duncan's Multiple Range Test). Means and standard erros (in parentheses) for $N = 5$.

Table 3. Effect of acetamido trichloro (VII), butyramido trichloro (I), and probenecid on uric acid excretion by *Cebus albifrons* monkeys after 0.2 mM/kg p.o. as the acids suspended in 0.1% gum tragacanth

	Postmedication clearance urate/GFR[a] / Premedication clearance urate/GFR							
	20 min	40 min	60 min	80 min	100 min	120 min	140 min	160 min
Acetamido trichloro (VII)	1.54 (0.33)	2.37[b] (0.50)	2.51[b] (0.42)	2.22[b] (0.46)	2.06 (0.36)	1.93[b] (0.26)	1.98[b] (0.20)	2.25 (0.57)
Butyramido trichloro (I)	1.42 (0.18)	1.54 (0.15)	1.65 (0.18)	1.69 (0.14)	1.78 (0.11)	1.81 (0.20)	1.81 (0.24)	1.83 (0.23)
Probenecid	1.09 (0.05)	1.43 (0.22)	1.60 (0.28)	2.06 (0.32)	2.25[b] (0.42)	2.19[b] (0.22)	2.30[b] (0.09)	2.48[b] (0.16)
Dextrose	1.13 (0.06)	1.12 (0.07)	1.19 (0.06)	1.23 (0.09)	1.28 (0.07)	1.20 (0.07)	1.30 (0.06)	1.34 (0.08)

[a]GFR (glomerular filtration rate) = clearance of inulin.
[b]$P < 0.05$; significantly different from corresponding dextrose mean (Duncan's Multiple Range Test). Means and standard errors (in parentheses) for $N = 5$.

The intravenous studies show that sodium tyropanoate has the highest uricosuric activity of all the compounds tested (Fig. 3, Table 1) and that its desiodo analog (compound III) is totally inactive. The chlorinated analog of tyropanoic acid (compound I) has uricosuric activity comparable with probenecid. Iopanoic acid and its chlorinated analogs showed little activity in our test (Fig. 4, Table 1).

From the intravenous studies it appeared that substitution in the amino group enhanced uricosuric activity. The 3-acetamido trichloro analog (compound VII) was therefore made and tested orally at a dose of 0.2 mM/kg. The results of the oral studies are shown in Fig. 5 and in Tables 2 and 3. The acetamido analog (VII) is well absorbed whether it is administered as the acid or as the sodium salt. The butyramido analog (I) is not as active when given as the acid, which means that particle size may play an important role on its absorption.

The data obtained from the intravenous and oral studies in *Cebus* monkeys indicate that, if an iodinated compound in the series had uricosuric activity, the chlorinated analog, although less active, retained sufficient activity. It is also apparent that acylation of the 3-amino group enhances the uricosuric activity, as does the addition of an ethyl group in the α position of the hydrocinnamic acid.

Two of the chlorinated analogs tested (I and VII) had uricosuric activity comparable with probenecid. We have expanded our studies with VII to preliminary toxicity evaluation and some ancillary pharmacological testing (unpublished data). The compound has low toxicity (oral $LD_{50} > 7000$ mg/kg in mice and $> 10{,}000$ mg/kg in rats) and it was inactive in a series of conventional CNS and cardiovascular tests. In addition, it has one-third the gastric irritancy-ulcerogenic potential of probenecid ($P < 0.01$) after three daily oral doses as high as 400 mg/kg to rats. Finally, on the basis of the clinical evidence with the iodinated analogs, the compound may have long duration of action in man, which may be a significant contribution to the management of gout.

SUMMARY

A series of 3-amino hydrocinnamic acid derivatives were tested for their uricosuric activity in *Cebus albifrons* monkeys. In general, if an iodinated compound (i.e., tyropanoic acid) had uricosuric activity, the chlorinated analog was less active. Acylation of the 3-amino group enhanced uricosuric activity. The trichloro acetamido analog of iopanoic acid was found to have uricosuric activity comparable with probenecid, very low toxicity, and, from clinical data on iopanoic acid, it may have long-lasting uricosuric activity in man.

REFERENCES

Bonsnes, R. W., Dill, L. V., and Dana, E. S. 1944. The effect of diodrast on the normal uric acid clearance. J. Clin. Invest. 23: 776–782.

Fanelli, G. M., Bohn, D., and Stafford, S. 1970. Functional characteristics of the renal urate transport in the *Cebus* monkey. Am. J. Physiol. 218: 627–636.

Gutman, A. B. 1966. Uricosuric drugs, with special reference to probenecid and sulfinpyrazone. Adv. Pharmac. 4: 91–142.

Henry, R. J., Sobel, C., and Kim, J. 1957. A modified carbonate-phosphotungstate method for the determination of uric acid and comparison with the spectrophotometric uricase method. Am. J. Clin. Pathol. 28: 152–160.

McChesney, E. W., and Banks, W. F. 1965. Urinary excretion of three oral cholecystographic agents in man. Proc. Soc. Exp. Biol. Med. 119: 1027–1030.

Mudge, G. H. 1971. Uricosuric action of cholecystographic agents. A possible factor in nephrotoxicity. New Engl. J. Med. 284: 929–933.

Postlethwaite, A. E., and Kelly, W. N. 1971. Uricosuric effect of radiocontrast agents. A study in man of four commonly used preparations. Ann. Internal Med. 74: 845–852.

Schreiner, G. E. 1950. Determination of inulin by means of resorcinol. Proc. Soc. Exp. Biol. Med. 74: 117–120.

Simkin, P. A. 1971. Uric acid metabolism in *Cebus* monkeys. Am. J. Physiol. 221: 1105–1109.

Skeith, M. D., and Healey, L. A. 1968. Urate clearance in *Cebus* monkeys. Am. J. Physiol. 214: 582–584.

Smith, H. W., Finkelstein, N., Aliminosa, B., Crawford, B., and Graber, M. 1945. The renal clearances of substituted hippuric acid derivatives and other aromatic acids in dog and man. J. Clin. Invest. 24: 388–404.

Choline and the Organic Cation Transport System

Barbara R. Rennick
Department of Pharmacology and Therapeutics
State University of New York Medical School
Buffalo, New York

The proximal renal tubule can actively excrete drugs and autopharmacologic agents that are organic cations. This transport from peritubular plasma to lumen is an active transport that requires energy and will be competitively inhibited by structural analogs. Some of the cations can be shown to have a maximum transport capacity (T_m). During transport, renal metabolism of the cations may occur.

In the case of choline, a biocation, net tubular excretion occurred when the plasma choline level was raised from the endogenous level of 2×10^{-5}M to 4×10^{-5}M in dogs and chickens. Further elevation of plasma choline increased tubular excretion until a T_m was reached at choline levels of 20×10^{-5}M.

At endogenous levels of plasma choline the renal clearance of choline was only 1/30th that of the glomerular filtration rate (GFR) in dogs and chickens. Since choline has a pKa at 13.4 it is always ionized in the body. For this reason it was concluded that the reabsorption of choline was an active transport process.

It is suggested that the kidney has a bidirectional transport system for choline which may offer a homeostatic mechanism to maintain a stable plasma choline.

Renal excretion of drugs and autopharmacologic agents which are strong organic bases (cations) is regulated by glomerular filtration of the nonprotein bound ions in the plasma and by tubular mechanisms. An active excretory transport from peritubular blood to urine has been demonstrated for many strong organic bases. The amount of the organic cation in the tubule fluid which will eventually arrive in the bladder urine may be altered by passive back-diffusion if a nonionized, lipid-soluble fraction of the molecule exists. In addition, active transport in the direction of reabsorption from lumen to plasma may occur. Another process to regulate the excretion of strong organic cations is intrarenal metabolism during the transport process. Metabolites may be polar as in the case of anionic conjugation products, which are then rapidly excreted by the tubule. On the other hand, certain renal metabolites of cations may be less well transported than the parent cation, as we shall see in the example of the oxidation product of choline.

The presence of these various mechanisms for transtubular movement presents a complex system to regulate excretion of cationic drugs and naturally occurring cations. In this discussion the regulation of the excretion of the naturally occurring organic cation, choline, will be used as the major example.

Several reviews dealing with the regulation of renal excretion of organic cations are available (Sperber, 1954, 1959; Peters, 1960; Weiner and Mudge, 1964; Weiner, 1967, 1971; Rennick and Quebbemann, 1971; Rennick, 1972).

METHODS TO DEMONSTRATE TUBULAR FUNCTION

Active Tubular Excretion

1. Active tubular excretion is present when the renal clearance of the cations exceeds the simultaneous glomerular filtration rate, provided lumenal trapping by nonionic diffusion is excluded.
2. The stop-flow technique will provide evidence for tubular excretion.
3. Tubular secretion may be studied *in vivo* in birds by the Sperber technique (Sperber, 1946, 1947, 1948a,b; Lindahl and Sperber, 1956). An accessory renal portal circulation in birds makes it possible to administer substances to the renal tubules of one kidney and to recognize tubular secretion rate without concern for plasma protein binding or glomerular filtration rate. Substrates are infused directly into a saphenous vein in the leg. The saphenous blood goes to the renal portal circulation and bathes the renal tubules (Fig. 1). Urine is collected separately from each kidney. Any infused substrate which enters the ipsilateral renal portal circulation and which is secreted by the renal tubules will appear in the urine from the ipsilateral kidney. The expression of the excess excreted from the infused kidney was described by Sperber in the following way: ATEF $= (E - C)/I$ where ATEF is the apparent tubular excretion fraction, E is the rate of excretion from the infused kidney, C is the rate of excretion from the control kidney, and I is the rate of infusion. If the infused substance is excreted by the renal tubules there will be a greater amount in the urine from the infused kidney than in the uninfused kidney. Any infused substance which escapes excretion from the infused kidney tubules will enter the systemic circulation and be circulated to both kidneys equally. The amount excreted by the control kidney is subtracted from the infused kidney excretion and the difference is the minimal amount excreted by the tubule of the infused kidney. The excess recovered from the infused

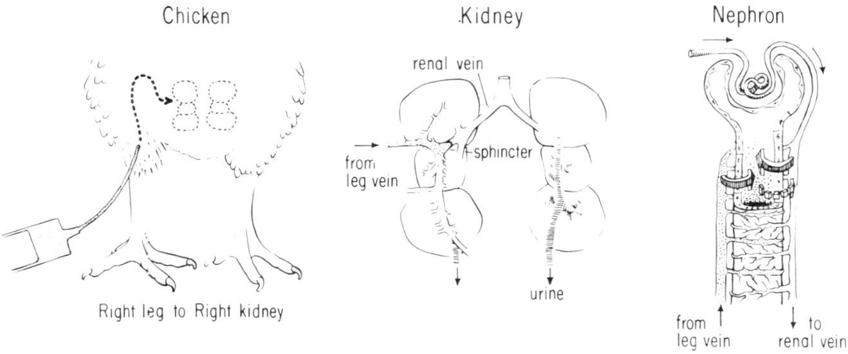

Fig. 1. Diagram of the renal-portal circulation in birds.

kidney was added by the tubule. Plasma protein binding will not alter the excretion. No plasma assays are necessary. It is necessary to coadminister a marker to determine the amount of the infusion reaching the kidney. For example, if one is studying the transport of an organic cation, the simultaneous transport of an organic anion such as p-aminohippuric acid (PAH) is measured. The ratio ATEF cation/ATEF PAH represents the transport efficiency (TE). A selective inhibition of the cation by a cation competitor, while the anion continues to be transported, indicates selective competition for the cation without any change in the renal perfusion. The Sperber technique provides some unique advantages. Studies can be performed to measure tubular transport with infusion of extremely small amounts of very potent pharmacologically active substances. For example, radioactively labeled norepinephrine can be administered at 10^{-9} moles/min and its tubular transport can be measured without complicating cardiovascular effects. Little of the infused material is available to the central circulation since it is being excreted on its first pass through the kidney. Another unique advantage of this technique is to study renal metabolism *in vivo*. When the urine is examined for the infused substrate and its metabolites, the metabolites found in excess in the urine from the infused kidney represent only the metabolites produced intrarenally. Furthermore, it is possible to secure information about the capacities *in vivo* of renal metabolic pathways, and to assess the effects of drugs and chemicals on the function of selected renal metabolic pathways *in vivo*.

4. Proximal tubule micropuncture samples which contain more concentrated cation when compared with simultaneous inulin values indicate active transport.
5. The perfused rat kidney can secrete cations as demonstrated by excretion in excess of simultaneous inulin clearance (M. E. Trimble, M. Acara, and B. Rennick, in press).
6. Excretion by *Lophius americanus*, an aglomerular fish, is taken as evidence for proximal tubular excretion (Forster, Berglund, and Rennick, 1958).

7. Infusion directly into the renal artery in mammals will allow the measurement of tubular excretion in cases such as choline where there is rapid disappearance of the infused substrate from the plasma upon intravenous administration.

Passive Nonionic Back Diffusion

1. A study of cation excretion during variation of urine pH and volume will indicate whether passive processes are present.

Active Tubular Reabsorption

1. Active tubular reabsorption is present when the renal clearance of the cations is less than the simultaneous filtered load, provided peritubular trapping by nonionic diffusion is excluded.
2. Proximal tubule micropuncture samples which contain less than the concentration which would have been filtered in relation to simultaneous inulin values indicate tubular reabsorption.
3. Enhanced excretion of a cation during administration of small amounts of a competitive inhibitor of transport may be evidence for inhibition of reabsorptive transport.

In Vitro Slice Uptake

The ability of slices of renal cortex to accumulate substrates against a concentration gradient may indicate a carrier mediated process (Cross and Taggart, 1950). The response to interference with energy sources and the effects of competitive inhibitors is readily measured.

PROXIMAL RENAL TUBULAR TRANSPORT OF ORGANIC CATIONS

Early evidence that the active tubular excretion of strong organic cations occurred was based on experiments which demonstrated virtually complete clearance of the synthetic organic cation tetraethylammonium (TEA) from the plasma on one circulation in dogs (Rennick *et al.,* 1947) and from experiments in the chicken by Sperber in which N'-methylnicotinamide (NMN), a naturally occurring metabolite, was rapidly excreted by the infused kidney (Sperber 1947, 1948b). Since these two substances are always ionized at body pH and could never be nonionized since their pKa's are so high, it seemed unlikely that these movements could occur by diffusion. A large number of organic cations are now known to be actively secreted by the proximal tubule (Table 1). The evidence has been gained in the several ways mentioned in the section on methods. Active transport mechanisms for cations have been supported also by the findings of competitive inhibition by analogs, inhibition by substances which interfere with energy sources and oxygen, and lack of inhibition by substrates for the organic anion transport system.

Table 1. Cationic drugs and autopharmacologic agents excreted by the proximal renal tubule

Autopharmacologic agents	Drugs
Acetylcholine	Atropine
Choline	Hexamethonium
Dopamine	Mecamylamine
Epinephrine	Mepiperphenidol
Histamine	Morphine
N′-methylnicotinamide	Neostigmine
Norepinephrine	Quinine
Serotonin	Tetraethylammonium
Thiamine	Triethylethanolamine
Tyramine	Tolazoline

FACTORS AFFECTING TRANSPORT RATE

The rate of tubular secretion of organic cations may vary from almost complete clearance, e.g., TEA which is cleared at the same rate as simultaneous PAH, to considerably lower clearances for choline and quinine. A number of mechanisms may be proposed to account for less than complete excretory transport of some cations by the tubule. Discussion of four of these follows.

Concurrent Metabolism of Substrate by the Renal Tubule

For some transportable cationic substrates the rate of tubular transport can be found to vary directly with the load of substrate offered. One explanation for this is metabolism by the renal parenchyma of some of the substrate to a nontransportable metabolite during renal transport. As the load of substrate offered is increased, the capacity of the metabolic pathway is exceeded, and more of the unmetabolized, transportable substrate is available for transport. An example of this mechanism was found in choline transport studies using the Sperber technique in hens (Acara and Rennick, 1972a). The ATEF for PAH at increasing infusion loads of PAH is demonstrated in Fig. 2. The ATEF is essentially 100% at all loads below the T_m. In the same type of experiment the pattern of the choline TE is different (Fig. 3). Choline TE is negligible at the lowest infusion rate and increases with increasing infusion loads to reach a peak at the T_m. Analysis of urine during choline infusion revealed that, at the lowest infusion loads, the infused choline had been partly converted to betaine (Fig. 4). Thus it was concluded that the lack of excretion of choline by the renal tubules at the low infusion loads was a result of renal metabolism of the infused choline as well as other, as yet undefined, dispositions.

The tubular transport of acetylcholine was found to increase as the load of acetylcholine was raised. This suggested that the renal tubule metabolized a portion of the acetylcholine being transported. The proportion metabolized decreased as the load was increased (Fig. 5) (Acara and Rennick, 1972b).

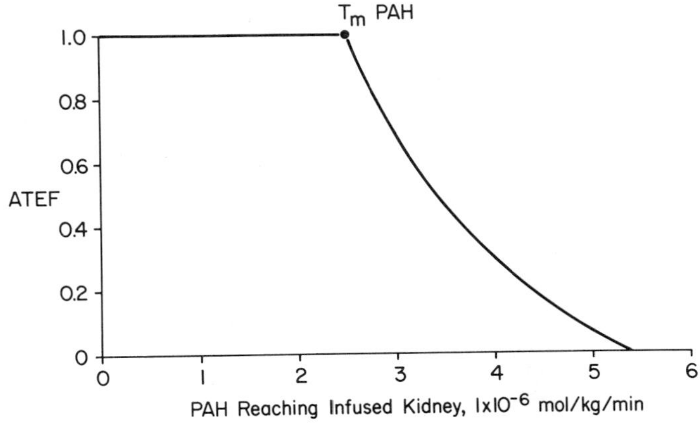

Fig. 2. Diagram of the ATEF of PAH at increasing loads of substrate to exceed the T_m.

In similar experiments in chickens it was found that all of the phenylethylamine reaching the kidney at infusion rates of 1×10^{-9} moles/kg/min was metabolized to phenylacetic acid and other metabolites (Quebbemann and Rennick, 1970). The phenylacetic acid formed in the renal cell was transported into the urine by a probenecid-sensitive step. In experiments using the Sperber technique in chickens, May, Fujimoto, and Inturrisi (1967) and Watrous, May, and Fujimoto (1970) studied the renal tubular transport of the cation morphine. They found that the cationic morphine was partially conjugated to anionic morphine ethereal sulfate during transport from blood to

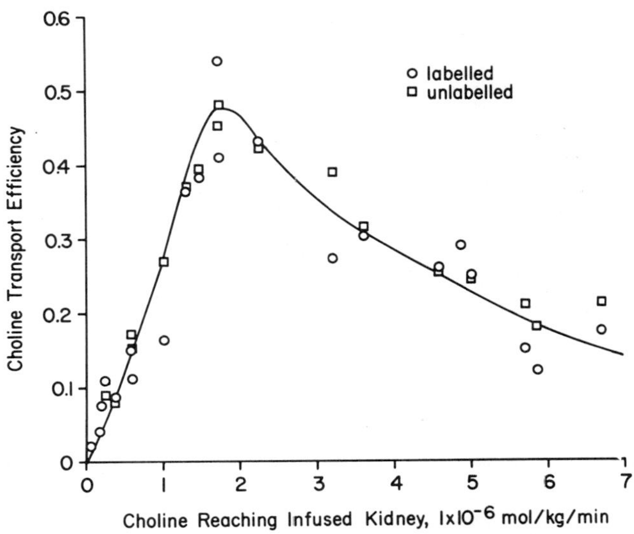

Fig. 3. Transport efficiency of choline at increasing infusion rates. PAH infusion rate, 0.4×10^{-6} moles/min throughout.

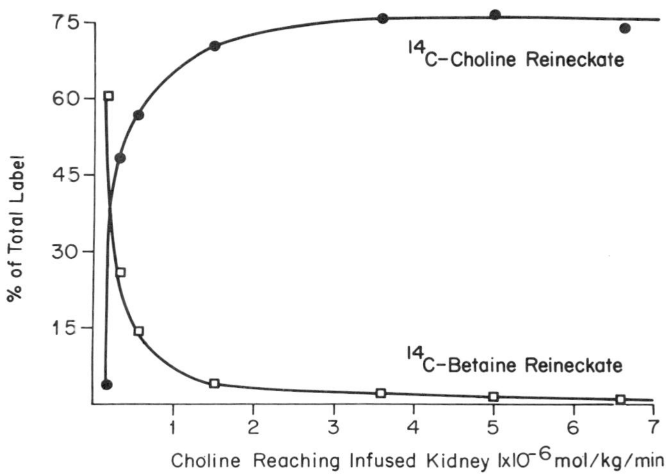

Fig. 4. Relative percentage of total excreted label recovered as [^{14}C] choline or [^{14}C] betaine reineckate at increasing infusion rates of choline. Each point represents a single determination.

urine across the proximal renal tubule. Such observations suggest a role for renal metabolism in altering the rate of renal tubular excretion of organic cations.

The tubular excretion of creatinine can be inhibited by either anionic or cationic competitors (O'Connell, Romeo, and Mudge, 1962; Rennick, 1967).

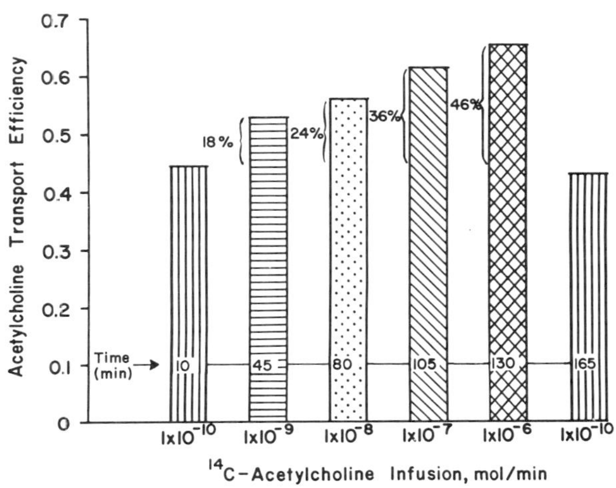

Fig. 5. Effect of increasing acetylcholine infusion rates on the TE of acetylcholine. Acetylcholine infusion rate appears below each bar; [^{3}H] PAH infusion rate, 3.5×10^{-10} moles/min. Consecutive time for each urine collection period is indicated for each infusion rate of acetylcholine. Each bar represent the mean of all 5-min urine collections during the time period shown. Percentage increase in acetylcholine transport is noted next to the upper portion of each bar.

Creatinine is an amphoteric substance and it has been suggested that this is the reason for the apparent bimodal transport. When [^{14}C] norepinephrine is infused in chickens in the Sperber technique, the transport of label can be inhibited by both anionic and cationic competitors (Rennick and Pryor, 1965). Renal tubular metabolism of norepinephrine to anionic metabolites was occurring simultaneously (Rennick, Pryor, and Basch, 1965). Although norepinephrine is amphoteric, it seems likely that the apparent bimodal transport of norepinephrine resulted from the stimultaneous presence of the cationic substrate and its anionic metabolites.

Affinity of Substrates for Transport Carrier and Maximum Transport Capacity

The affinity of a series of organic cations for the cationic transport system has been assessed indirectly in two major ways. Using the Sperber technique in chickens, the ability of a series of bases to inhibit the transport of NMN has been measured. The ability to inhibit may reflect the affinity for the carrier (Volle *et al.*, 1959). In studies with renal cortical slice uptake, inhibitor potency has been similarly measured against NMN uptake (Farah, Frazer, and Porter, 1959). Great variation in competitor potency was found. The review by Peters (1960) carefully records the findings in this area. No conclusions can be made about structure-inhibition potency that are helpful for understanding the carrier mediation. A protein has been isolated from kidney tissue which has great affinity for the transported cations (Ross, Pessah, and Farah, 1969; Magour, Farah, and Sroka, 1969). It is suggested that this is the transport protein which acts as a carrier for organic cations.

The maximum transport capacity (T_m) for these transportable cations should be a factor in determining excretion characteristics of these substrates. Unfortunately it has not been possible to obtain T_m's for many of the cations owing to their toxic side effects. Some values for T_m's expressed on the basis of body weight in kilograms for one kidney in units of 10^{-6} moles/kg/min are as follows: TEA, dog, 0.4 (Rennick and Farah, 1956); choline, chicken, 1.2 (Acara and Rennick, 1972a); NMN, chicke, 2.5 (Sperber, 1954); priscoline, 0.6–0.75 (Orloff, Aronow, and Berliner 1953).

Passive Back Diffusion

The apparent rate of tubular excretion of some cations can be modified by the simultaneous process on nonionic back diffusion. A cationic substrate previously transported into the lumen of the proximal tubule may be non-ionized at the pH of the distal tubule fluid and diffuse out of the lumen along its concentration gradient. Torretti, Weiner, and Mudge (1962) studied the tubular excretion of several organic cations using competitive inhibitors and modifying urine pH in dogs. In their well-controlled studies they were able to conclude that some organic ions are excreted by a three-component mechanism, i.e., filtration, active tubular excretion, and passive reabsorption. Quinine and tolazoline were substrates whose transport was characterized by these three renal mechanisms.

Active Tubular Reabsorption

Active tubular reabsorption of organic cations may occur at a site beyond the site of simultaneous active tubular excretion. Such a model for bidirectional transport of some cations would resemble the currently accepted model for uric acid excretion. Such bidirectional transports could account for excretion rates of cations that are less than 100%. The pattern of tubular transport of the naturally occurring cation choline suggests the possibility of bidirectional transport. Choline is a cation with a high pKa and would be ionized at any body pH, thus nonionic back diffusion would not occur. As was mentioned earlier, choline is excreted by the renal tubule when a load of choline is infused into the peritubular blood. The tubular excretion of choline has demonstrated a maximum capacity (T_m) (Fig. 6). It was found that the addition of small amounts of hemicholinium-3 (HC-3) would produce a 30%

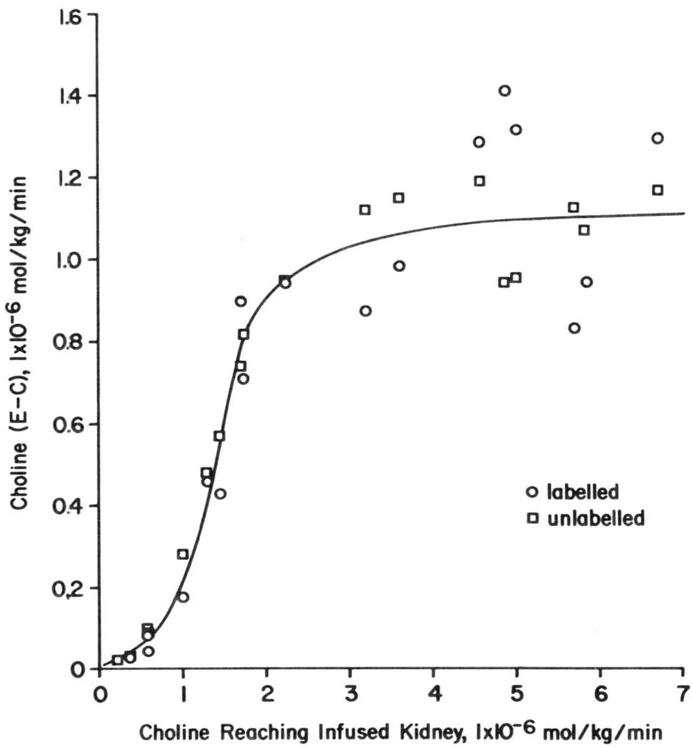

Fig. 6. Excretion (E–C) of choline at increasing choline infusion rates. E excretion from infused kidney; C, excretion from control kidney. PAH infusion rate, 0.4 × 10^{-6} moles/min.

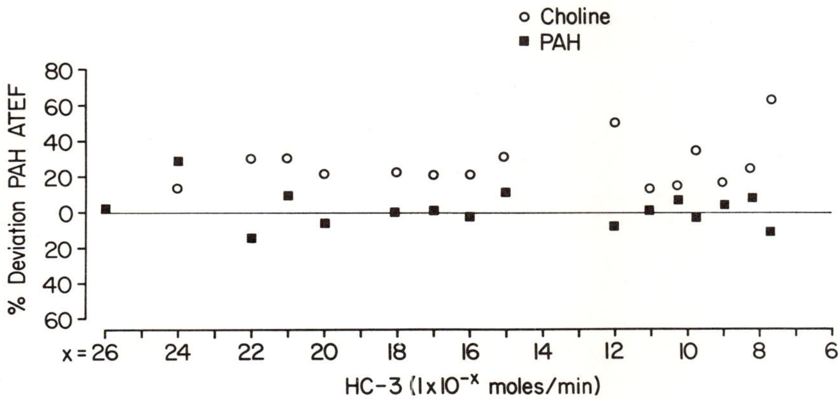

Fig. 7. Percentage increase in choline excretion during choline loading caused by increasing infusions of HC-3. Simultaneous PAH ATEF is noted.

increase in the tubular excretion fraction of choline during net secretion (Fig. 7) (Acara, Kowalski, and Rennick, 1973). It is unusual to find something that increases tubular transport, and it was particularly unexpected here because HC-3 was thought to inhibit the membrane transport of choline into nerves. One interpretation of the mechanism of this enhancement of choline tubular transport is that reabsorptive transport of choline is more sensitive to inhibition by HC-3 than the secretory transport. This resembles the reasoning that is used to explain the biphasic effect of salicylates at high and low doses on uric acid transport.

Reabsorptive transport of choline is suggested by another piece of evidence. The renal clearance of choline at endogenous plasma levels of 2×10^{-5}M is only 1/30th that of the simultaneous glomerular filtration rate in

Table 2.

	Endogenous plasma choline (1×10^{-5} M)	Endogenous renal clearance of choline[a] (ml/kg/min)
Dog	1.97 ± 0.338 (3)	0.02 ± 0.005 (3)
Chicken	2.12 ± 0.190 (18)	0.03 ± 0.003 (26)
	With exogenous choline	
Dog[b]	20.0	2.0
Chicken[c]	31.5	5.0

Number of samples given by number in parentheses.
[a]One kidney.
[b]Renal artery infusion.
[c]Intravenous infusion.

dogs and chickens (Table 2). Since choline diffusion seems unlikely, the above two observations suggest that the renal tubule may have the capacity to transport choline actively in the direction of reabsorption.

HOMEOSTATIC REGULATION OF PLASMA CHOLINE CONCENTRATION BY BIDIRECTIONAL TRANSPORT ACROSS THE RENAL TUBULE AND TUBULAR METABOLISM OF CHOLINE

Endogenous plasma levels of free choline were found to be maintained at an extremely stable value of about 2×10^{-5}M in several species (Bligh, 1952). The concentration of free choline in plasma showed no variation following strenuous exercise and ingestion of food. Injected choline disappeared rapidly from the circulation (Gardiner and Paton, 1972). The mechanisms which maintain the very stable plasma free choline have not been determined. Choline is a biologically active cationic substance which has three major biologic roles to play: (1) the synthesis of acetylcholine by neurons is dependent on a supply of choline entering from plasma and being acetylated by choline acetyltransferase; (2) choline is a component of membranes in the form of phosphatidylcholine; (3) betaine, which is formed by the oxidation of choline by choline oxidase, is a major methyl donor. We have attempted to determine the role of the kidneys in the homeostatic regulation of plasma choline levels. We measured the renal clearance of choline in the endogenous state in dogs and chickens. Plasma and urine choline were measured by an enzymatic radiochemical microassay using choline kinase and measuring the production of [^{32}P]phosphorylcholine in the presence of added AT^{32}P. The plasma choline levels in anesthetized dogs and unanesthetized hens agreed with those of Bligh (1952) (Table 2.) The renal clearance of choline at endogenous levels was only 1/50th–1/30th that of the glomerular filtration rate in dogs and chickens. Thus the freely filtered choline was reabsorbed by the tubule. This suggested active reabsorption of the filtered choline. Thus at the usual level of plasma choline of 2×10^{-5}M the kidney conserves plasma choline by returning the filtered choline to the body (Acara and Rennick, 1973).

I have mentioned earlier in another context that when choline is infused into the peritubular blood of the chicken kidney at low levels the kidney converts choline to metabolites, but with increasing infusion load the tubule begins to excrete the choline into the tubule fluid. At infusion loads of about 2×10^{-6} moles/kg/min a transport maximum for choline of 1.2×10^{-6} moles/kg/min is attained.

Similar experiments were performed in dogs with the choline being infused into a renal artery to avoid pharmacologic complications arising from systemic infusion of large amounts of choline. Choline disappears rapidly from the blood when administered intravenously. Figure 8 shows the renal clearance of choline from the infused kidney plotted against the plasma concentrations resulting from the increasing choline infusions. The renal

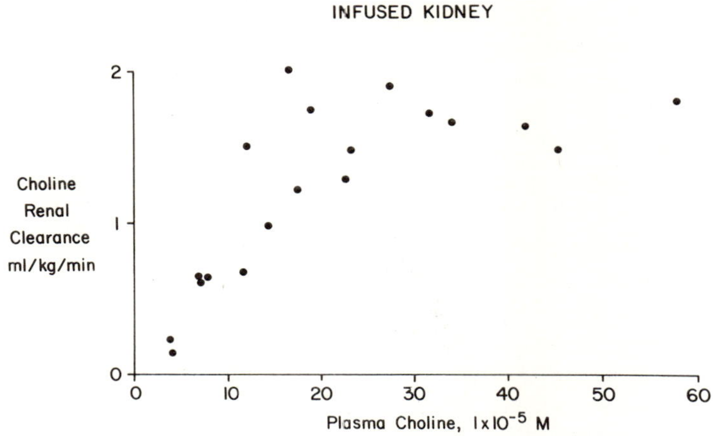

Fig. 8. Renal clearance of choline from the infused kidney during increasing rates of choline infusion into the renal artery of three dogs.

clearance of choline rose to values above the 1 ml/kg/min which would represent glomerular filtration at plasma levels of choline which were about five times greater than the endogenous levels. At plasma levels over 20×10^{-5}M, or 10-fold greater than the endogenous levels, a plateau of clearance was reached suggesting that the transport maximum had been reached for this experimental situation (Acara and Rennick, 1973).

Clearances were plotted for the uninfused kidney where the recirculated choline was elevating the plasma level (Fig. 9). Here the renal clearance rose when the plasma level was doubled over the endogenous level. These data support the idea that a rise in the plasma choline level in the peritubular blood results in an active transport of choline from blood to urine. A rise in plasma level from 2 to 4×10^{-5}M initiates tubular excretion of choline. At this level the metabolic and storage processes for choline may be saturated and choline remains in the cell to be transported. In parallel studies in the chicken, tubular transport of choline began at exactly the same value of 4×10^{-5}M (Acara and Rennick, 1973).

Figure 10 shows a stop-flow picture for choline. Choline was infused into the renal artery in dogs during occlusion of the ureter. Release of occlusion revealed a urine concentration curve that was superimposed on the curve for simultaneous PAH transport, and thus indicated secretion into the proximal tubule. The proximal tubule localization for organic cation transport had previously been shown for TEA (Rennick and Moe, 1960). Similar stop-flow data for choline had been shown by Vander (1962) (Acara and Rennick, 1973).

These results are interpreted to mean that the kidney has a major role to play in the homeostatic regulation of the level of choline in the plasma (Fig. 11). At endogenous levels of plasma choline which are $1{-}2 \times 10^{-5}$M, choline is freely filtered at the glomeruli and this cationic choline in the

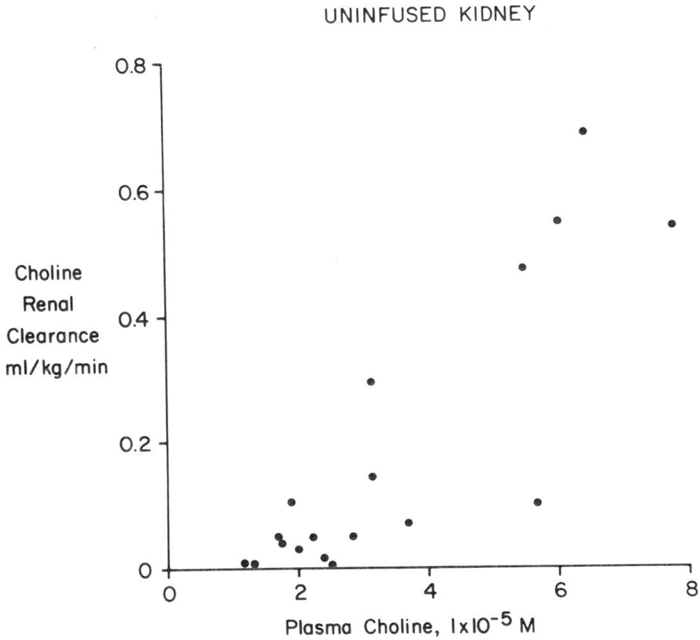

Fig. 9. Renal clearance of choline from the uninfused kidney of three dogs during infusion into the contralateral renal artery.

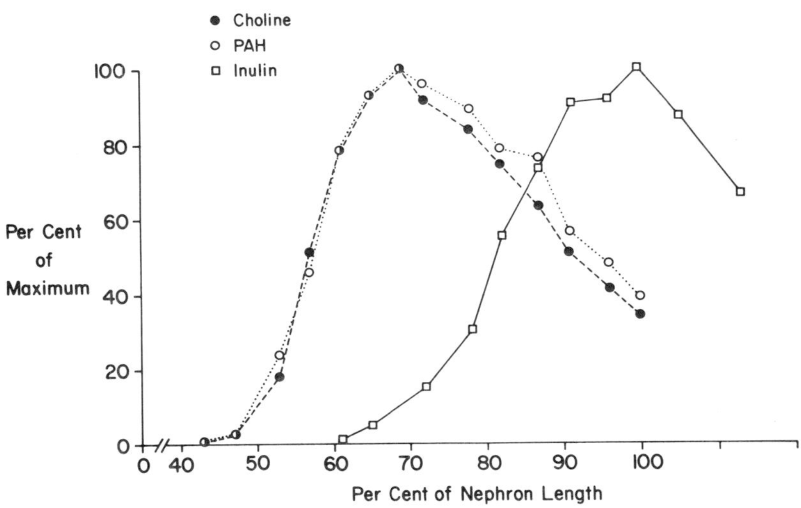

Fig. 10. Excretion of choline, PAH, and inulin in stop-flow experiments in dogs following injection into the renal artery. The recovery of choline in the urine obtained from the injected kidney after release of occlusion was 29% of that injected. Similar recovery of PAH was 48% of that injected.

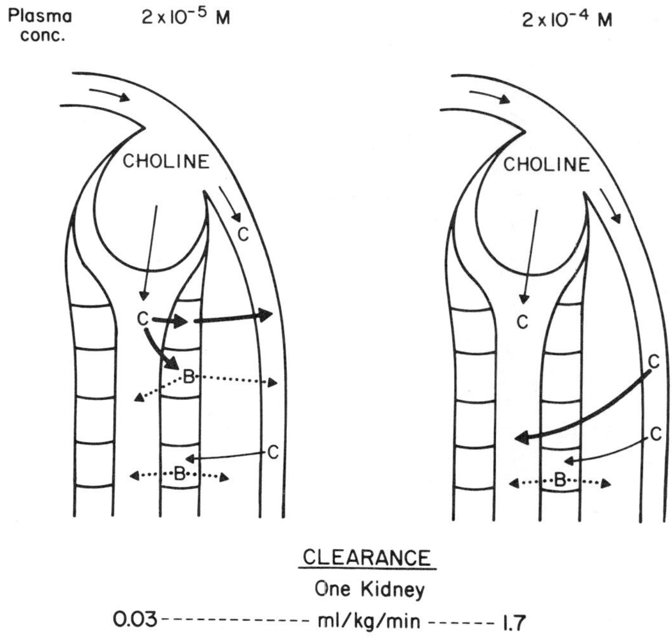

Fig. 11. Diagram of nephron to demonstrate proposed bidirectional transports of choline. The pathway of choline transport at plasma choline concentrations of 2×10^{-5}M (endogenous level) is by filtration and net reabsorption by an active process in nephron on left. At plasma concentrations of 2×10^{-4}M the excretion of choline is by glomerular filtration and net tubular excretion by an active process in nephron on right. Betaine formed in tubule cell diffuses from site of production. C, choline; B, betaine.

filtrate is largely reabsorbed by an active process as it moves down the tubule. At the same time choline entering the peritubular side of the proximal tubule cell is metabolized to betaine which is not transported into the lumen, but only diffuses to the extent of a few percent. Thus at endogenous levels of plasma choline the kidney acts to conserve body stores of choline by preventing the loss of filtered choline (Acara and Rennick, 1973).

As the concentration of choline is raised in the peritubular plasma, active tubular excretion of choline begins at levels only twice that of the endogenous choline levels in dog and chicken. This indicates the sensitivity of the feedback mechanism that regulates excretion. As plasma choline levels increase, tubule secretion increases to reach a maximum at peritubular plasma choline concentration of about 20×10^{-5}M in both dog and chicken, concentrations 10 times that of the endogenous plasma choline levels. Thus the kidney acts to reduce the body load of choline by active tubular transport.

These data suggest that the renal tubule conserves plasma choline by active reabsorption of filtered choline and metabolism of choline reaching the kidney to nontransportable betaine. On the other hand, the kidney can enhance excretion of plasma choline when the plasma concentration rises by activating an excretory tubular transport mechanism when the plasma choline doubles in concentration. This tubular excretion increases until plasma choline rises to 10 times the endogenous concentration, at which time a tubular maximum transport capacity is reached. Thus choline excretion is regulated by bidirectional active transports coupled with renal metabolism.

SUMMARY AND DISCUSSION

The proximal renal tubule has the capacity to transport actively endogenous cations such as choline in either the direction of excretion or reabsorption. Such transport mechanisms may be homeostatic mechanisms to regulate the body load of autopharmacologic agents. In addition the renal tubule may metabolize such transported substrates. It seems increasingly clear that some common transport carrier in tubule membranes is available to cationic drugs and naturally occurring cations such as choline and catecholamines to regulate excretion.

These transports for cations in the proximal renal tubule cells may have counterparts in other epithelial tissues. The choroid plexus has an active transport step for cations to move these substrates from the cerebrospinal fluid in an outward direction, presumably into blood. Choline is transported by the choroid plexus in this way (Aquilonius and Winbladh, 1972).

Although the mechanisms are not so amenable to proof, it is widely suggested that the reaccumulation of norepinephrine released from nerve terminals is an active process. In a review of the transport of biogenic amines, Murphy and Kopin (1972) discuss these transports of biogenic amines in many tissues. Thus the many translocations of endogenous cations may result from transport processes similar to those which are so readily quantitated in the proximal renal tubule.

ACKNOWLEDGMENTS

Dr. Margaret Acara has been an active collaborator in the work on choline transport and metabolism. This investigation was supported by USPHS Grants AM 10420 and HL 14092. M.A. was supported in part by United Health Foundation Fellowship FTF-12-UB-71.

REFERENCES

Acara, M., and B. R. Rennick. 1972a. Renal tubular transport of choline: modifications caused by intrarenal metabolism. J. Pharmac. Exp. Ther. 182: 1–13.

Acara, M., and B. R. Rennick. 1972b. Renal tubular transport of acetylcholine and atropine: enhancement and inhibition. J. Pharmac. Exp. Ther. 182: 14–26.

Acara, M., and B. R. Rennick. 1973. Regulation of plasma choline by the renal tubule; bidirectional transport of choline. Am. J. Physiol. 225: 1123–1128.

Acara, M., M. Kowalski and B. R. Rennick. 1973. Enhancement by hemicholinium - 3 of choline and acetylcholine excretion by the renal tubule of the chicken. J. Pharmac. Exp. Ther. 185: 254–260.

Aquilonius, S. M., and B. Winbladh. 1972. Cerebrospinal fluid clearance of choline and some other amines. Acta Physiol. Scand. 85: 78–90.

Bligh, J. 1952. The level of free choline in plasma. J. Physiol. 117: 234–240.

Cross, R. J., and J. V. Taggart. 1950. Renal tubular transport: accumulation of p-aminohippurate by rabbit kidney slices. Am. J. Physiol. 161: 181–190.

Farah, A., M. Frazer, and E. Porter. 1959. Studies on the uptake of N'-methylnicotinamide by renal slices of the dog. J. Pharmac. Exp. Ther. 126: 202–211.

Forster, R. P., F. Berglund, and B. R. Rennick. 1958. Tubular secretion of creatine, trimethylamine oxide, and other organic bases by the aglomerular kidney of *Lophius americanus*. J. Gen. Physiol. 42: 319–327.

Gardiner, J. E., and W. D. M. Paton. 1972. The control of the plasma choline concentration in the cat. J. Physiol. 227: 71–86.

Lindahl, K. M., and I. Sperber. 1956. Tubular excretion of histamine in the hen. Acta Physiol. Scand. 36: 13–16.

Magour, S., A. Farah, and A. Sroka. 1969. The partial purification of a carrier-like protein for organic bases from the kidney. J. Pharmac. Exp. Ther. 167: 243–252.

May, D. G., J. M. Fujimoto, and C. E. Inturrisi. 1967. The tubular transport and metabolism of morphine-N-methyl-C^{14} by the chicken kidney. J. Pharmac. Exp. Ther. 157: 626–635.

Murphy, D. L. and J. Kopin. 1972. The transport of biogenic amines. *In* L. E. Hokin (ed.), Metabolic Pathways (3rd edn), vol. 6, Metabolic Transport, Academic Press, New York, chap. 13.

O'Connell, J. M. B., J. A. Romeo, and G. H. Mudge. 1961. Renal tubular secretion of creatinine in the dog. Am. J. Physiol. 203: 985–990.

Orloff, J., L, Aronow, and R. W. Berliner. 1953. Transport of priscoline by renal tubules. J. Pharmac. Exp. Ther. 109: 214–217.

Peters, L. 1960. Renal rubular excretion of organic bases. Pharmac. Rev. 12: 1–35.

Quebbemann, A., and B. R. Rennick. 1970. Inhibition of renal tubular transport of catecholamines by cocaine: an organic base mechanism. J. Pharmac. Exp. Ther. 175: 248–258.

Rennick, B. R. 1967. Transport mechanisms for renal tubular excretion of creatinine in the chicken. Am. J. Physiol. 212: 1131–1134.

Rennick, B. R. 1972. Renal excretion of drugs: tubular transport and metabolism. Ann. Rev. Pharmac. 12: 141–156.

Rennick, B. R., and A. Farah. 1956. Studies on the renal tubular transport of tetraethylammonium ion in the dog. J. Pharmac. Exp. Ther. 116: 287–295.

Rennick, B. R., and G. K. Moe. 1960. Stop-flow localization of renal tubular excretion of tetraethylammonium. Am. J. Physiol. 198: 1267–1270.

Rennick, B. R., G. K. Moe, R. H. Lyons, S. W. Hoobler, and R. Neligh. 1947. Absorption and renal excretion of the tetraethylammonium ion. J. Pharmac. Exp. Ther. 91: 210–217.

Rennick, B. R., and M. Z. Pryor. 1965. Effects of autonomic drugs on renal tubular transport of catecholamines in the chicken. J. Pharmac. Exp. Ther. 148: 262–269.

Rennick, B. R., M. Z. Pryor, and B. G. Basch. 1965. Urinary metabolites of epinephrine and norepinephrine in the chicken. J. Pharmac. Exp. Ther. 148: 270–276.
Rennick, B. R., and A. J. Quebbemann. 1971. Renal tubular excretion of drugs: proximal tubule secretion and metabolism. *In* J. W. Fisher and E. J. Cafruny (eds.), Renal Pharmacology, Appleton-Century-Crofts, New York.
Ross, C. R., N. I. Pessah, and A. Farah. 1969. Attempts to label the renal carrier for organic bases with dibenamine. J. Pharmac. Exp. Ther. 167: 235–242.
Sperber, I. 1946. A new method for the study of renal tubular excretion in birds. Nature (Lond.) 158: 131.
Sperber, I. 1947. The mechanism of renal excretion of some detoxication products in the chicken. Proceedings of the 17th International Physiological Congress, Oxford University Press, London, pp. 217–218.
Sperber, I. 1948a. The excretion of some glucuronic acid derivatives and phenol sulphuric esters in the chicken. Lantbr-Högsk. Ann. 15: 317–349.
Sperber, I. 1948b. The excretion of piperidine, guanidine, methylguanidine and N'-methylnicotinamide in the chicken. Lantbr-Högsk. Ann. 16: 49–64.
Sperber, I. 1954. Competitive inhibition and specificity of renal tubular transport mechanisms. Archs Internat. Pharmacodyn. 97: 221–231.
Sperber, I. 1959. Secretion of organic anions in the formation of urine and bile. Pharmac. Rev. 11: 109–134.
Torretti, J., I. M. Weiner, and G. H. Mudge. 1962. Renal tubular secretion and reabsorption of organic bases in the dog. J. Clin. Invest. 41: 793–804.
Vander, A. J. 1962. Renal excretion of choline in the dog. Am. J. Physiol. 202: 319–324.
Volle, R. L., C. G. Huggins, G. A. Rodriques and L. Peters. 1959. Inhibition of the renal tubular transport of N'-methylnicotinamide (NMN) by 1.1-dialkylpiperidinium compounds in the avian kidney. J. Pharmac. Exp. Ther. 126: 190–194.
Watrous, W. M., D. G. May, and J. M. Fujimoto. 1970. Mechanism of the renal tubular transport of morphine and morphine ethereal sulfate in the chicken. J. Pharmac. Exp. Ther. 172: 224–229.
Weiner, I. M. 1967. Mechanisms of drug absorption and excretion. The renal excretion of drugs and related compounds. Ann. Rev. Pharmac. 7: 39–56.
Weiner, I. M. 1971. Sites of drug excretion. Chap. 18. Excretion of drugs by the kidney. *In* B. B. Brodie and J. R. Gillette (eds.), Concepts in Biochemical Pharmacology, Part 1, Handb. Exp. Pharmac. 28/1, Springer-Verlag, Berlin.
Weiner, I. M., and G. H. Mudge. 1964. Renal tubular mechanisms for excretion of organic acids and bases. Am. J. Med. 36: 743–762.

The Mechanism of Action of Diuretics in Renal Tubules

Maurice B. Burg
Laboratory of Kidney and Electrolyte Metabolism
National Heart and Lung Institute
Bethesda, Maryland

The cortical portion of the thick ascending limb of Henle's loop was dissected from rabbit kidneys and perfused *in vitro*. There was active chloride transport resulting in net NaCl reabsorption from the lumen with the electrical p.d. oriented lumen positive. Furosemide, mersalyl, and ethacrynic acid in the tubule lumen each caused a large and reversible decrease in the electrical potential difference (p.d.) and net chloride flux, indicating inhibition of the active chloride transport. Furosemide in the bath had no effect. Ethacrynic acid and mersalyl in the bath caused the p.d. to decrease, but the inhibition of the p.d. was not reversible. Evidence is presented that the reversible inhibition of chloride transport by the drugs in the lumen of the thick ascending limb of Henle's loop is related to their diuretic effect *in vivo,* whereas the irreversible inhibition by ethacrynic acid and mersalyl in the bath is more likely a nonspecific toxic effect which is normally prevented *in vivo* by binding of the drugs to plasma proteins or complexing to amino acids. The action of the diuretic drugs is specific to individual tubule segments as indicated by the results of additional studies in which furosemide in the lumen inhibited electrolyte transport in the thick ascending limb of Henle's loop but not the cortical collecting tubule, or proximal convoluted tubule and amiloride in the lumen inhibited electrolyte transport in the collecting tubule but not in the ascending limb.

The development of effective and safe diuretic drugs was empirical, the result of synthesis and testing of chemicals with molecular structures similar to previously known diuretics. Without any direct evidence, it was generally assumed that diuretics inhibit active Na transport in the renal tubules so that, of the salt and water filtered at the glomerulus, less is reabsorbed by the tubules and more appears in the urine. Investigation had been aimed at defining the effect of diuretics on active Na transport in renal and other tissues, and it remained unexplained why the diuretics greatly inhibited Na transport in the kidney with so little effect elsewhere in the body.

The present studies provide evidence that the previous emphasis on inhibition of active Na transport was misdirected and that a basic understanding of the mechanism of action of diuretics requires a different approach.

METHODS

The most effective diuretics inhibit net NaCl reabsorption in the thick ascending limb of Henle's loop, as determined by micropuncture and clearance studies. In order directly to study their action at this site fragments of the cortical portion of the thick ascending limb were dissected from rabbit kidneys and perfused *in vitro,* using the method described previously (Burg and Green, 1973a).

In previous studies of the thick ascending limb, using this method, there was net reabsorption of NaCl from the tubule lumen, but the driving force was active chloride transport, not active Na transport as previously believed. The active chloride transport caused an electrical p.d. which was positive in the lumen, and the p.d. was responsible for the net Na transport which was passive (Burg and Green, 1973a). The magnitude of the positive p.d. is related under some conditions to the rate of NaCl transport. In the present studies the effects of diuretic drugs on the p.d. and on the net Cl transport (measured chemically) was determined.

RESULTS AND DISCUSSION

In Table 1 are listed three important diuretics previously known to act in the ascending limb of Henle's loop. It can be seen that, when the drugs were placed in the tubule lumen, each caused the electrical p.d. and net Cl transport to decrease. Therefore, all three drugs inhibit active Cl transport in this segment, not active Na transport as was previously believed. The fall in the p.d., secondary to inhibition of active Cl transport, accounts for the accompanying decrease in the passive transport of Na. It should be noted that whereas low concentrations of furosemide and mersalyl (on the order of 10^{-5}M) in the lumen were effective, a much higher concentration of ethacrynic acid (10^{-3}) was used. The reason for this will be apparent later.

Figure 1 demonstrates the reversibility of the effect of furosemide. Furosemide in the lumen caused the p.d. to decrease within a few seconds. When the furosemide was removed, the p.d. immediately returned to the control level. The diuretic effect of furosemide *in vivo* is similarly characterized by rapidity of onset and reversibility. It should be noted that the effective concentration of furosemide in the tubule lumen is 10^{-5}M. Ten

Table 1. Effect of diuretics in the lumen on the thick ascending limb of Henle's loop

	Potential difference (mV)			Net chloride transport ($pEq cm^{-1} sec^{-1}$)		
Drug	Control	Experi-mental	*n*	Control	Experi-mental	*n*
Furosemide (10^{-5}M)	5.5	1.0	(29)	8.7	2.3	(3)
Mersalyl (3×10^{-5}M)	6.8	2.9	(12)	8.1	4.6	(8)
Ethacrynic acid (10^{-3}M)	6.7	2.3	(6)	10.1	4.3	(2)

Results taken from Burg *et al.* (1973) and Burg and Green (1973, b, c).

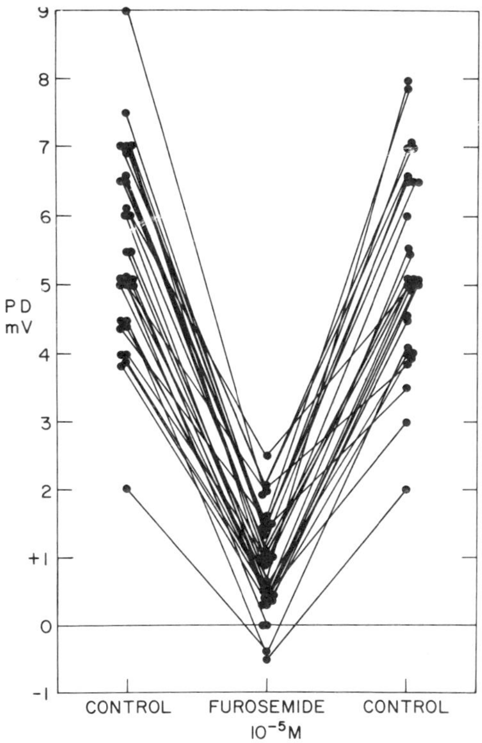

Fig. 1. Effect of furosemide in the lumen on the p.d. across the thick ascending limb of Henle's loop. (From Burg *et al.*, 1973.)

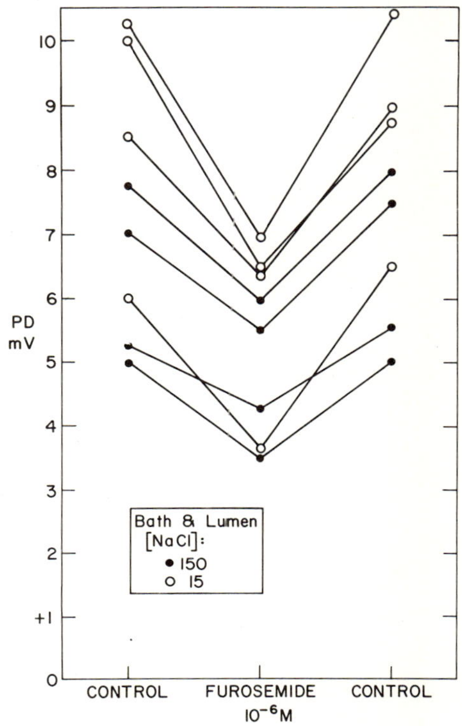

Fig. 2. Lack of effect of furosemide in the bath on the p.d. across the thick ascending limb of Henle's loop. (From Burg *et al.*, 1973.)

times that concentration of furosemide (10^{-4}M) had essentially no effect when placed in the bath (Fig. 2). Furosemide is filtered at the glomerulus and is also secreted into the tubule fluid by the proximal tubule cells (Deetjen, 1966). Most likely accumulation in the tubule fluid is necessary for the action of furosemide, as well as of the other drugs mentioned.

Since both mersalyl and ethacrynic acid inhibit numerous sulfhydryl-catalyzed reactions, they might have nonspecific toxic effects. Therefore, caution is required in relating any *in vitro* effect of the drugs to the diuretic effect *in vivo.* In order to test the specificity of the effect of mersalyl, the additional effect of p-chloromercuribenzoate (PCMB) was determined. The sulfhydryl reactivity of PCMB is similar to that of mersalyl, as are most of its biological effects. A striking exception is that, as discovered by Miller and Farah (1962), PCMB reverses the diuretic effect of mersalyl *in vivo.*

The interaction between PCMB and mersalyl was examined in the experiments shown in Fig. 3. Mersalyl in the lumen caused the p.d. to decrease. The effect with mersalyl was slower, however, than with the nonmercurial diuretic furosemide, requiring 5–10 min rather than a few seconds. After removal of

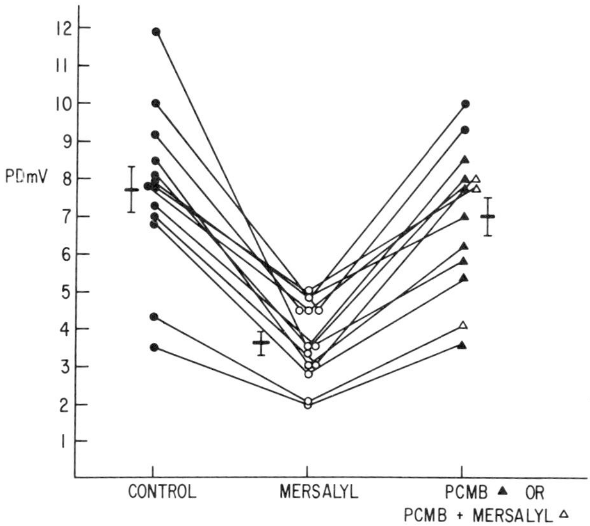

Fig. 3. Effect of mersalyl and PCMB in the lumen on the thick ascending limb of Henle's loop. Control (no drug) •, mersalyl (3×10^{-5}M) ○, PCMB ($1–3 \times 10^{-5}$M) ▲, PCMB + mersalyl △. (From Burg and Green, 1973b.)

the mersalyl, the p.d. recovered spontaneously. This also was a relatively slow process requiring 10–20 min. With PCMB, however, the recovery was immediate, whether it was substituted for the mersalyl or added to the mersalyl in the lumen. Net chloride transport was similarly affected (Burg and Green, 1973b).

Thus, PCMB reversed the effect of mersalyl. Since the unique antagonism between the drugs applies both to the inhibition of Cl transport *in vitro* and to the diuretic action *in vivo,* the two effects are most likely related.

In the experiments shown in Fig. 4 and Table 2, mersalyl was added to the bath rather than the lumen. Addition of 3×10^{-5}M, which caused inhibition when placed in the lumen, had no effect in the bath. Addition of 10^{-4}M caused the p.d. to decrease gradually, but the effect did not reverse spontaneously when the drug was removed, nor with addition of PCMB to the lumen or bath. Most likely, this is a nonspecific toxic effect of mersalyl, different from the diuretic effect of the drug in the lumen.

Although other mercurials also caused the p.d. to decrease, the effect differed from that of mersalyl in the lumen. It had been proposed that mercuric ions are released from the organic mercurial diuretics and that the mercuric ions are the actual effective form of the drug (Weiner and Farah, 1968). The effect of $HgCl_2$ added to the perfusate is shown in Table 3. Addition of 10^{-6}M in the lumen had no effect on the p.d. Addition of 3×10^{-6}M of $HgCl_2$ did cause the p.d. to fall, but the fall was slow, requiring

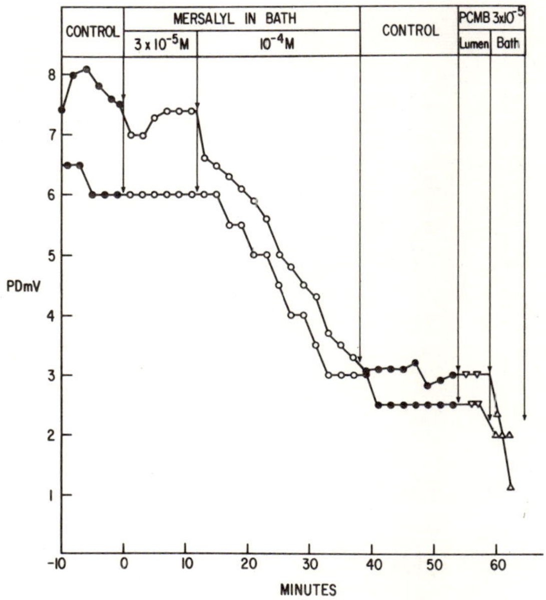

Fig. 4. Effect of mersalyl and PCMB in the bath on the thick ascending limb of Henle's loop. (From Burg and Green, 1973b.)

15–30 min compared with 5–10 min for a comparable effect of mersalyl. When PCMB was placed in the lumen, it did not reverse the effect of $HgCl_2$ which was progressive, as shown by the further decrease in p.d. in the after control periods when PCMB had been substituted for $HgCl_2$. Therefore, release of mercuric ion into the tubule fluid cannot account for the action of the mercurial diuretics. Either mercuric ion is released within the tissue, or, more likely, the intact molecule of the organic mercurial itself is the effective

Table 2. Effect of mercurials in the bath on the thick ascending limb of Henle's loop.

Drug	Concentration (M)	Bath	Potential difference (mV) Control	Potential difference (mV) Experimental	*n*
PCMB	3×10^{-5}	Saline	5.2	1.3	(2)
PCMB	3×10^{-5}	Serum	4.6	4.5	(3)
Mersalyl	3×10^{-5}	Saline	6.4	6.0	(3)
Mersalyl	10^{-4}	Saline	6.4	2.5	(3)
Mersalyl	3×10^{-4}	Serum	5.0	5.6	(2)

Taken in part from Burg and Green (1973b).

form of the drug rather than the mercuric ion, as proposed by Kessler, Lozano, and Pitts (1957). Cysteine protected against the effect of mercuric ion in the lumen. Mercuric cysteine in the lumen had no effect on the p.d. in concentrations as high as 10^{-3}M (Table 3).

PCMB in the bath also caused the p.d. to decrease slowly, as shown in Table 2. This effect was prevented by the presence of serum proteins. When the bath was serum, rather than the usual saline buffer (without added protein), PCMB in the bath had no effect on the p.d. (Table 2). Serum also protected against the effect of mersalyl in the bath. The presence of 10^{-4}M of mersalyl in the bath caused the p.d. to decrease when there was no protein added to the bath (Fig. 4, Table 2). With serum in the bath, however, an even higher concentration of mersalyl (3×10^{-4}M) had no effect (Table 2).

Why did PCMB reverse the effect of mersalyl in the lumen, but not of $HgCl_2$ in the lumen, nor of mersalyl in the bath? A possible explanation is that mercurials have at least two different sites of action in the thick ascending limb of Henle's loop. The first is the site associated with the diuresis *in vivo* and may be located at or near the lumen membrane, explaining why the effect of mersalyl is so rapidly reversed by PCMB in the lumen. The second site may be inside the tubule cells. The slow and irreversible effects of the various mercurials ($HgCl_2$ in the lumen, and mersalyl or PCMB in the bath) could result from gradual entry of these compounds into the cells and subsequent toxic inhibition of the cellular metabolic processes. *In vivo* the cells could be protected from this toxic effect by binding of mercurials by protein in the plasma or complexing of mercuric ions with cysteine in the tubule fluid. Although the mercurial diuretics may reach the tubule fluid by glomerular filtration, this process is limited by binding to serum proteins, and

Table 3. Effects of mercurials in the lumen on the thick ascending limb of Henle's loop

	Potential difference (mV)			
Drug	Control	Experimental	After control	*n*
$HgCl_2$ (10^{-6}M)	5.3	5.0		(2)
$HgCl_2$ (3×10^{-6} M)	7.3	2.3	0.3[a]	(4)
Hg cysteine (10^{-3}M)	6.8	6.4	6.9	(4)

[a]Replacement by $1–3 \times 10^{-5}$ PCMB.
From Burg and Green, 1973b.

secretion into the lumen by proximal tubule cells may be important for their action (reviewed by Cafruny, 1968).

The presence of 10^{-3}M ethacrynic acid in the lumen caused the p.d. and chloride transport to fall (Table 1). A lower concentration (10^{-4}M) had no effect on the p.d. (Table 4). In contrast, the ethacrynic-cysteine complex, shown by Beyer *et al.* (1965) to be a major excretory product of ethacrynic acid in the urine, was an effective inhibitor at a much lower concentration (3×10^{-6}M) in the lumen (Table 4). Net Cl transport was similarly affected (Table 4). The ethacrynic-cysteine complex may be formed in the proximal tubule cells during the process of secretion into the tubule lumen. It is proposed that this complex rather than ethacrynic acid itself is the principal effective form *in vivo.*

Ethacrynic acid was previously found to have numerous biological actions, including inhibition of respiration and glycolysis, inhibition of Na and K fluxes, and inhibition of Na- and K-activated ATPase (reviewed by Burg and Green, 1973c). The effects were associated with the sulfhydryl reactivity of ethacrynic acid and were prevented by premixing of the drug with dithiothreitol or cysteine. Also, high concentrations of ethacrynic acid (usually 10^{-4}–10^{-3}M) were required for these effects both in renal and nonrenal tissue. It is difficult to associate any of these effects with that of ethacrynic acid in the present studies since the ethacrynic-cysteine complex was a more, rather than a less, active inhibitor in the thick ascending limb of Henle's loop, and active Cl transport rather than active Na or K transport was inhibited. It is even questionable whether the diuretic effect of ethacrynic acid involves inhibition of sulfhydryl-catalyzed reactions at all, since the ethacrynic-cysteine adduct was more effective, although it should have less sulfhydryl reactivity.

It is possible that, like the mercurials, ethacrynic acid has more than one site of action in the thick ascending limb of Henle's loop. The presence of 10^{-3}M ethacrynic acid in a bath free of protein caused the p.d. to decrease

Table 4. Effect of diuretics in the lumen on the p.d. across the thick ascending limb of Henle's loop

	Potential difference (mV)			Net chloride transport ($pEq\,cm^{-1}sec^{-1}$)		
Drug	Control	Experimental	*n*	Control	Experimental	*n*
Ethacrynic acid (10^{-4}M)	5.1	5.0	(3)			
Ethacrynic-cysteine (3×10^{-6}M)	8.0	2.7	(11)	9.9	2.4	(4)

From Burg and Green, 1973c.

Table 5. Effect of diuretics in the bath on the thick ascending limb of Henle's loop

Drug	Bath	Potential difference (mV)			
		Control	Experimental	After control	*n*
Ethacrynic cysteine (10^{-5}M)	Saline buffer	8.1	7.8	7.4	(3)
Ethacrynic acid (10^{-3}M)	Saline buffer	6.5	1.6	1.0	(3)
Ethacrynic acid (10^{-3}M)	Serum	7.8	7.4	7.2	(3)

From Burg and Green, 1973c.

(Table 5). (In other studies lower concentrations in the bath had no definite effect on the p.d.) The decrease in p.d. was slower than with ethacrynic acid in the lumen and did not reverse when the ethacrynic acid was removed from the bath. Serum in the bath prevented this effect of ethacrynic acid (Table 5), presumably by binding the drug. Ethacrynic-cysteine in the bath had no effect (Table 5) even at a higher concentration (10^{-5}M) than that effective in the lumen (3×10^{-6}M, Table 4) and without added protein. Thus, entry of ethacrynic acid from the bath into the cells of the thick ascending limb of Henle's loop might cause an irreversible toxic inhibition of cellular metabolism which differs from the diuretic effect in the tubule lumen.

Ethacrynic acid is a highly reactive compound which has many biological effects in the high concentrations generally used in *in vitro* studies. When used as a diuretic, the toxicity may be mitigated by binding of the drug to serum proteins or to amino acids such as cysteine. In the kidney the drug might be secreted into the tubule fluid by proximal tubule cells (Beyer *et al.*, 1965). The ethacrynic-cysteine adduct (and possibly other similar complexes) might be formed prior to or during this transport process by proximal tubule cells. Consistent with the latter, Duggan and Noll (1972) observed that, when ethacrynic acid was incubated with kidney cells *in vitro,* adducts of ethacrynic acid were formed and released into the bath. This mechanism explains how a compound as reactive as ethacrynic acid can greatly reduce NaCl reabsorption in the thick ascending limb of Henle's loop without causing greater toxic effects than it does in renal and other tissues. Not only is the ethacrynic-cysteine complex less toxic, but lower concentrations suffice for the diuretic effect than of ethacrynic acid itself.

Another interesting aspect of the effect of diuretics is their marked specificity to certain nephron segments. The effects of amiloride and furosemide on different segments are compared in Table 6. As indicated earlier,

Table 6. Effects of diuretics in the lumen of kidney tubules

Drug	Concentration (M)	Segment[a]	Potential Difference (mV) Control	Potential Difference (mV) Experimental	n
Furosemide	10^{-5}	TAL	+ 6	+ 1	(29)
Furosemide	10^{-4}	CCT	−75	−82	(4)
Furosemide	10^{-4}	PCT	− 4	− 4	(4)
Amiloride	10^{-5}	CCT	−39	+ 5	(6)
Amiloride	10^{-4}	TAL	+ 5.8	+ 5.4	(4)

[a]TAL, thick ascending limb of Henle's loop; CCT, cortical collecting tubule; PCT, proximal convoluted tubule.
From Burg *et al.*, 1973; Burg and Green, 1973 b,c.

furosemide in the tubule lumen inhibits active Cl transport in the thick ascending limb of Henle's loop. With 10^{-5}M concentration in the tubule lumen the p.d. fell from 5.5 to 1.0 mV (Table 6). There was a similar fall in net NaCl transport (Burg *et al.*, 1973). Ten times the concentration of furosemide (10^{-4}M) had no effect on the p.d. of the cortical collecting tubule (Table 6), and net Na and K transport similarly were unaffected (Burg *et al.*, 1973). The presence of 10^{-4}M furosemide in the lumen also had no effect on the p.d. of the proximal convoluted tubule (Table 6), and the net Na transport and fluid absorption in the proximal tubule also were not significantly changed (Burg *et al.*, 1973). Thus, the effect of furosemide in the lumen was limited to the thick ascending limb of Henle's loop, where it inhibited active Cl transport. It had no effect on the other segments which lack a comparable active Cl transport system.

The presence of 10^{-5}M amiloride in the lumen of the cortical collecting tubule (Table 6) caused the p.d. in that segment to reverse polarity. The active Na and K transport measured simultaneously were virtually completely inhibited (Stoner and Burg, 1974). In contrast, ten times that concentration of amiloride (10^{-4}M) had no significant effect on the p.d. across the thick ascending limb of Henle's loop (Table 6), and it also did not affect the net NaCl transport measured in the same experiments (Stoner and Burg, 1974). Thus, the effect of amiloride was limited to the cortical collecting tubule where it inhibited active Na and K transport. It had no effect on the thick ascending limb of Henle's loop which lacks a comparable Na and K transport system.

CONCLUSION

Three major diuretic drugs (furosemide, mersalyl, and ethacrynic acid) act in the lumen of the thick ascending limb of Henle's loop by inhibiting an active chloride transport system, not active Na transport as previously believed. This explains how the drugs can profoundly inhibit NaCl transport in the kidney with so little effect on the active Na transport systems which are common elsewhere in the body. Further progress in understanding these drugs may depend on studying their action in model Cl- rather than Na-transporting systems.

REFERENCES

Beyer, K. H., J. E. Baer, J. K. Michaelson, and H. F. Russo. 1965. Renotropic characteristics of ethacrynic acid: A phenoxyacetic saluretic-diuretic agent. J. Pharm. Exp. Ther. 147: 1.

Burg, M., and N. Green. 1973a. Function of the thick ascending limb of Henle's loop. Am. J. Physiol. 224: 659.

Burg, M., and N. Green. 1973b. Effect of mersalyl on the thick ascending limb of Henle's loop. Kidney Internat. 4: 245.

Burg, M., and N. Green. 1973c. Effect of ethacrynic acid on the thick ascending limb of Henle's loop. Kidney Internat. 4: 301.

Burg, M., L. Stoner, J. Cardinal, and N. Green. 1973. Furosemide effect on isolated perfused tubules. Am. J. Physiol. 225: 119.

Cafruny, E. J. 1968. The site and mechanism of action of mercurial diuretics. Pharm. Rev. 20: 89.

Deetjen, P. 1966. Micropuncture studies on site and mode of diuretic action of furosemide. Ann. N.Y. Acad. Sci. 139: 408.

Duggan, D. E., and R. M. Noll. 1972. Effects of ethacrynic acid upon membrane ATPase of dog kidney *in vivo* and *in vitro*. Proc. Soc. Exp. Biol. Med. 139: 762.

Kessler, R. H., R. Lozano, and R. F. Pitts. 1957. A comparison of the pharmacological behavior of chlormerodrin, meralluride, mersalyl, and mercuric chloride in the dog. J. Pharm. Exp. Ther. 121: 432.

Miller, T. B., and A. E. Farah. 1962. Inhibition of mercurial diuresis by nondiuretic mercurials. J. Pharm. Exp. Ther. 135: 102.

Stoner, L., and M. Burg. 1974. Am. J. Physiol. In press.

Weiner, I., and A. Farah. 1968. Pharmacology of mercurial diuretics. Proceedings of the 3rd International Pharmacology Meeting, Vol. 8, Salt and Water Balance, Pergamon Press, New York, pp. 15–36.

Interrelationship of Renal Handling of Sodium, Calcium, and Phosphate

Martin Goldberg, Zalman S. Agus, and Laurence H. Beck
Renal-Electrolyte Section, Department of Medicine
University of Pennsylvania School of Medicine
Philadelphia, Pennsylvania

There has been a recent resurgence of interest among investigators in the regulation of calcium and phosphate excretion by the kidney. In particular, since several observations have demonstrated a correlation between the renal handling of these two ions with sodium transport, it should be of interest to attempt to define the mode and mechanism of the interrelationships of these three ion species. Aside from changes in the plasma levels of these specific ions, there are three categories of physiological or pharmacological experiments which have been shown to affect calcium and phosphate excretion, in most cases associated with a natriuresis. First, it has long been known that parathyroid hormone produces a phosphaturia, and some experiments have suggested that elevations in the plasma level of this hormone result in a lowering of urinary calcium excretion. More recently, some evidence has suggested that the renal tubular effects of this hormone might be mediated through cyclic adenosine monophosphate. The specific renal tubular sites of these effects and their mechanisms have until recently not been elucidated. Secondly, acute expansion of the extracellular fluid volume with saline solutions characteristically produces phosphaturia and calciuria along with the increased sodium excretion. Finally, in the group of diuretic drugs, acetazolamide, the inhibitor of carbonic anhydrase, appears to be the most potent and most consistently phosphaturic agent, whereas the loop blockers, ethacrynic acid and furosemide, cause marked increases in calcium excretion with variable changes in phosphate excretion.

METHODS

Work in our laboratory during the past three years has involved the use of the micropuncture technique to study some of the factors involved in the renal regulation of calcium and phosphate excretion. Most of the data which will now be summarized is derived from the use of the recollection technique in the dog. With this method, a site in the tubule is punctured, fluid is aspirated for subsequent analyses, and an experimental procedure is performed. During the steady state the identical site is repunctured and fluid is reanalyzed for inulin and the appropriate elements to evaluate the effects of the procedure on the transport of the ions under study. (Agus *et al.,* 1971). Inulin is analyzed with a fluorimetric technique, and calcium and phosphate in tubular fluid were analyzed utilizing a recently developed method employing the electron microprobe. With this technique 0.3-nl quantities of tubular fluid can be analyzed in replicate for several elements simultaneously. Highly linear curves are reproducibly obtained, and appropriate recoveries and comparisons with other methods were performed (Agus *et al.,* 1973).

RESULTS AND DISCUSSION

In Fig. 1 are summarized data obtained from the proximal tubule of the dog. The upper portion of this graph contains values for the ratio of tubular fluid to plasma ultrafiltrate (TF/UF) calcium concentration plotted against corresponding values for tubular fluid over plasma (TF/P) inulin used as an index

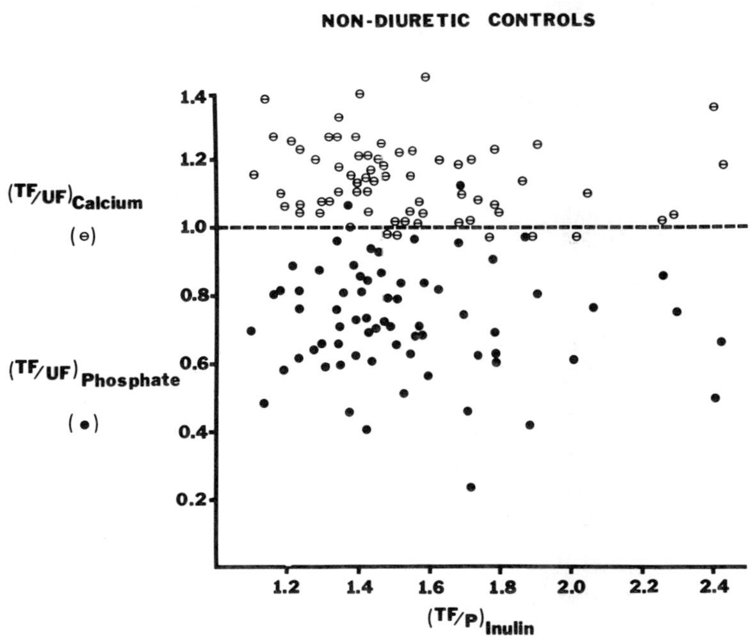

Fig. 1. Relationship between proximal tubular fluid/plasma ultrafiltrate calcium (TF/UF calcium) and TF/UF phosphate and TF/P inulin during hydropenia in individual tubules from 16 dogs. (From Agus *et al.,* 1973.)

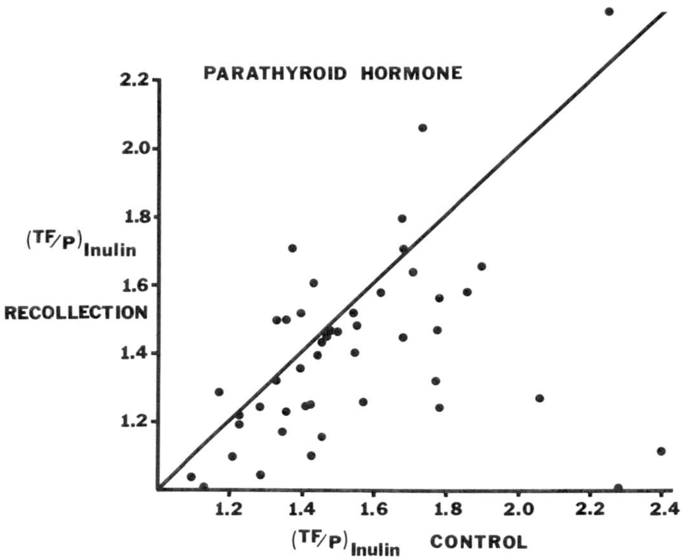

Fig. 2. Effects of parathyroid hormone on tubular fluid/plasma inulin concentration (TF/P) inulin in single proximal tubules of 11 dogs. Mean values fell from 1.57 during initial (control) observations to 1.38 during parathyroid hormone (recollection). (From Agus *et al.*, 1971, 1973.)

of fluid reabsorption; in the lower portion simultaneously obtained values for TF/UF phosphate concentration are illustrated. It should be noted that the mean value for TF/UF calcium is slightly greater than 1 and does not change with TF/P inulin, whereas the mean value for TF/UF phosphate is significantly less than 1 at a value of approximately 0.65. It should also be noted that in these intact animals there is no tendency for a change in the ratio of tubular fluid to ultrafiltrate phosphate concentration with increasing fluid reabsorption along the proximal tubule. Thus, in the hydropenic state, after initial adjustments are made early in the proximal tubule establishing equilibrium ratios for these ions, both calcium and phosphate reabsorption closely parallel sodium and fluid reabsorption.

Our initial series of experiments was designed to evaluate the effects of purified parathyroid hormone (PTH) on the proximal tubule of the dog. Figure 2 illustrates the effects of the hormone on proximal tubular sodium and fluid reabsorption. The initial or control values for TF/P inulin ratio are shown on the abscissa and the corresponding recollection values after PTH are plotted on the ordinate. The diagonal line represents the line of no change. It can be clearly seen that the majority of the points lie below the line, indicating that parathyroid hormone significantly inhibits proximal tubular sodium and fluid reabsorption, the mean change being approximately 30%.

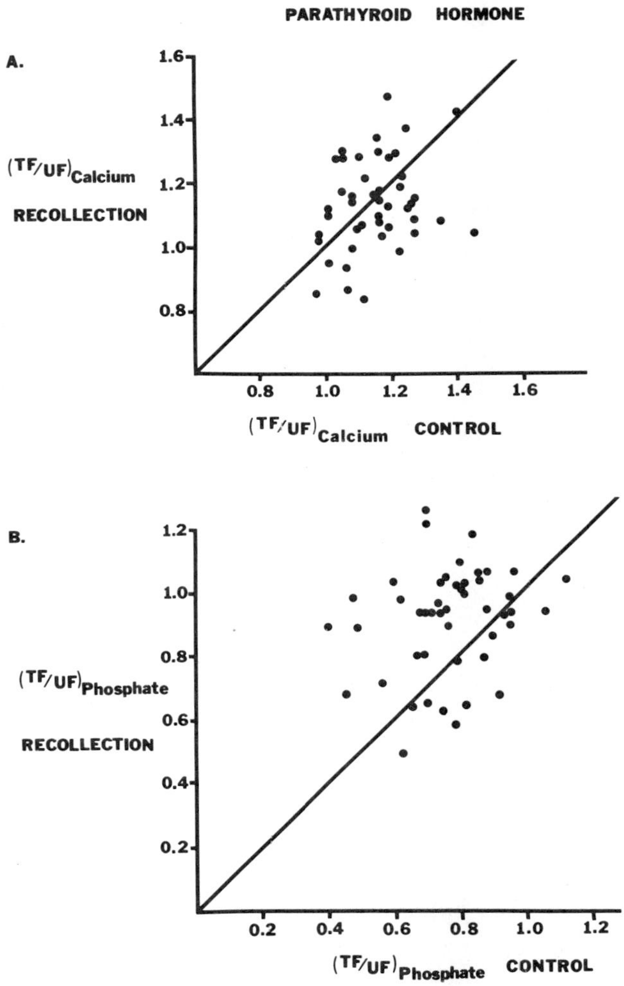

Fig. 3. Effects of parathyroid hormone on proximal tubular fluid/plasma ultrafiltrate calcium (TF/UF calcium) and (TF/UF) phosphate in individual tubules from 11 dogs. (From Agus *et al.*, 1971, 1973.)

Figure 3 summarizes the changes in tubular fluid calcium and phosphate concentrations factored for their corresponding plasma ultrafiltrate levels following PTH. As seen in the upper graph, the points scatter about the line of no change for calcium, indicating that calcium reabsorption was inhibited in parallel with the inhibition of sodium and fluid. On the other hand, as illustrated in the lower graph, tubular fluid to ultrafiltrate phosphate concentration ratios were significantly elevated by parathyroid hormone, rising from an initial value of approximately 0.65 to a value of 0.85. Therefore, phosphate reabsorption was inhibited proportionately greater than that of sodium, fluid, and calcium. All of these observations with parathyroid hormone are summarized in Fig. 4. Here the mean regression lines for fractional reabsorption of phosphate and calcium *versus* fractional reabsorption of fluid in the proximal tubule are plotted before and after administration of the hormone; the broken lines are the results after hormone administration. With regard to calcium, PTH does not change the relationship between fractional reabsorption of this ion and fluid reabsorption. The administration of PTH not only produces an inhibition of phosphate reabsorption associated with the depression of fluid reabsorption, but in addition alters the relationship such that at any level of fluid reabsorption there is less phosphate reabsorbed than prior to the administration of the hormone.

In Table 1 the changes in fractional reabsorption of sodium, phosphate, and calcium in the proximal tubule are compared with changes in the clearances of these ions for the whole kidney. The clearance data are summarized at the bottom of the table. It is obvious that the final urine does not quantitatively reflect the marked alterations in the transport of sodium, phosphate, and calcium in the proximal tubule. Thus, despite the major alteration in sodium reabsorption proximally, there is only a minimal increase

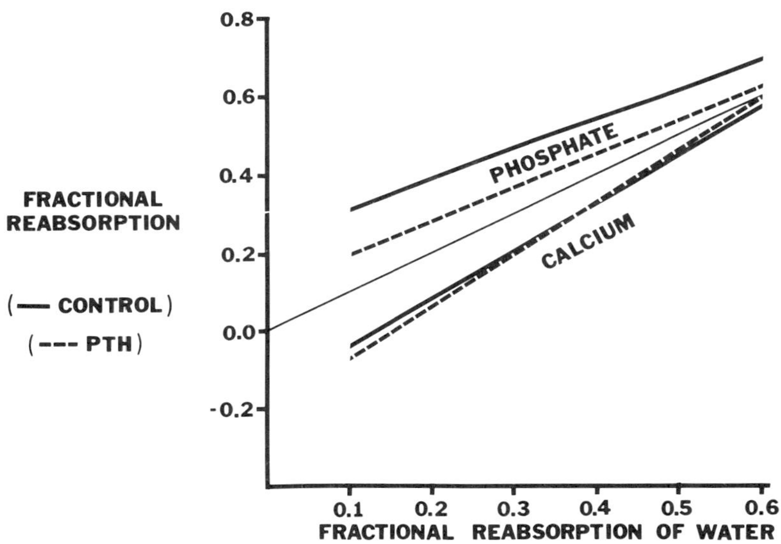

Fig. 4. Effects of parathyroid hormone on proximal fractional reabsorption of calcium and phosphate versus fractional reabsorption of water. The regression lines for these relationships in the proximal tubule before (solid lines) and after (broken lines) PTH administration in 11 dogs are illustrated. The slopes of these regression lines are not significantly different before and after PTH for both calcium and phosphate, but the difference in the intercept on the ordinate of the regression lines relating fractional water (sodium) and phosphate reabsorption is significantly different ($p < 0.005$). The thin solid line represents fractional reabsorption of sodium assuming isotonic reabsorption.

Table 1. Effects of parathyroid hormone on proximal tubule (micropuncture) and final urine (clearance)

	Micropuncture ($N = 11, n = 47$)			Clearance			
	Fractional sodium reabsorption	Fractional phosphate reabsorption	Fractional calcium reabsorption	GFR	C_{Na}	C_P	C_{Ca}
Control	0.34 ± 0.03	0.51 ± 0.02	0.25 ± 0.04	32 ± 3	0.09 ± 0.03	2.7 ± 0.6	0.13 ± 0.03
Recollection	0.25 ± 0.03	0.31 ± 0.04	0.15 ± 0.06	33 ± 3	0.16 ± 0.05	9.6 ± 1.1	0.06 ± 0.01
P	< 0.02	< 0.005	< 0.05	n.s.	< 0.002	< 0.001	< 0.05

Abbreviations: control, values (mean ± s.e.m.) before PTH; recollection, values during infusion of PTH; GFR, glomerular filtration rate; C_{Na}, C_P, C_{Ca}, clearances of sodium, phosphate, and calcium, respectively.

in sodium clearance, indicating that most of the proximally rejected sodium was reabsorbed at sites in the distal nephron. In contrast, a major rise in phosphate clearance is manifest, indicating that the bulk of the proximally rejected phosphate is not reabsorbed distally. Finally, with regard to calcium, there actually occurs a significant decrease in calcium clearance following the administration of the hormone, despite the fact that the distal nephron was presented with an increased load of calcium. This indicates that the hypocalciuric effect of parathyroid hormone is probably mediated somewhere in the distal nephron.

Since the adenylate cyclase system has been proposed as the mediator of the target organ effects of parathyroid hormone, we performed a series of experiments evaluating the effects of dibutyryl cyclic AMP on proximal tubular transport. Some of these data are illustrated in Fig. 5. The observations on TF/P inulin are shown at the top and those on TF/UF phosphate at the bottom. It is apparent that dibutyryl cyclic AMP has virtually the same effect on the proximal tubule as does PTH, that is, a significant inhibition of proximal sodium and fluid reabsorption associated with a significant rise in tubular fluid phosphate concentration. As with PTH there were no changes in proximal tubular calcium concentration, and the alterations in the final urine were also similar to those with PTH.

Our conclusions from this initial series of experiments were as follows. The action of parathyroid hormone appears to involve the concomitant inhibition of sodium and phosphate reabsorption as well as calcium in the proximal tubule. Sodium and calcium are inhibited in proportion to each other, whereas phosphate is disproportionately inhibited. The rejected sodium is mostly reabsorbed in the distal nephron, whereas the proximally rejected phosphate is mostly unreabsorbed distally. Furthermore, there is a distal stimulation of calcium reabsorption resulting in a reduction in calcium excretion. These events therefore result in an apparent selective phosphaturia and hypocalciuria. From these observations it was apparent that there was a correlation between the proximal tubular reabsorption of phosphate and sodium, which raises the question that at least a portion of phosphate transport may be dependent on sodium transport. On the other hand, it was clear that parathyroid hormone was capable of modifying or altering the sodium-phosphate relationship. The mode or mechanism of this PTH-induced alteration was, of course, unclear.

In order to probe these mechanisms further, we next embarked on a series of experiments in intact and parathyroidectomized dogs in which agents known to have primary effects on sodium and fluid transport were administered. First we evaluated the effects of removal of PTH *per se* on the pattern of proximal tubular phosphate reabsorption. In Figure 6 are plotted TF/UF phosphate *versus* TF/P inulin in the proximal tubule. In the intact animals there was no significant trend of alteration in TF/UF phosphate with progressive fluid reabsorption, and the 95% confidence bands and mean regression

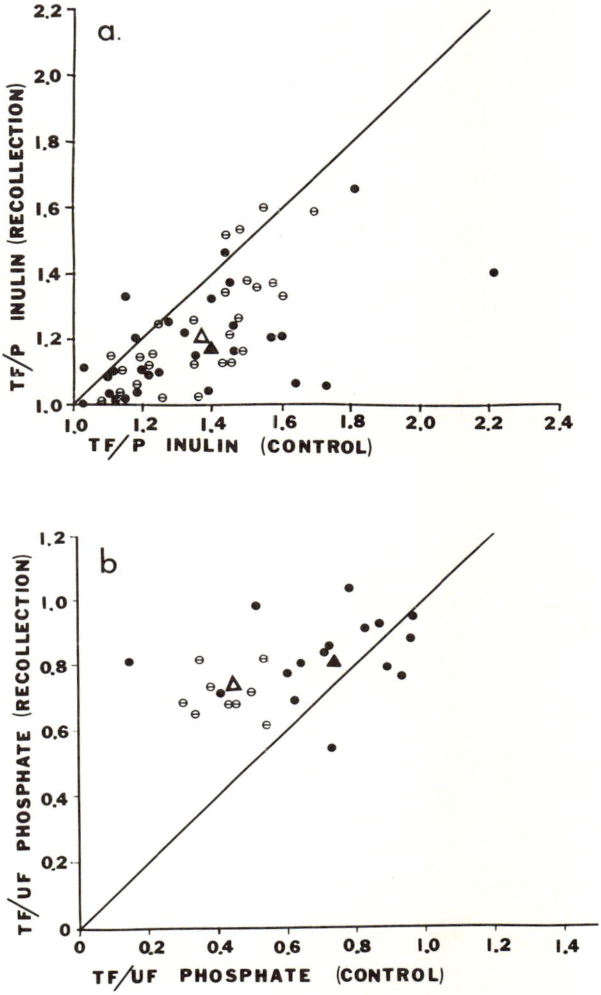

Fig. 5. Effects of intravenous (solid symbols) and intra-arterial (open symbols) dibutyryl cyclic AMP on proximal tubular fluid reabsorption and TF/UF phosphate. See text.

line for the intact animals are indicated in the area enclosed by the two broken lines. The slope of the line is not different from zero. The data points and the solid regression line are taken from proximal tubular samples of animals less than 24 hr after thyroparathyroidectomy (TPTX). It should be noted that, in contrast to the intact group, there is indeed a trend for progressive reduction in tubular phosphate concentration with increasing fluid reabsorption along the nephron, so that the values for end proximal TF/UF phosphate are significantly different from the values in the intact animals at corresponding rates of fluid reabsorption. This suggests that in the

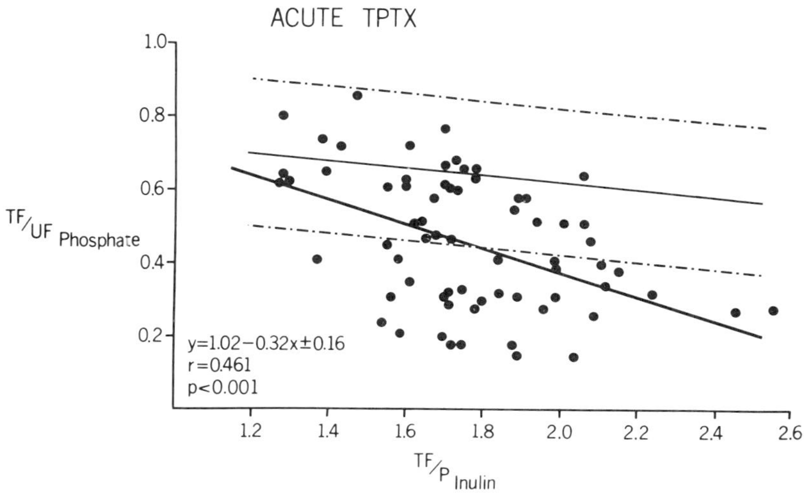

Fig. 6. Relationship between TF/UF phosphate and TF/P inulin in single proximal tubules of acutely thyroparathyroidectomized dogs. The data points and mean regression line are superimposed on the 95% confidence limits of the relationship in intact animals. See text. (From Beck and Goldberg, 1973b.)

absence of parathyroid hormone there is some fixed relationship between phosphate and sodium concentrations in the tubular reabsorbate and that phosphate concentration in this reabsorbate is greater than that in the tubular fluid. PTH therefore must in some way modulate or alter the relationship of sodium to phosphate in the reabsorbate to allow for a relatively constant tubular fluid phosphate concentration in the latter portion of the proximal tubule.

In the next series of experiments the carbonic adhydrase inhibitor acetazolamide was administered to both intact and parathyroidectomized animals. In Fig. 7 the initial and recollection values for TF/P inulin are shown on the left-hand panel and the corresponding values for TF/UF phosphate are illustrated on the right. Solid circles represent intact animals and open circles TPTX animals. First, it is clear that acetazolamide is an extremely potent proximal tubular inhibitor of sodium and fluid. Furthermore, whether or not PTH was present or absent, this inhibition of proximal sodium reabsorption was associated with a significant elevation of proximal tubular phosphate concentration, as demonstrated on the right-hand side of Fig. 7. The only difference between the intact animals (solid circles) and the parathyroidectomized animals (open circles) is that the phosphate load at the end of the proximal tubule following the drug was lower because the original baseline load was lower. Hence, it is clear (from these data) that PTH is not necessary for inhibition of at least a portion of proximal phosphate reabsorption when sodium and fluid transport are inhibited. It should also be noted that when

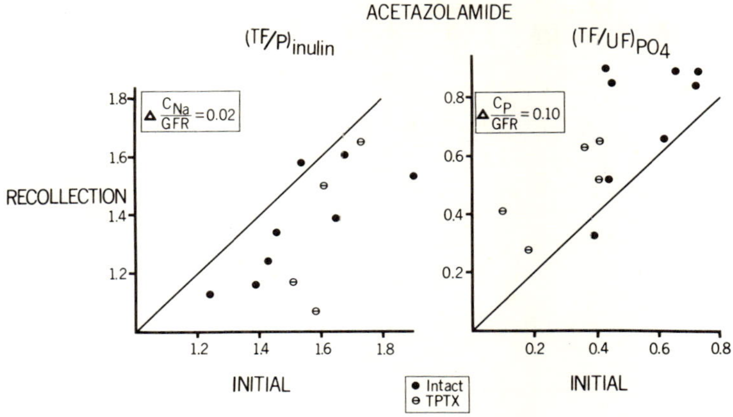

Fig. 7. Effects of acetazolamide on TF/P inulin and TF/UF phosphate in intact and thyroparathyroidectomized (TPTX) dogs. See text. (From Beck and Goldberg, 1973a.)

phosphate reabsorption is inhibited, even with acetazolamide, this occurs disproportionately to the inhibition of sodium reabsorption. In contrast, as seen in Fig. 8 which summarizes the data on the ratio of tubular fluid to ultrafiltrate calcium concentration, this calcium ratio is unaltered by acetazolamide, indicating that inhibition of proximal calcium reabsorption by the drug occurs in direct proportion to the inhibition of sodium and fluid reabsorption with or without PTH. Table 2 summarizes the clearance data for the whole kidney in the acetazolamide experiments. In the intact animals acetazolamide produced only a modest natriuresis, reflecting the large distal

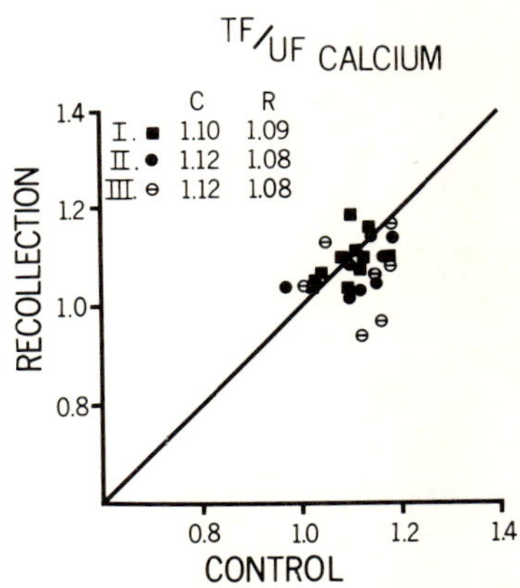

Fig. 8. Control *versus* recollection values for TF/UF calcium in nondiuretic control animals that received no acetazolamide (I), and in intact (II) and thyroparathyroidectomized animals (III) which had received an infusion of acetazolamide. (From Beck and Goldberg, 1973a.)

Table 2. Effects of acetazolamide on fractional excretion of sodium, calcium, and phosphate in intact and thyroparathyroidectomized (TPTX) dogs

C_{Na}/GFR × 100 (%)		C_p/GFR × 100 (%)		C_{Ca}/GFR × 100 (%)	
Control	Recollection	Control	Recollection	Control	Recollection
		Intact ($N = 8$)			
0.2 ± 0.1	*1.8 ± 0.2	1.3 ± 0.3	*11.0 ± 3.2	0.5 ± 0.1	0.5 ± 0.1
		TPTX ($N = 7$)			
0.2 ± 0.1	*1.5 ± 0.3	0.8 ± 0.6	*3.4 ± 1.8	0.8 ± 0.2	0.6 ± 0.1

Abbreviations as in Table 1.

*Recollection value is significantly different ($P < 0.01$) from the corresponding control value.

reabsorptive capacity for sodium. The major portion of the proximally rejected phosphate, on the other hand, was excreted in the urine, resulting in a fractional excretion of 11% of filtered load. Of additional interest is the observation that, despite the large proximal inhibition of calcium, there was *no* increase in renal calcium excretion. This suggests that the distal calcium reabsorptive mechanism is dissociated from that of sodium, and furthermore that the intrinsic response of the distal nephron to increased loads from the proximal tubule is to reabsorb all of the incremental calcium delivery. Hence the proximal tubule does not appear to be an important regulator of final calcium excretion.

Now let us look at the data in the TPTX animals. The magnitude of the natriuresis produced by acetazolamide was comparable with the intact animals. The phosphaturia, on the other hand, was significantly less than that in the intact animals. This was in part due to the smaller load of phosphate present at the end of the proximal tubule following the drug, but in addition the degree of this blunted phosphaturia suggests that a significant portion of the proximally rejected phosphate load may have been reabsorbed in the distal nephron, in contrast to the intact animals. Again, acetazolamide caused no significant alteration in urinary calcium excretion, despite the changes in the proximal tubule.

Our next series of experiments involved the administration of acute saline loads to both intact and TPTX animals, since clearance studies by Frick and Slatopolsky (personal communication) have revealed that saline-induced phosphaturia is markedly blunted in acutely parathyroidectomized animals. Figure 9 summarizes the proximal tubular micropuncture data in saline-loaded intact animals as well as animals studied either shortly after parathyroidectomy or 24 hr after the surgical procedure. In each of the groups

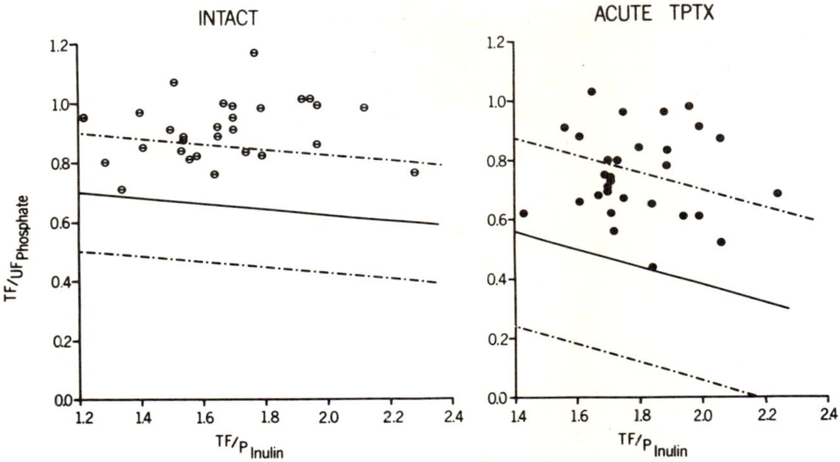

Fig. 9. Effects of acute saline loading on the relationship between TF/UF phosphate *versus* TF/P inulin in intact and acutely thyroparathyrodectomized animals. The data points in each group are superimposed on the 95% confidence limits of the presaline values for each group. See text. (From Beck and Goldberg, 1973b.)

saline produced the familiar marked fall in proximal tubular fluid reabsorption as reflected by the decrease in the value for TF/P inulin. With regard to phosphate, although the baseline values for TF/UF phosphate were lower in the two parathyroidectomized groups as compared with the intact animals, the postsaline level of TF/UF phosphate was no different in the three groups. Therefore, the load of phosphate present at the end of the proximal tubule following saline expansion was comparable in intact and TPTX animals. In the final urine, however, striking differences were present, as illustrated in Fig. 10 in which the fractions of filtered phosphate remaining at the end of

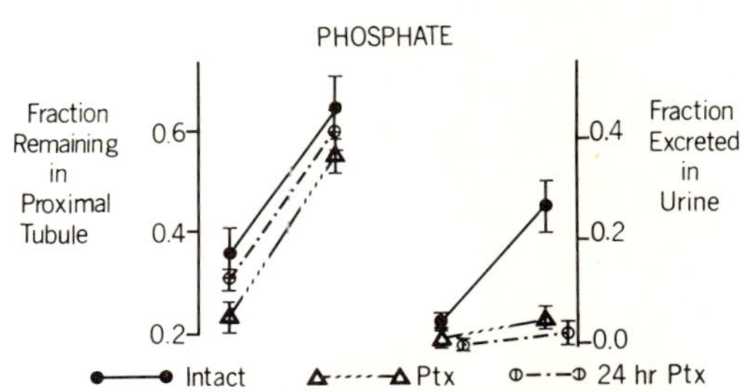

Fig. 10. Effects of acute saline loading on proximal tubular fractional rejection of phosphate compared with fractional excretion of phosphate in three groups of animals: intact dogs; acutely thyroparathyroidectomized dogs (4-6 hr); animals that were parathyroidectomized 24 hr prior to study. It should be noted that saline produced comparable inhibition of phosphate reabsorption in the proximal tubule in all three groups of animals, but only in the intact animals was there a significant phosphaturia. See text. (From Beck and Goldberg, 1973b.)

the proximal tubule in both the intact and parathyroidectomized groups are shown on the left (the lines connect the points before and after saline administration), and the fractions of filtered phosphate excreted in the urine before and after saline in both groups of animals are shown on the right. The change in proximal tubular phosphate reabsorption, in both intact and TPTX animals, were comparable (approximately 30% of filtered load after saline).

CONCLUSIONS

Phosphate

1. Filtered phosphate is mostly reabsorbed in the proximal tubule and most of the phosphate escaping proximal reabsorption is excreted in the urine in intact animals. Therefore, phosphaturia in these animals parallels changes in proximal tubular phosphate reabsorption.
2. In the absence of parathyroid hormone, that is, in parathyroidectomized animals, a large distal reabsorptive capacity for phosphate appears to be present, resulting in a blunted phosphaturia, even with major inhibition of proximal tubular phosphate reabsorption.
3. There appear to be two components to proximal tubular phosphate transport. One appears to be sodium-dependent in that alterations in proximal sodium reabsorption are associated with parallel changes in phosphate transport, but a second component to proximal phosphate reabsorption is influenced by parathyroid hormone, which seems to affect or modulate the relationship between sodium and phosphate in the reabsorbate. Whether or not this influence of PTH is directly on an independent phosphate pump or merely produces an alteration in a linked sodium-phosphate transport pathway is unclear at this time. In actuality it appears that high levels of PTH affect both components of proximal phosphate transport, that is, have some direct influence on sodium transport as well as producing an alteration in the sodium-phosphate relationship.

Calcium

1. Calcium appears to be reabsorbed both in the proximal and distal nephron, roughly in parallel to sodium.
2. Parathyroid hormone, via its effects on proximal sodium transport, also inhibits proximal calcium reabsorption in this nephron segment, but in the final urine a reduction in urinary calcium occurs because of the PTH-induced stimulation of distal calcium reabsorption.
3. Calcium and sodium appear to be intimately related in the proximal tubule, such that maneuvers which primarily inhibit sodium reabsorption cause parallel and proportional changes in calcium transport. In the distal nephron, however, the two ions appear to be dissociated.
4. Calcium excretion is probably *regulated* in the distal nephron, since large loads of calcium delivered out of the proximal tubule can be quantitatively

reabsorbed without producing any change in urinary calcium excretion. The nature of the complex relationship between sodium and calcium in the distal portions of the nephron of course remains to be elucidated.

ACKNOWLEDGMENTS

This work was supported by Research Grant HL-00340 from the National Heart and Lung Institute and from Training Grant AM-05634 from the National Institute of Arthritis, Metabolic, and Digestive Diseases, National Institutes of Health. We are especially indebted to Dorothy Senesky for her important role in the development of the technique of specimen processing for electron microprobe, to Norman Walters for his support and cooperation in the operation and maintenance of the microprobe instrument and for his helpful suggestions, to Marta McCusker for her technical assistance in the micropuncture laboratory, and to Carmen D'Angelo, Lidia Kosolopous, Leonids Kosolopous, Elizabeth Colonna, and Frances McKee for the laboratory analyses.

REFERENCES

Agus, Z.A., J.B. Puschett, D. Senesky, and M. Goldberg. 1971. Mode of action of parathyroid hormone and cyclic adenosine 5'-monophosphate on renal tubular phosphate reabsorption in the dog. J. Clin. Invest. 50: 617–626.

Agus, Z.S., L.B. Gardner, L.H. Beck, and M. Goldberg. 1973. Effects of parathyroid hormone on renal tubular reabsorption of calcium, sodium and phosphate. Am. J. Physiol. 224: 1143–1148.

Beck, L.H., and M. Goldberg. 1973a. Effects of acetazolamide and parathyroidectomy on renal transport of sodium, calcium and phosphate. Am. J. Physiol. 224: 1136–1142.

Beck, L.H., and M. Goldberg. 1973b. Mechanism of blunted phosphaturia in saline-loaded parathyroidectomized (PTX) dogs. Clin. Res. 23: 676 (abstr.).

Some Recent Developments in Renal Electrolyte Transport[1]

A. N. Richards Memorial Lecture

Gerhard Giebisch
Department of Physiology
Yale University School of Medicine
New Haven, Connecticut

It is a fitting tribute to Richards' achievements that he is being remembered on the occasion of this Symposium on Advances in Renal Physiology and Pharmacology. A.N. Richards spent his most productive years in Philadelphia as Professor of Pharmacology at the University of Pennsylvania. Here he and Wearn initiated and developed the powerful methods for execution of the well-known and incisive micropuncture experiments on the nephron. It was also here that one of the most successful kidney research projects flourished under Richards' forceful leadership by improving the techniques for microscopy of the amphibian kidney and by developing the chemical methods necessary to measure accurately the main constituents of glomerular and tubular fluid. It was also in Richards' laboratory that, as a crowning achievement, the direct chemical studies of glomerular and tubular fluid were extended to the mammalian kidney.

Renal physiology is greatly indebted to A.N. Richards. He and his associates carried out a series of remarkably simple, direct, and clear-cut experiments on the single nephron level which, by comparing the composition of glomerular and tubular fluid with plasma, defined many glomerular and tubular functions. During his most productive period Richards was responsible, primarily, for transforming renal physiology from a largely speculative to a more rational discipline. Many deductions from more indirect approaches to the study of renal function, in particular those based on clearance

[1]Work carried out in the author's laboratory was supported by grants from the National Institutes of Health and the American Heart Association.

methods, began to rely more and more heavily on the functional structure of the nephron as defined by Richards' school.

It was the author's privilege to learn the micropuncture approach to renal physiology in Philadelphia during a six-months stay in the early 1950's from Dr. Phyllis A. Bott, a former associate of Dr. Richards. Dr. Bott had worked in A.N. Richards' department, collaborated with him on several studies, and carried on many of his laboratory traditions. Dr. Bott was deeply devoted to Richards and described him as a hard taskmaster, a first-rate and exemplary scientist, and an investigator with an unflinching devotion to the kidney.

In this presentation some recent work on proximal and distal tubular ion and fluid transport will be discussed. Problems of particular interest have to do with (1) newer aspects of the functional organization of the proximal tubular epithelium, (2) the mechanisms of coupling individual ion transfer processes, and (3) the elucidation of some of the mechanisms by which ion translocation across individual cell membranes is controlled within the renal epithelium.

In view of the fundamental role of the proximal tubular epithelium in the preservation and maintenance of the extracellular fluid volume, it is not surprising that the process of proximal tubular fluid and ion transport has been under continuous scrutiny. The thesis that proximal tubular sodium transport is active in nature was first proposed by Wesson and Anslow (1948), and later confirmed by the demonstration that net movement of sodium ions can occur uphill, that is to say, against an electrochemical potential gradient as these ions pass across the proximal tubular epithelium (Windhager and Giebisch, 1961; Giebisch and Windhager, 1964; Kashgarian *et al.*, 1963). It is generally believed that such solute reabsorption generates an osmotic concentration difference which drives water passively from the lumen to the peritubular fluid.

Figure 1 summarizes some essential points of the fundamental organization of proximal tubule cells (Giebisch, 1972). This epithelial cell schema is supported by a considerable body of evidence (Giebisch, 1972; Diamond, 1964; Curran and Macintosh, 1962; Windhager, Lewy, and Spitzer, 1969). Proximal tubule cells are luminally linked to each other by a junctional complex, the tight junction. An extracellular compartment is interposed between neighboring cells and constitutes a transport path parallel to the cellular transport route. In view of the overall isosmotic character of the proximal fluid transport operation, it is thought that sodium chloride is pumped into the interspace compartment at a rate sufficiently high to generate a fluid pool of local hypertonicity. Fluid moves from lumen to the interspace compartment in response to this osmotic pressure gradient. In a terminal step the reabsorbate is transferred from the interspaces across the basal membrane and the capillary wall by a force determined by the balance between hydrostatic and oncotic pressure difference across these barriers.

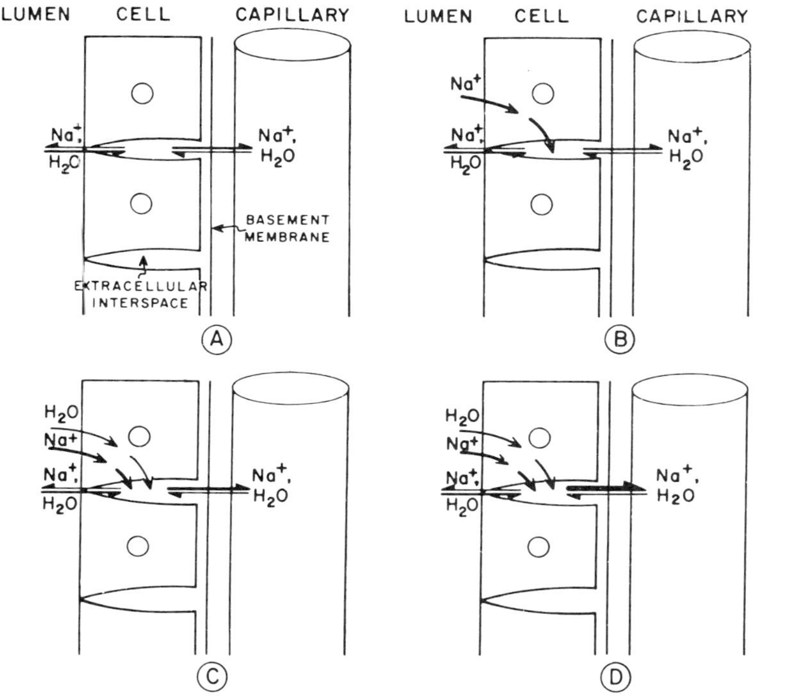

Fig. 1. Schematic representation of renal tubule cell, including routes of sodium and water movement. In A the tubular cell has a luminal and peritubular (antiluminal) cell membrane. Adjacent cells are joined luminally by tight junctions which are very short in the proximal tubule. Located between tubule cells is an extracellular interspace. This latter system (i.e., the tight junction, interspace, and basement membrane) constitutes a separate, low-resistance, extracellular pathway for water movement. In B sodium is actively pumped from the cells into the extracellular interspaces, making them hypertonic and setting up an area of local hypertonicity. In C water follows sodium passively along an osmotic gradient but can very probably also enter the interspace via the tight junction. In D the intercellular compartment is hypertonic in the region close to the tubular lumen but becomes isosmotic because of water equilibration along the antiluminal portion of the channel. Fluid and sodium movement out of the interspaces towards the capillary is achieved by slight elevation of the hydrostatic pressure in this compartment. A final transfer step is that of capillary uptake of sodium and water achieved by the net balance of hydrostatic and oncotic pressure across the capillary wall. (From Giebisch, 1972.)

The extracellular compartment between proximal tubule cells has emerged as a major determining factor of the passive permeability properties of the proximal tubular epithelium. In addition, changes in the properties of tubular interspaces have been shown to be fundamentally involved in coupling net proximal sodium and fluid reabsorption to peritubular events.

It is mainly on the basis of electrophysiological studies that we may conclude that proximal tubular interspaces represent a low-resistance shunt path in parallel with cell membrane resistances (Boulpaep, 1971; Frömter, Müller, and Wick, 1971; Windhager, Boulpaep, and Giebisch, 1967). The transepithelial resistance of the proximal tubular epithelium is not only unusually low but also much too low if the proximal tubules were lined with membranes having the electrical resistance of proximal tubular cell membranes. The low overall resistance of the epithelium can only be explained by assuming a low-resistance fluid path in parallel to that of the tubular cell membranes. Such a functional organization of the proximal tubular epithelium is consistent with the actual transepithelial resistance values observed.

The importance of the intraepithelial but extracellularly located shunt path in determining the overall transepithelial permeability properties is also underscored by comparing the ionic selectivity of single proximal tubule cells with that of the whole epithelium. Boulpaep (1971) and Frömter *et al.* (1971) have carried out electrophysiological experiments which have clearly shown that the membranes of individual tubule cells show high ionic selectivity. By discriminating sharply between individual ion species they control the entry of various ions into the cell. For instance, the permeability of the peritubular membrane to potassium ions is some 25 times higher than to sodium ions (Giebisch, 1961). In contrast, the permeability of the tubular epithelium as a whole is such that the transepithelial mobility ranking of various ions is very similar to that predicted from ion mobilities in free solution, with the sole exception that anion mobility is less than that of cations (Boulpaep, 1971; Frömter *et al.,* 1971; Boulpaep and Seely, 1971). From such studies it is safe to conclude that the permeability of the proximal tubular epithelium is determined little by the properties of tubular cell membranes and almost exclusively by the properties of low-resistance fluid paths between tubular cells. This is a consequence of the fact that a very large fraction of the transepithelial ion movement takes place via intercellular transport pathways. The assumption of fixed negative charges lining these fluid paths explains the observation that cation movement across the proximal tubular epithelium is faster than that of anions.

The relatively high permeability of the proximal tubular epithelium has prompted a search for additional driving forces of proximal transepithelial fluid movement. We agree with others (Windhager *et al.,* 1969; Brenner and Troy, 1971; Perrson, Agerup, and Schnermann, 1972; Green, Windhager, and Giebisch, 1972) that these do exist in the form of the oncotic pressure difference across the proximal tubular epithelium. However, these forces do not play a major role as a direct and essential force for reabsorptive fluid movement. They act only to modify proximal fluid movement in the presence of active sodium transport.

As an example, it has become apparent that changes in the transepithelial oncotic pressure difference affect proximal fluid transport only to a relatively small degree by exerting a direct osmotic effect across the epithelium. Rather they appear to modulate the efficiency of proximal sodium transport by

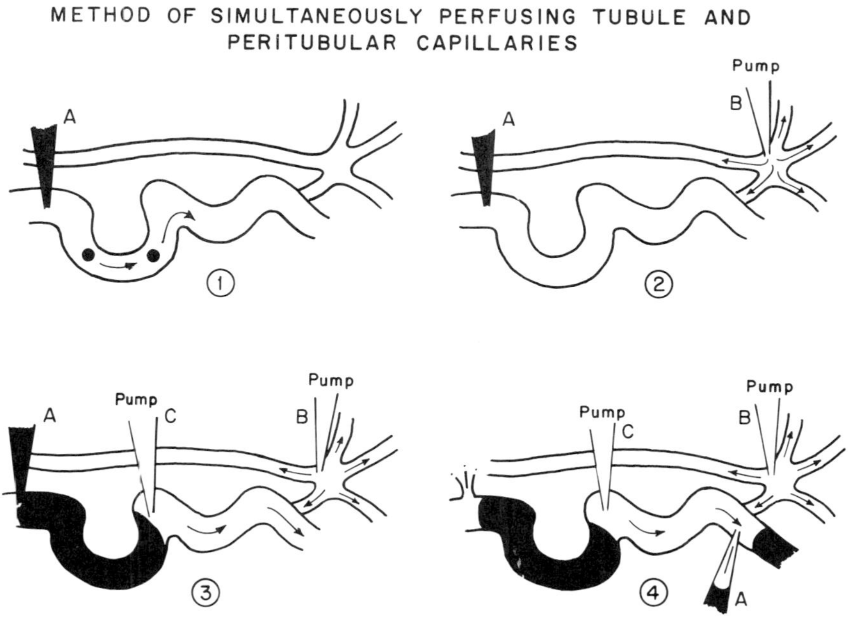

Fig. 2. Method of simultaneously perfusing tubule and peritubular capillaries: (1) oil-filled pipette A placed in tubule; (2) pipette B, connected to perfusion pump, placed in vascular star; (3) pipette C, connected to perfusion pump, placed in tubule and interspace between A and C filled with oil; (4) pipette A removed and placed distally in tubule, and distal oil block placed and collection begun. (Green *et al.*, 1972.)

changing the conductance of the intercellular transport path. The following experiments support this view.

By the use of continuous luminal and peritubular perfusion methods it is possible to expose segments of proximal tubule to well-defined fluid media. Figure 2 is a schematic description of the method used in our laboratory (Green *et al.*, 1972). A proximal tubule, some distance away from a vascular star, was punctured and small oil droplets allowed to flow down the tubule to outline its course. Pipette B was then positioned in a vascular star. It contained Ringer's solution with different amounts of albumin. The pump for the tubular perfusion was set uniformly to deliver 25 nl/min, that for the peritubular perfusion at 1μ/min. The tubular perfusion pipette B was placed just distal to pipette A. Oil was then injected through pipette A to fill the segment between the pipettes. Pipette A was then withdrawn and used for collection of tubular fluid from the most distal loop of the proximal convolution.

The effect of altering the colloid-oncotic pressure difference across the tubulo-capillary barrier on proximal tubular fluid transfer is shown in Fig. 3. Reabsorptive rate, expressed as nlmin^{-1} mm^{-1}, is plotted against the osmotic

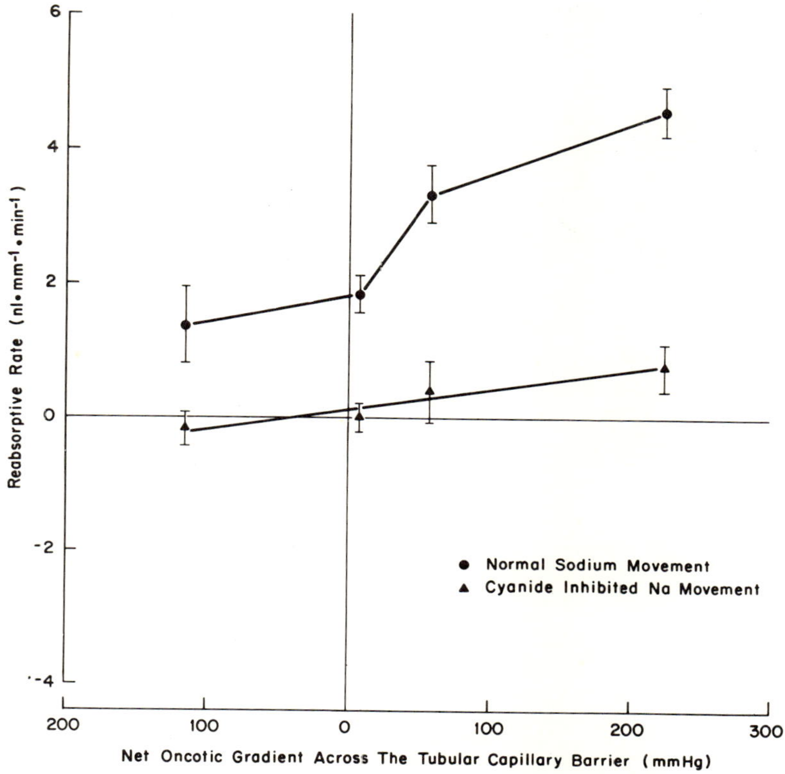

Fig. 3. Effect of human serum albumin on fluid movement across the tubulo-capillary barrier. Reabsorptive rate, calculated in $nl min^{-1} mm^{-1}$, is plotted against the net oncotic pressure difference across the tubulo-capillary barrier: series 1, normal sodium movement; series 2, net sodium movement inhibited by poisoning the sodium pump with 4 mM cyanide. The apparent 'negative' net oncotic pressure difference was produced with human serum albumin in the tubular lumen. Vertical bars are ± s.e. (Green *et al.*, 1972.)

pressure difference. Two series of experiments were done. One group in each series, having 15 gm% human serum albumin (HSA) within the tubule, had a net oncotic force tending to draw water into the tubule. Hence, the results of these experiments are plotted against a 'negative' net oncotic pressure.

The lower set of data was obtained under conditions in which sodium reabsorption had been abolished. This was achieved by perfusing the functionally isolated segment of the proximal tubule with Ringer's solution containing 4 mM cyanide, a concentration which blocks the sodium pump (Giebisch *et al.,* 1964). In both series the capillaries were perfused with Ringer's solution containing 2.5, 10, or 20 g% HSA.

In the series of experiments in which cyanide was used the sodium concentration was equal in both tubule and peritubular capillaries. Under these conditions varying the amount of HSA in peritubular capillaries produced only a small effect on the amount of fluid reabsorbed from the tubule. The slope was significant and allowed for the calculation of a hydraulic conductance value (L_p). It is quite similar to that derived from hydraulic conductance measurements in which a raffinose concentration difference was used to induce osmotic water movement. The magnitude of the fraction of filtrate which could be moved if the full osmotic effect of the protein were to take place across the tubular wall is some 8%. Thus, based on these perfusion studies in which the protein concentration was selectively changed in the lumen and in peritubular capillaries in order to measure the osmotically induced water flow it appears that the normal transepithelial protein concentration difference does not act as a major primary driving force for fluid movement across the proximal tubular epithelium. This confirms previous results obtained in our and other laboratories (Giebisch *et al.*, 1964; Kashgarian *et al.*, 1964; Ullrich, Rumrich, and Fuchs, 1964).

Inspection of Fig. 3 also shows that, in contrast to the situation just described, changes in the transepithelial protein concentration difference had a dramatic effect on fluid movement when the tubule was perfused with normal Ringer's solution, that is, when net sodium transport was present and proceeded at a normal rate.

The line connecting the experimental points can be divided into three portions; there was only a small difference between the values of transepithelial fluid movement when 15 g% albumin was present in the tubule and when it was not, both groups having 2½ g% albumin in the capillary circulation. In contrast there is a marked difference between 2.5 and 10 g% albumin in the peritubular capillaries. The latter difference is highly significant. From these results it can be concluded that, over a range from 2.5 to about 10 g%, albumin can regulate the amount of fluid reabsorbed across the proximal tubular epithelium but that such movement is primarily dependent on sodium transport. Inspection of the right-hand side of Fig. 3 also shows that the presence of 20 g% albumin in the capillary fluid causes a further significant increase in fluid reabsorbed but that the effect is smaller.

It appears from these experiments that sodium transport is primarily responsible for fluid transfer across the tubule, and that proteins, over a physiological range, have a regulatory effect on the amount of fluid reabsorbed into the capillaries. Neither the low L_p data nor the perfusion data, in which net sodium movement was almost abolished while the transepithelial albumin gradient was changed, support the idea that proteins exert a large osmotic effect across the tubular wall.

The following sequence of events has been suggested to explain the effects of peritubular protein concentration changes and Fig. 4 summarizes some relevant features of the proximal tubular epithelium (Windhager *et al.*, 1969; Green *et al.*, 1972; and Boulpaep, 1972a). If the oncotic pressure in peritubular capillaries were lowered, the hydrostatic pressure in the intercellular compartment might increase since removal of fluid from the interspaces is

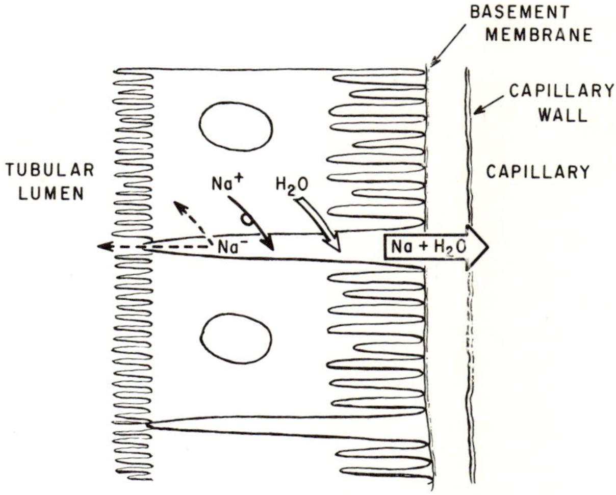

Fig. 4. Schematic presentation of some properties of single proximal tubule cells. (Modified from Giebisch, 1969.)

reduced. Transitorily, there would be disequilibrium between the rate of sodium accumulation and its removal until a new steady state at higher intercellular pressure levels is achieved. The increased hydrostatic pressure is thought to result in enhanced back-leakage of sodium ions from interspaces into the tubular lumen via an intercellular route across the apical 'tight' junction thus rendered less efficient. The prediction from such a cell model would be an increase of the intercellular back-leak component, and not in active pumping rate. Stated in electrical terms, a decline of the electrical resistance of the intercellular transport path would be expected with decreasing extratubular protein concentration.

Experiments which Boulpaep and Grandchamp carried out on a doubly perfused *Necturus* kidney confirm this thesis (Grandchamp and Boulpaep, 1972). The methods used have been described in detail elsewhere (Boulpaep, 1972b). Essentially the approach consists of comparing the transepithelial resistance with that across the cell membranes of tubule cells at different peritubular oncotic pressures. Impalement of a tubule cell with double-barreled micropipettes and injection of a small current through one barrel allows a voltage drop to be measured across the cell membrane. For a given current the magnitude of the voltage drop recorded is proportional to the resistance of the cell membrane. A similar arrangement can be employed with respect to the tubular wall as a whole, and allows for the measurement of transepithelial resistance. An alternative method for the latter measurement utilizes the principle of cable analysis in which current is injected from a point source placed in the tubular lumen and the voltage decline, i.e., its attenuation, is measured by probing microelectrodes along the tubule. The extent to which the voltage drops along the tubule is a measure of its resistance. If a large fraction of the injected current leaks across the tubular wall, the voltage will drop sharply along the tubule. On the other hand, a tight epithelial arrangement will permit less current to leak across the tubular wall. As a consequence, voltage attenuation will be less and the length constant, that is, the distance by which the voltage has declined to about one-third of its initial value, longer.

In Grandchamp and Boulpaep's (1972) experiments the colloid-osmotic pressure of the peritubular fluid was altered and, at the same time, measurements were made of the electrical resistance across both cell membranes of single tubule cells and the tubular wall. The cellular resistance of proximal tubule cells was not affected by changes in peritubular oncotic pressure, whereas there was a significant fall in transepithelial resistance with the lowering of the protein concentration. Thus, the transepithelial specific transverse resistance, as measured by changes in the length constant, fell conspicuously with the lowering of the colloid-osmotic pressure in peritubular capillaries. These results support the idea that changes in the transepithelial colloid-oncotic pressure difference affect the efficiency of proximal sodium reabsorption by acting primarily on the intercellular sodium back-leak component.

It would also be expected that, with the rise in peritubular protein concentration, there ought to be a limit to the amount of fluid which can be reabsorbed. The limit would be set by the capacity of the sodium pump. The data shown in Fig. 3 support this notion since with 20 g% albumin in peritubular capillaries the protein effect tails off. It is also consistent with the described functional organization of the proximal tubular epithelium that the albumin effect be asymmetrical. It would be expected that changes in the luminal protein concentration would be small and limited by the hydraulic conductance of the whole tubulo-capillary barrier. We have indeed observed only a small effect of increasing the luminal protein concentration on transepithelial fluid movement, whereas the protein effect was of much greater magnitude in the opposite direction, that is, when changes were effected in the peritubular fluid compartment.

The idea that a sizeable passive component of sodium chloride transport is responsible for proximal tubular fluid movement has recently been suggested in a different manner (J. Kokko and F.C. Rector, unpublished). On the basis of studies on isolated perfused tubules of the rabbit, Kokko and Rector present the following hypothesis. Preferential sodium bicarbonate reabsorption in the earliest part of the proximal tubule increases the luminal chloride concentration significantly above plasma levels. This concentration gradient establishes a driving force for passive chloride transport from lumen to peritubular fluid and, at the same time, renders the lumen electrically positive by generating a diffusion potential. The slight positivity within the lumen is thought to provide a main driving force for passive sodium and fluid reabsorption. In perfusion studies on the isolated rabbit proximal tubule it was also demonstrated that glucose is electrogenic in the sense that its presence is necessary to make the lumen electrically negative (Kokko and Rector, 1971; Frömter and Lüer, 1973; Maruyama and Hoshi, 1972). Its absence in the middle and late portions of the proximal tubule is thought to contribute importantly to the development of the luminal positivity. This would put primary importance in the process of proximal fluid reabsorption upon tubular hydrogen ion secretion and glucose reabsorption, since these would ultimately be responsible for making the lumen positive and for generating a driving force for sodium reabsorption.

Together with Green we have carried out a series of luminal and peritubular perfusion experiments to assess the role of bicarbonate, chloride, and glucose in the process of proximal tubular fluid transport (R. Green and G. Giebisch, unpublished). Tubular and peritubular fluids were balanced, phosphate-buffered, isosmotic solutions having a pH between 7.39 and 7.42. The peritubular fluid contained 10 g% albumin.

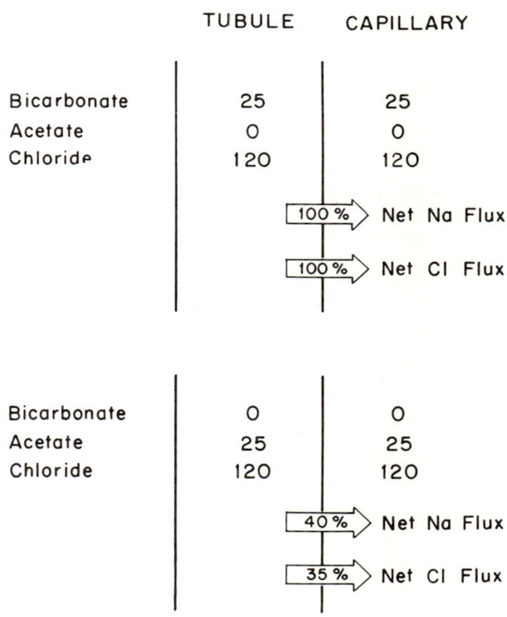

Fig. 5. Summary of tubular and peritubular perfusion experiments on proximal tubules of the rat. The effect of varying bicarbonate concentrations. Experimental techniques were similar to those schematically shown in Fig. 2. Tubular perfusion solutions contained 155 mM Na, 5 mM K, 2 mM Ca, and 17 mM PO_4. pH ranged between 7.39 and 7.42. The peritubular solutions always contained 10 g% albumin. Each net flux average corresponds to 9–14 individual observations.

Figure 5 summarizes relevant data. In this and the following two figures the transepithelial fluxes are given as percentages of the flux of that ion when bicarbonate-containing Ringer's solution was used. The average sodium flux of 100%, shown in the upper panel, corresponds to 500 pM $min^{-1}mm^{-1}$, and the 100% chloride flux to 330 pM $min^{-1}mm^{-1}$. Glucose was absent from both luminal and peritubular perfusion fluids. The flux rates of sodium and water across the perfused tubules were not different from those found in normal blood-supplied proximal tubules of rats. Not shown in this figure are the transepithelial chloride concentration differences. When bicarbonate-containing Ringer's solution was used the chloride concentration in the collected perfusate was 2.8 mEq/liter higher than that in the perfusion fluid.

The lower part of Fig. 5 shows that leaving bicarbonate out of the perfusion solutions results in a 60% reduction of sodium and a 65% reduction of chloride flux. The chloride concentration difference between collected perfusate and the peritubular perfusion fluid was 2.6 mEq/liter, thus not different from that perfusion series in which fluid reabsorption proceeded at a normal rate. The absence of bicarbonate did not mean that the solutions were unbuffered since they all contained 17 mEq/liter phosphate. It is also noteworthy that acetate concentration changes in the perfusion experiments did not affect transepithelial fluid movement.

We would conclude from these experiments, in agreement with Ullrich, Radtke, and Rumrich (1971), that bicarbonate ions augment net sodium and fluid transport across the proximal tubular epithelium. Apparently, this effect is not solely related to the establishment of transepithelial chloride concentration gradients. It is of interest that addition of bicarbonate to the lumen alone raises sodium and fluid transport from 40% to some 70%. For the full restoration of fluid movement, however, it is necessary to have bicarbonate present in both luminal and peritubular perfusion fluid.

The stimulatory effect of bicarbonate on net sodium and fluid transport is also observed in intestine (Turnberg *et al.,* 1970), gall bladder (Diamond, 1968), and choroid plexus epithelium (Wright, 1972). The mechanism of this effect is not known. The possible role of hydrogen ion secretion in the bicarbonate effect is presently being explored.

Figure 6 summarizes data from experiments designed to test the effect of chloride gradients on transepithelial sodium, fluid, and chloride fluxes in the absence of bicarbonate. With an artificially induced normal chloride gradient (see upper panel) the chloride flux returns to a value of 100% but sodium and water fluxes are still only 55% of control. Fluid movement in the presence of a favorable chloride concentration difference, i.e., 135 mEq/liter in the lumen and 120 mEq/liter in the capillaries, is sensitive to the inhibitory effect of 4 mM cyanide. Its addition to the perfusion fluids reduced sodium fluxes to some 18% of controls. If inhibition of active sodium transport were complete, it could be argued that this fraction of sodium transfer could be driven by the transepithelial chloride concentration gradient.

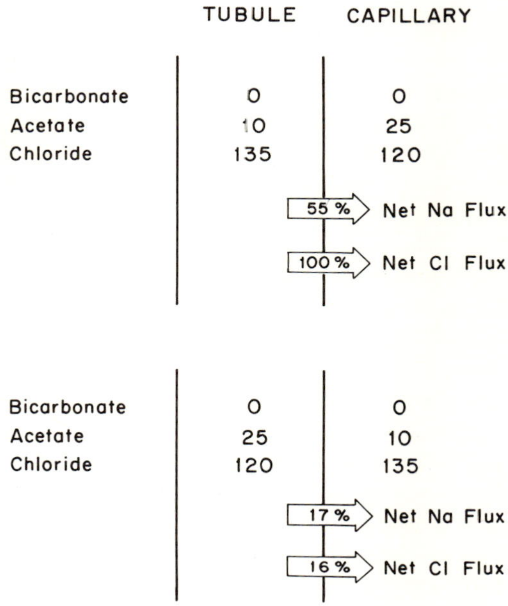

Fig. 6. Summary of tubular and peritubular perfusion experiments on proximal tubules of the rat. The effect of varying chloride concentrations.

The lower panel shows that with an adverse chloride concentration gradient, even in the absence of bicarbonate, the sodium and chloride fluxes, particularly that of sodium, are diminished but not abolished. However, these fluxes are significantly augmented when bicarbonate is added both to lumen and capillary fluid. This is shown in Fig. 7. In the presence of a reversed chloride gradient (luminal chloride lower than peritubular chloride concentration) chloride fluxes remain low, but sodium and fluid movement return, now with bicarbonate present, to some 50% of normal. Analysis of the collected perfusate for chloride ions proved that the chloride concentration had remained below that of plasma throughout the perfusion. This experiment is best explained by coupling of chloride to active sodium transport. Finally, as indicated by the data in the lower panel, when glucose was added to bicarbonate-containing Ringer's solution, sodium chloride fluxes were not found to be higher than those of controls when no glucose was present.

We present the following conclusions from these data: (1) active sodium transport plays the key role in proximal sodium and fluid reabsorption; (2) bicarbonate ions augment this process by an unknown mechanism; (3) the presence of a transepithelial chloride concentration gradient favoring reabsorption ($Cl_{lum} > Cl_{peritub}$) plays a small but significant role in augmenting proximal tubular fluid reabsorption. As the main permeant ion species the rate of active sodium movement is affected by the ease with which chloride follows. A high luminal chloride concentration augments and a low chloride concentration in the lumen retards net fluid movement. However, we do not believe that chloride is primarily responsible for fluid and sodium reabsorption. Two lines of evidence support this view. First, proximal tubular fluid reabsorption in the presence of a favorable chloride gradient is sensitive to metabolic inhibition. Secondly, the reabsorption of sodium continues against a transepithelial concentration gradient of chloride. Thus, the increase in tubular chloride concentration augments, but is not a main driving force for, tubular fluid transfer. Finally, it also appears that glucose is not directly responsible for a large fraction of sodium transport. If the electrogenic effects of glucose are significant (we have not made potential measurements in our perfusions), it appears doubtful that small differences in electrical polarization across the proximal tubular epithelium have a profound effect on proximal sodium transport. The results of our perfusion studies with and without glucose point in this direction. Also, evidence that glucose affects sodium transport by a mechanism other than that of an osmotic diuretic is sparse. It seems from our experiments that the control and maintenance of the extracellular fluid volume is not primarily regulated by passive driving forces. Rather, active sodium transport is entrusted with this vital function. Factors such as changes

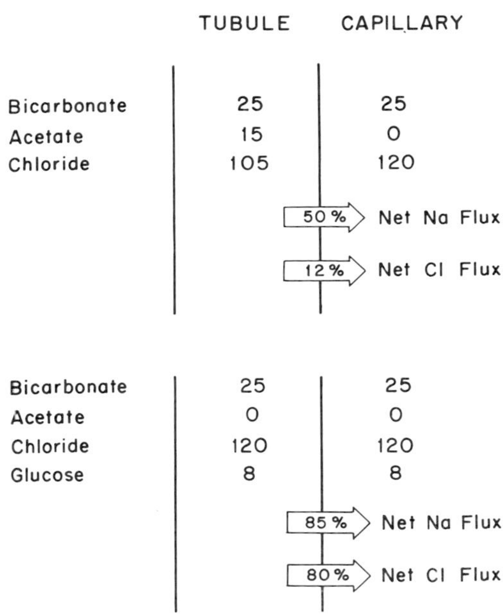

Fig. 7. Summary of tubular and peritubular perfusion experiments on proximal tubules of the rat. The effect of bicarbonate and chloride concentration changes and of changing glucose.

in intercellular back-leak and in chloride and bicarbonate concentration only modulate the efficiency of active tubular sodium transport.

In the following some distal tubular transport phenomena will be considered. At the level of the distal tubule several cationic exchange operations between lumen and cell account for the well-established interrelationship between sodium, potassium, and hydrogen ion movement. Since it has been studied most extensively in our laboratory, special attention will be directed to the role of potassium ions in tubular ion exchange, especially its interaction with sodium and hydrogen ion transport.

Specifically, two problems will be analyzed in some detail. First, how does the rate of sodium excretion affect urinary potassium excretion and what is the mechanism of this ionic interdependence? A second problem to be considered is the effect of acid-base disorders on potassium transport. Again, an attempt will be made to explore the mechanism of the ionic interdependence between distal tubular hydrogen and potassium ion transport.

In the rat, it can be shown that under almost all conditions net secretion of potassium along the distal tubule accounts for most of the excreted potassium (Malnic, Klose, and Giebisch, 1964, 1966a; Malnic, de Mello-Aires, and Giebisch, 1971; Giebisch, 1971). Measurements of the respective electrochemical potential differences across individual cell membranes led to the definition of the transport elements incorporated in the cell schema shown in Fig. 8 (Giebisch, 1971; Malnic, Klose and Giebisch, 1966b).

According to our view potassium entry into the distal tubular lumen across the luminal membrane is passive and driven by the combined electrical and chemical potential difference. Changes in the activity of the peritubular potassium uptake mechanism control the intracellular potassium concentration and thus, in part, the driving force acting on potassium as it crosses the luminal cell membrane. Potassium entry into the lumen across the luminal cell membrane is opposed by active potassium reabsorption. The electrical negativity in the distal tubule and in the cortical collecting tubule as well is dependent upon the luminal sodium concentration (Giebisch *et al.,* 1966;

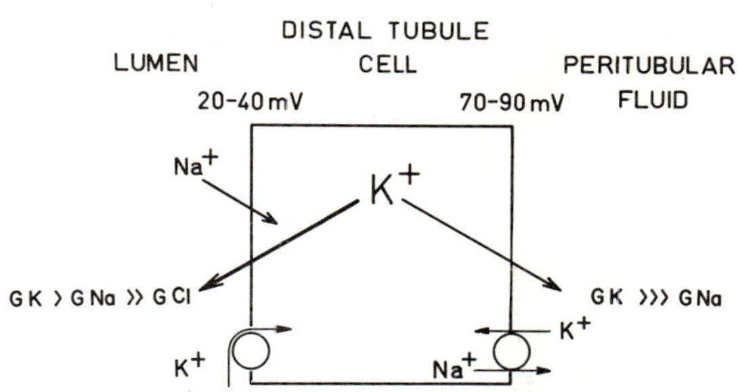

Fig. 8. Schematic presentation of some properties of single distal tubule cells.

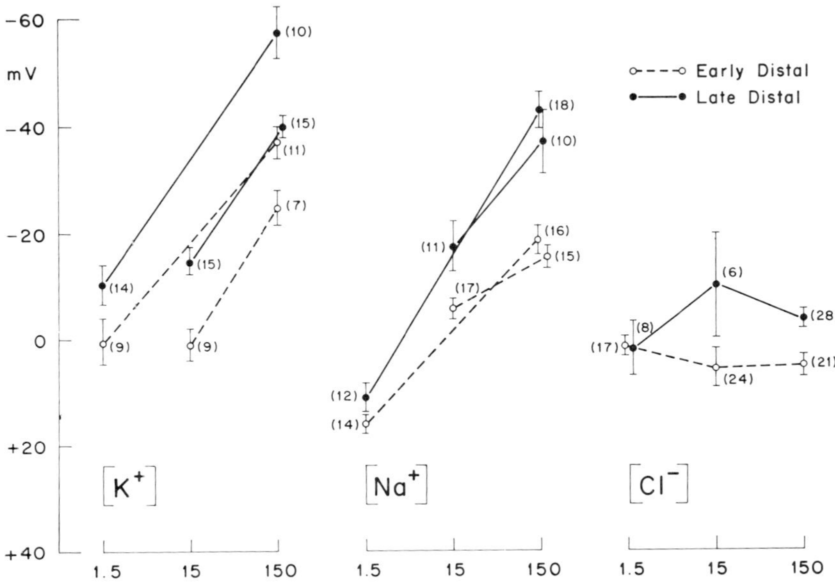

Fig. 9. Summary of effects on distal transepithelial potential differences of various luminal ion substitutions. Solutions containing 1.5, 15.0, and 150.0 mEq/liter of K_2SO_4 and Na_2SO_4, or of choline chloride, were used and isotonicity with plasma was achieved by addition of mannitol. (From Malnic and Giebisch, 1972a.)

Malnic and Giebisch, 1972a; Grantham, Burg, and Orloff, 1970). In Fig. 9 the effects of changes in the luminal potassium, sodium, and chloride concentrations on the distal transepithelial potential difference (p.d.) are shown. It is clear that the magnitude of the transepithelial p.d. is proportional to the luminal sodium concentration. Hence, with a fall in the luminal sodium concentration, the luminal negativity declines. The sequence of events after dietary sodium restriction which lowers urinary potassium excretion may be a relevant example. This is a situation which results in a dramatic fall of sodium excretion. With the fall in tubular sodium concentration and the decline in the transepithelial potential difference, the potassium secretory mechanisms along the distal tubule and the collecting ducts will be rendered less efficient. Along the distal tubule this leads to moderately reduced secretion, as observed by Malnic *et al.* (1966a). Along the collecting duct, where the fall in sodium concentration is more pronounced, potassium secretion ceases and this is a consequence of the fact that, with the fall in luminal negativity, the driving force for potassium entry into the tubular lumen declines, leaving unopposed the active potassium reabsorption mechanism which resides both along the distal tubules and the collecting ducts (Giebisch, 1971; Malnic *et al.*, 1966b; Diezi *et al.*, 1973). In support of this view, enhanced potassium reabsorption along the collecting ducts has been demonstrated during dietary sodium depletion by both indirect and direct methods. In view of the clear-cut evidence obtained by micropuncture experiments done in low sodium states that the amount of sodium at the distal tubular level is adequate for Na-K exchange to proceed at a rate far in excess of the observed one (Malnic *et al.,* 1966a), we propose that a major part of the interrelationship between sodium and potassium transport is due to changes in the electrical driving force acting on the latter. The delivery of sodium to the distal tubule, and particularly to the collecting duct, must be sufficient to exceed the total amount which can be reabsorbed. Unless an adequate concentration of sodium is maintained at the most distal tubular site capable of secreting potassium, the p.d. will fall and the unopposed reabsorptive process will remove potassium from the lumen. The process of potassium secretion is an exchange for sodium which is conditioned by the necessity to maintain electroneutrality on the one hand and by the low chloride permeability of the distal tubular epithelium on the other. This exchange, however, is a fairly unspecific one and, in contrast to most pump and carrier mechanisms, is not governed by a fixed stoichiometric exchange ratio.

In addition, it is possible that a mechanism suggested by Grantham *et al.* (1970) may also be involved in the sodium sensitivity of potassium secretion along the collecting tubule. These investigators showed evidence supporting the presence of active sodium for potassium exchange, a mechanism different from that at the distal tubular level. The fall of potassium secretion with the fall in sodium concentration might be attributed here to an inadequate supply of the counter-ion, that is, of sodium for exchange with potassium. It is clear, however, that this mechanism of active sodium-dependent potassium secretion could at best account for complete suppression of potassium secretion, but not for the reversal of the direction of potassium transport, i.e., active potassium reabsorption. The latter has been observed to be present during dietary sodium deprivation along the papillary collecting ducts (Diezi *et al.,* 1973).

How does the delivery of increased amounts of tubular fluid and sodium to the distal tubule enhance tubular potassium secretion? Evidence obtained by Morgan and Berliner (1969) in perfusion experiments of single distal tubules in the rat, and evidence obtained in our laboratory by Wiederholt *et al.* (1970) is consistent with the view that the distal tubular transport system of potassium is flow-limited. This means that it responds under many, but not all, conditions to the delivery of increased fluid loads unspecifically with an increased rate of potassium secretion. The following observations support this view. The potassium concentrations in free-flow samples of distal tubules are quite similar to concentrations in the steady state in stop-flow microperfusions, and they remain virtually unchanged over a several-fold increment of distal tubular flow rates (Malnic *et al.,* 1964, 1966a,b, 1971; Wiederholt *et al.,* 1970). Obviously, if the distal tubular potassium concentrations are independent of flow rate, the amount of potassium secreted at each point

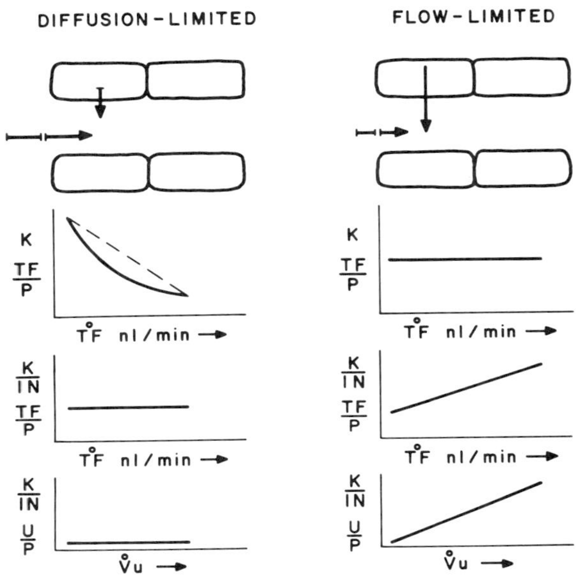

Fig. 10. Schematic presentation of expected behavior of distal transepithelial potassium concentration differences and of fractional distal tubular and urinary potassium excretion in a diffusion-limited and flow-limited system. (From Giebisch, 1971.)

varies directly with volume flow. Other factors remaining constant, net secretion into the distal tubule increases with volume flow past the secretory site.

Figure 10 summarizes the expected behavior of distal transepithelial potassium concentration ratios and of fractional distal tubular and urinary potassium excretion in a diffusion (transport)-limited and flow-limited system. When the concentration differences in experimental conditions such as graded saline diuresis, or after furosemide administration, are measured, the excretion rate of potassium varies directly with distal tubular flow rate without any significant changes of tubular potassium concentrations (Giebisch, 1971; Morgan and Berliner, 1969; Wiederholt *et al.*, 1970). Over more than a ten-fold change in distal tubular flow rate no change was observed in tubular potassium concentration. Thus, it appears that similar transepithelial concentration differences are maintained across the distal tubular epithelium at increasingly higher distal tubular flow rates. Only subsequent to dietary potassium deprivation have we observed a fall of transepithelial potassium concentration differences with increasing distal tubular flow rates keeping constant the amount of potassium secreted per unit time (Wiederholt *et al.*, 1970). From clearance experiments it is also safe to conclude that potassium excretion is not augmented during the induction of water diuresis. Although it is presently not clear which functional transport parameters are responsible for transforming a flow-limited into a transport-limited transport system, it is clear that changes in distal tubular flow rate *per se* are a powerful factor determining urinary excretion rate of potassium. Under many conditions, net secretion is proportional to flow and limited only by the volume flow rate past the secretory site within the tubule.

The kaliuresis of saline loading or that observed after administration of diuretics (Malnic *et al.,* 1966b; Duarte, Chomety, and Giebisch, 1971) is probably a consequence of this flow phenomenon. In view of the uniquely electrogenic role of sodium ions, a greater efficacy of a distal sodium load as compared with a fluid load of nonelectrolytes, such as mannitol or urea, is not surprising. Potassium secretion would be more effectively stimulated by fluid loads containing sodium. This is due to the supportive role of sodium in maintaining the lumen at optimally negative electrical potential levels.

It is also the distal tubule which is responsible for the wide range of potassium secretion associated with acid-base disturbances. Figure 11 summarizes relevant results. Changes of fractional potassium secretion are plotted as function of distal tubular length and show that alkalosis stimulates and

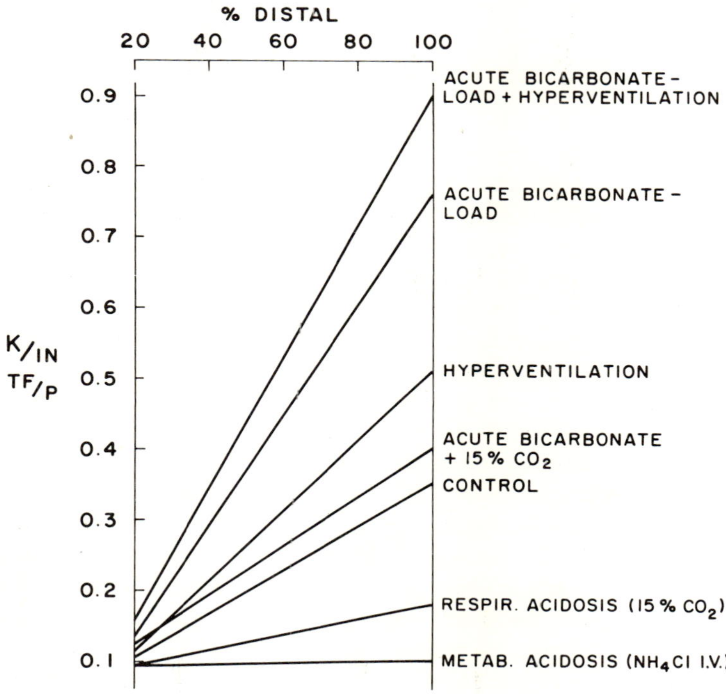

Fig. 11. Summary of distal tubular potassium secretion, plotted as a function of tubular length, during control conditions and during various acid-base disturbances. (Modified from Giebisch, 1971.)

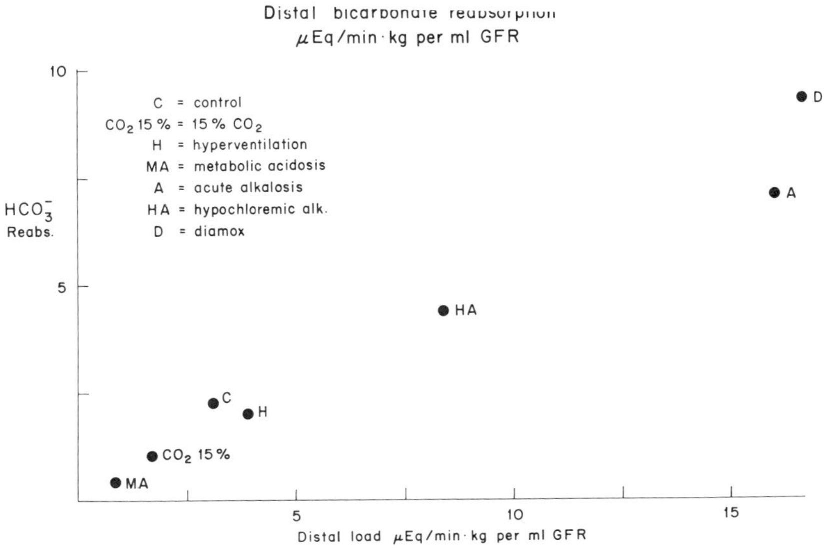

Fig. 12. Relationship between distal load of bicarbonate and amount of bicarbonate reabsorbed along the distal tubule. (Data from Malnic *et al.*, 1972a,b; Vieira and Malnic, 1968; Malnic and Vieira, 1972.)

acute acidosis depresses distal tubular potassium secretion (Malnic *et al.*, 1971; Giebisch, 1971).

It is interesting to compare the simultaneous rates of potassium secretion with those of hydrogen ions to gain information concerning the relationship between these individual flux rates. In general, the rate of distal tubular bicarbonate reabsorption and, by implication, that of hydrogen ion secretion, is found to increase with the delivery of increased amounts of bicarbonate to the distal tubule. The bicarbonate reabsorptive mechanism, or that of distal tubular hydrogen ion secretion, appears in the rat, at least, to be highly unsaturated.

Figure 12 summarizes results of several series of experiments in which the rate of distal tubular bicarbonate reabsorption was measured by comparing early and late distal tubular inulin and bicarbonate concentrations (Malnic, de Mello-Aires, and Giebisch, 1972a,b). The latter were measured by means of an antimony electrode system (Vieira and Malnic, 1968; Malnic and Vieira, 1972). It is clear that distal tubular net bicarbonate reabsorption increases with the distal load. Compared with control and acidotic situations bicarbonate reabsorption in the distal tubule increases during bicarbonate loading, after dismox, and during hypochloremic alkalosis (de Mello-Aires and Malnic, 1972). Since the available evidence indicates that tubular bicarbonate reabsorption is mediated via hydrogen ion secretion (Rector, 1971), it follows that, in almost all experimental situations, potassium and hydrogen ion secretion rates rise in parallel. It is also clear that the rate of the distal tubular hydrogen ion secretion rate is very tightly dependent on the luminal bicarbonate (buffer) load. For instance, at a *constant* luminal buffer load, it can be shown in split-drop experiments that the absolute rate of distal tubular bicarbonate reabsorption (i.e., hydrogen ion secretion) is diminished during metabolic alkalosis (Malnic *et al.,* 1972a,b; Malnic and Giebisch, 1972b). Nevertheless, in free-flow situations bicarbonate reabsorption (i.e. hydrogen ion secretion) is dramatically increased during the very significantly higher tubular bicarbonate load which reaches the distal tubule under such conditions (Malnic and Vieira, 1972; Vieira and Malnic, 1968).

In view of these findings we suggest that intracellular pH changes, and not the rate of tubular hydrogen ion secretion, play a key role in the linkage between acid-base disturbances and potassium transport (Malnic *et al.,* 1971). We have also carried out a number of tracer flux studies concerned with the kinetics of distal transepithelial potassium movement, and observed that alkalosis stimulates the rate of uptake of potassium across the peritubular cell membrane (Wiederholt *et al.,* 1971; de Mello-Aires *et al.,* 1973).

Figure 13 gives an overall view of the transport elements residing within a distal tubule cell. At the top a distal tubule cell is shown with asymmetrical

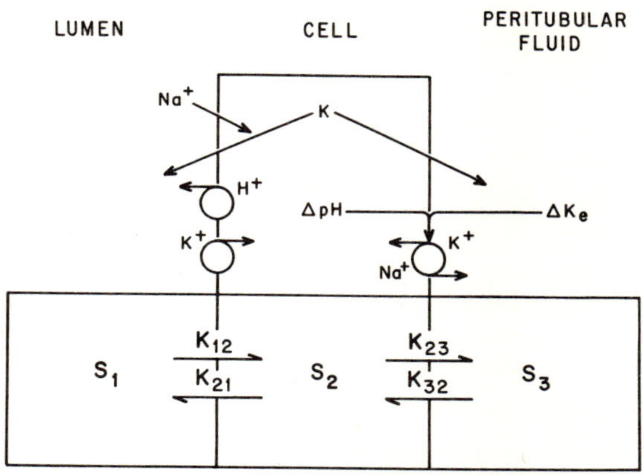

Fig. 13. Upper part. Schematic presentation of some properties of a single distal tubule cell. The different electrical polarization across the luminal and peritubular cell boundaries should be noted. Sodium entry across the luminal cell membrane is facilitated by a higher sodium permeability at this site than across the peritubular cell membrane. The coupling ratio of Na-K at the peritubular membrane is unknown. It is also unknown whether active K uptake across the luminal cell membrane is coupled to other ion transport. Lower part. Schematic illustration of three-compartment system consisting of tubular lumen, the cell compartment, and the peritubular fluid compartment. S_1, S_2, and S_3 denote amount of solute in individual compartments. k_{12}, k_{21}, k_{23}, and k_{32} are rate coefficients defining unidirectional solute movement across the luminal and peritubular cell membrane, respectively. (From Giebisch and Malnic, 1973.)

electrical polarization and an active sodium-potassium exchange pump located within the peritubular membrane. With stimulation of potassium secretion, either by alkalosis or by exogenous potassium loading, the cellular potassium transport pool increases. This increase in the amount of potassium partaking in the transport process is due to stimulation in active uptake of potassium across the peritubular cell border. It appears that it is the driving force acting on passive potassium movement across the luminal cell membrane which is regulated by changes in the intracellular potassium content rather than by primary changes in the transport properties of the luminal cell border. It is this variable which is subject to modulation by changes in peritubular potassium uptake. In view of the evidence surveyed, it appears likely that pH changes act directly on the potassium pump at the peritubular cell membrane.

The cell schema also includes relatively 'uncoupled' individual flux components (K^+, Na^+, H^+) across the luminal cell membrane. We believe that the relative rates of potassium, hydrogen, and sodium movement are coupled loosely by mechanisms which involve changes in cellular concentrations, electrical potential, and luminal buffer loads.

REFERENCES

Boulpaep, E.L. 1971. Electrophysiological properties of the proximal tubule: importance of cellular and intercellular transport pathways. *In* G. Giebisch (ed.), Electrophysiology of Epithelial Cells, F.K. Schattauer Verlag, New York, pp. 91–112.

Boulpaep, E.L. 1972a. Permeability changes of the proximal tubule of Necturus during saline loading. Am. J. Physiol. 222: 517–531.

Boulpaep, E.L. 1972b. Electrophysiological techniques in kidney micropuncture. Yale J. Biol. Med. 45: 397–413.

Boulpaep, E., and J.F. Seely. 1971. Electrophysiology of proximal and distal tubules of the autoperfused dog kidney. Am. J. Physiol. 221: 1084–1096.

Brenner, B.M., and J.L. Troy. 1971. Postglomerular vascular protein concentration: evidence for a causal role in governing fluid reabsorption and glomerulo-tubular balance by the renal proximal tubule. J. Clin. Invest. 50: 336–349.

Curran, P.F., and J.R. Macintosh. 1962. A model system for biological water transport. Nature (Lond.) 193: 347–348.

de Mello-Aires, M., G. Giebisch, G. Malnic, and P.F. Curran. 1973. Kinetics of potassium transport across single distal tubules of rat kidney. J. Physiol. 232: 47–70.

de Mello-Aires, M., and G. Malnic. 1972. Micropuncture study of acidification during hypochloremic alkalosis in the rat. Pflügers Arch. Ges. Physiol. 331: 13–24.

Diamond, J.M. 1964. The mechanism of isotonic water transport. J. Gen. Physiol. 48: 15–42.

Diamond, J.M. 1968. Transport mechanisms in the gall-bladder. *In* Handbook of Physiology. Alimentary Canal, section 6, Vol. V, American Physiological Society Washington, D.C., pp. 2451–2482.

Diezi, J., P. Michoud, J. Aceves, and G. Giebisch. 1973. Micropuncture study of electrolyte transport across papillary collecting duct of the rat. Am. J. Physiol. 224: 623–634.

Duarte, C., F. Chomety, and G. Giebisch. 1971. The effects of amiloride, ouabain and furosemide upon distal tubular function in the rat. Am. J. Physiol. 221: 632–640.

Frömter, E., and K. Lüer. 1973. Free flow potential profile along rat proximal tubule. Pflügers Arch. Ges. Physiol. 339: R47.

Frömter, E., C.W. Müller, and T. Wick. 1971. Permeability properties of the proximal tubular epithelium of the rat kidney studied with electrophysiological methods. *In* G. Giebisch (ed.), Electrophysiology of Epithelial Cells, F.K. Schattauer Verlag, New York, pp. 119–146.

Giebisch, G. 1961. Measurement of electrical potential difference on single nephrons of the perfused Necturus kidney. J. Gen. Physiol. 44: 659–678.

Giebisch, G. 1969. Functional organization of proximal and distal tubular electrolyte transport. Nephron 6: 260–281.

Giebisch, G. 1971. Renal potassium excretion. *In* C.L. Rouiller and A.F. Muller (eds.), The Kidney, Morphology, Biochemistry and Physiology, vol. 3, Academic Press, New York, pp. 329–382.

Giebisch, G. 1972. Coupled ion and fluid movement in the kidney. New Engl. J. Med. 287: 913–919.

Giebisch, G., R.M. Klose, G. Malnic, W.J. Sullivan, and E.E. Windhager. 1964. Sodium movement across single perfused proximal tubules of rat kidneys. J. Gen. Physiol. 47: 1175–1194.

Giebisch, G., and G. Malnic. 1973. Coupled ion movement across the renal tubule. *In* H.H. Ussing and N. A. Thorn (eds.), Alfred Benzon Symposium V: Transport Mechanism in Epithelia, Munksgaard, Copenhagen, pp. 537–552.

Giebisch, G., G. Malnic, R.M. Klose, and E.E. Windhager. 1966. Effect of ionic substitutions upon distal transtubular potential differences in rat kidney. Am. J. Physiol. 211: 560–568.

Giebisch, G., and E.E. Windhager. 1964. Renal tubular transfer of sodium, chloride and potassium. Am. J. Med. 36: 643–669.

Grandchamp, A., and E.L. Boulpaep. 1972. Effect of intrarenal pressures on the permeability of the intercellular shunt pathway and proximal Na reabsorption. Proceedings of 5th International Congress on Nephrology, Mexico City, p. 149.

Grantham, J.J., M.B. Burg, and J. Orloff. 1970. The nature of transtubular Na and K transport in isolated rabbit renal collecting tubules. J. Clin. Invest. 49: 1815–1826.

Green, R., E.E. Windhager, and G. Giebisch. 1972. Effects of transepithelial oncotic pressure difference on proximal tubular fluid movement in the rat. Proceedings of 5th International Congress on Nephrology, Mexico City, p. 145.

Kashgarian, M., H. Stöckle, C.W. Gottschalk, and K.J. Ullrich. 1963. Transtubular electrochemical potentials of sodium and chloride in proximal and distal renal tubules of rats during antidiuresis and water diuresis (diabetes insipidus). Pflügers Arch. Ges. Physiol. 277: 89–106.

Kashgarian, M., Y. Warren, R.L. Mitchell, and F.H. Epstein. 1964. Effect of protein in tubular fluid upon proximal tubular reabsorption. Proc. Soc. Exp. Biol. Med. 117: 848–850.

Kokko, J.P., and F.C. Rector. 1971. Flow dependence of transtubular poten-

tial difference in isolated perfused segments of rabbit proximal convoluted tubule. J. Clin. Invest. 50: 2745–2750.
Malnic, G., M. de Mello-Aires, and G. Giebisch. 1971. Influence of acid-base equilibrium on distal tubular potassium transport in the rat. Am. J. Physiol. 221: 1192–1208.
Malnic, G., M. de Mello-Aires, and G. Giebisch. 1972a. Micropuncture study of renal tubular hydrogen ion transport during alterations of acid-base equilibrium in the rat. Am. J. Physiol. 222: 147–158.
Malnic, G., M. de Mello-Aires, and G. Giebisch. 1972b. Acidification of phosphate buffers in cortical tubules of rat kidney. Pflügers Arch. Ges. Physiol. 331: 275–278.
Malnic, G., and G. Giebisch. 1972a. Some electrical properties of distal tubular epithelium in the rat. Am. J. Physiol. 223: 797–808.
Malnic, G., and G. Giebisch. 1972b. Mechanism of renal hydrogen ion secretion. Kidney Internat. 1: 280–296.
Malnic, G., R.M. Klose, and G. Giebisch. 1964. Micropuncture study of renal potassium excretion in the rat. Am. J. Physiol. 206: 674–686.
Malnic, G., R.M. Klose, and G. Giebisch. 1966a. Micropuncture study of distal tubular potassium and sodium transport in rat nephron. Am. J. Physiol. 211: 529–547.
Malnic, G., R.M. Klose, and G. Giebisch. 1966b. Microperfusion study of distal tubular potassium and sodium transfer in rat kidney. Am. J. Physiol. 211: 548–559.
Malnic, G., and F.L. Vieira. 1972. The antimony microelectrode in kidney micropuncture. Yale J. Biol. Med. 45: 356–367.
Maruyama, T., and T. Hoshi. 1972. The effect of d-Glucose on the electrical potential profile across the proximal tubule of newt kidney. Biochim. Biophys. Acta 282: 214–225.
Morgan, T., and R.W. Berliner. 1969. A study by continuous microperfusion of water and electrolyte movements in the loop of Henle and distal tubule of the rat. Nephron 6: 388–405.
Persson, A.E.G., B. Agerup, and J. Schnermann. 1972. The effect of luminal application of colloids on rat proximal tubular net fluid flux. Kidney Internatn. 2: 203–213.
Rector, F.C., Jr. 1971. Renal secretion of hydrogen. *In* C.L. Rouillier and A. Muller (eds.), The Kidney, Morphology, Biochemistry and Physiology, vol. 3, Academic Press, New York, pp. 209–253.
Turnberg, L.A., J.S. Fordtran, N.W. Carter, and F.C. Rector. 1970. Mechanism of bicarbonate absorption and its relationship to sodium transport in the human jejunum. J. Clin. Invest. 49: 548–556.
Ullrich, K.J., H. Radtke, and G. Rumrich. 1971. The role of bicarbonate and other buffers on isotonic fluid absorption in the proximal convolution of the rat kidney. Pflügers Arch. Ges. Physiol. 330: 149–161.
Ullrich, K.J., G. Rumrich, and G. Fuchs. 1964. Wasserpermeabilität und transtubulärer Wasserfluss corticaler Nephronabschnitte bei verschiedenen Diuresezuständen. Pflügers Arch. Ges. Physiol. 280: 99–119.
Vieira, F.L., and G. Malnic. 1968. Hydrogen ion secretion by rat renal cortical tubules as studied by an antimony microelectrode. Am. J. Physiol. 214: 710–718.
Wesson, L.G., Jr., and W.P. Anslow. 1948. Excretion of sodium and water during osmotic diuresis in the dog. Am. J. Physiol. 153: 465–474.
Wiederholt, M., N. Strieder, R.N. Khuri, and G. Giebisch. 1970. The kinetics

of potassium transport in the renal tubules of the rat. Pflügers Arch. Ges. Physiol. 319: R74.

Wiederholt, M., J.W. Sullivan, G. Giebisch, A.K. Solomon, and P.F. Curran. 1971. Measurement of unidirectional K and Na fluxes on single distal tubules of Amphiuma kidney. J. Gen. Physiol. 57: 495–525.

Windhager, E.E., E.L. Boulpaep, and G. Giebisch. 1967. Electrophysiological studies of single nephrons. Proceedings of 3rd International Congress on Nephrology, Washington, D.C., Vol. 1, S. Karger, New York, pp. 35–47.

Windhager, E.E., and G. Giebisch. 1961. Micropuncture study of renal tubular transfer of sodium chloride in the rat. Am. J. Physiol. 200: 581–590.

Windhager, E.E., J.E. Lewy, and A. Spitzer. 1969. Intrarenal control of proximal tubular reabsorption of sodium and water. Nephron 6: 247–259.

Wright, E.M. 1972. Mechanism of ion transport across the choroid plexus. J. Physiol. 226: 545–571.

Effects of Acute Changes in Renal Cortical Blood Flow Distribution on Renal Function in Dogs

Richard L. Riley
Department of Physiology and Biophysics
Hahnemann Medical College and Hospital, and The Merck Institute
West Point, Pennsylvania

The development of a technique for induction of experimental hypertension in laboratory animals by Goldblatt *et al.* (1934) was an initial and singularly important contribution to both basic and clinical researchers in hypertension. Subsequently, numerous new methods and modifications have been developed in an attempt to simulate specific hypertensions seen in man. Most of these methods involve stimulation of renin secretion at some point in the development of the high blood pressure. Recently, Ayers, Harris, and Lefer (1969) demonstrated that the initial events following partial renal artery constriction are decreased intrarenal arteriolar resistance and stimulation of renin secretion. Later, as renal vascular resistance rises during the development of high blood pressure, renin secretion returns to or below normal. More recently Gutmann *et al.* (1973) reported an immediate increase in renal venous plasma renin activity (RVPRA) following partial renal artery constriction in *conscious* dogs. A decrease in intrarenal vascular resistance, with no alteration of intrarenal distribution of blood flow, was also reported in these dogs.

In these studies the significance of the vasodilator response is uncertain since renin secretion induced by partial renal artery or suprarenal aortic constriction may also result from stimulation of juxtaglomerular cell baroreceptors (Skinner, McCubbin, and Page, 1964). In view of this uncertainty we developed an interest in the contribution of vasodilatation *per se* to the distribution of renal cortical blood flow (RCBF) and to renin secretion.

A vast number of techniques are available for assessment of individual components of renal function in the anesthetized dog. Our primary objective was to develop and test a reliable anesthetized-dog model capable of evaluating total renal function in a single dog. This paper substantiates the stability of all parameters in such a model for the duration of an experimental period, and then cites the responsiveness of the preparation to significant renal vasodilation. The intent is not to offer interpretations of vasodilator-induced effects on renal function, but to present a method and demonstrate its potentials and limitations.

METHODS

Lean, conditioned, female mongrel dogs, 20–30 kg, with bilateral single renal arteries were used. Dogs were fed commercial dog chow during the conditioning period with no attempt to stimulate or reduce RVPRA with low or high salt diet, respectively. Pan water was allowed *ad lib.* Anesthesia was induced with 20 mg/kg Nembutal i.v. and surgical anesthesia maintained with a constant i.v. infusion of 0.5% α-chloralose solution (in normal saline with 5% dextrose at 1–2 ml/min).

An i.v. catheter (PE-90) was inserted into the abdominal vena cava via the right medial saphenous vein (Fig. 1). This catheter was used for infusion of α-chloralose and/or saline venoclysis, and for sampling of caval blood. An aortic catheter (PE-90) was inserted via the right medial saphenous artery and secured with the distal tip at the level of the renal arteries. Mean aortic pressure, pulsatile pressure, and heart rate were recorded using standard techniques on a Hewlett-Packard recording system.

Ureters were catheterized bilaterally (PE-90) with the catheter tips near the renal hilus. Independent urine samples were collected in calibrated tubes. Urine collection periods were uniformly of 5 min duration. A PE-90 catheter was introduced in the vena cava through the left medial saphenous vein and the distal tip manually deflected into the right renal vein. The catheter was advanced an additional 1–2 cm to prevent its return to the vena cava. A PE-50 catheter was introduced into the left ovarian vein and secured with the tip in the left renal vein. Following assurance of bilateral catheter placement and patency, the midline incision was closed.

A left laparotomy was performed at the level of the left kidney and both renal arteries manually exposed and isolated. Care was taken to manipulate the kidneys and adjacent tissues no more than necessary. The renal nerves were left intact. Micron electromagnetic flow probes of the appropriate size were placed around both renal arteries. The probes were calibrated *in vitro* and *in vivo,* and pulsatile and mean blood flows were recorded from both kidneys simultaneously. After confirming the integrity of blood-flow recordings, a 23-g infusion unit (Abbott Butterfly Infusion Set) was carefully inserted into the left renal artery proximal to the electromagnetic flow probe according to the method of McNay, McDonald, and Goldberg (1965). This needle was not secured in place and great care was taken to assure its position in the artery.

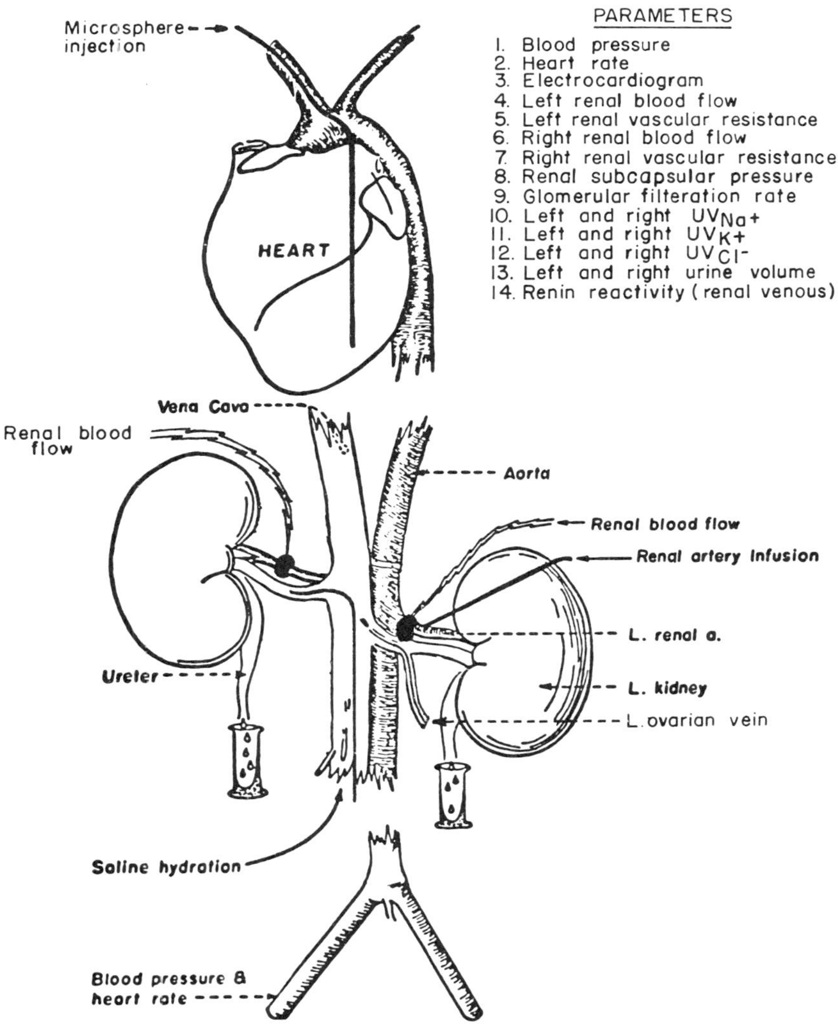

Fig. 1. Diagram of the experimental model in the studies reported. Parameters monitored are noted.

A 30-sec duration bilateral carotid artery occlusion was performed to test the integrity of the autonomic nervous system. In the chloralose anesthetized dog the procedure produced immediate, reversible reductions in total renal blood flow (RBF) and increases in mean aortic blood pressure, pulse pressure, and heart rate. Renal autoregulatory mechanisms remained intact during all tests. A PE-90 catheter was then inserted into the right common carotid artery and advanced retrograde so the tip resided within the left ventricle or in the aortic arch. This catheter was used solely for arterial injections of microsphere boli. Intraventricular localization of the catheter is desired to assure complete mixing of microspheres with blood and to reduce axial streaming of the spheres. The 15γ-diameter microspheres are completely cleared from the blood in one circulation time and those entering the renal circulation are localized only in glomerular capillaries (Fig. 2). Since initial blood flow in the canine kidney is predominantly cortical (Selkurt, 1963) and the microspheres are entrapped in glomerular capillaries, this method is useful only for estimating cortical distribution of RBF. It is not satisfactory for estimation of medullary or papillary flow distribution since sphere distribution in these areas is not proportional to blood flow. Under these conditions, intrarenal concentration (or density) of microspheres following aortic injections is proportional to the percentage of cardiac output distributed to each kidney (Katz *et al.*, 1971; McNay and Abe, 1971; Rudolph and Heymann, 1967; Slotkoff *et al.*, 1971; Stein *et al.*, 1971). Sequential injections of four different isotopically labeled microsphere boli (one injection prior to, two injections during, and one injection following intrarenal arterial infusion) are

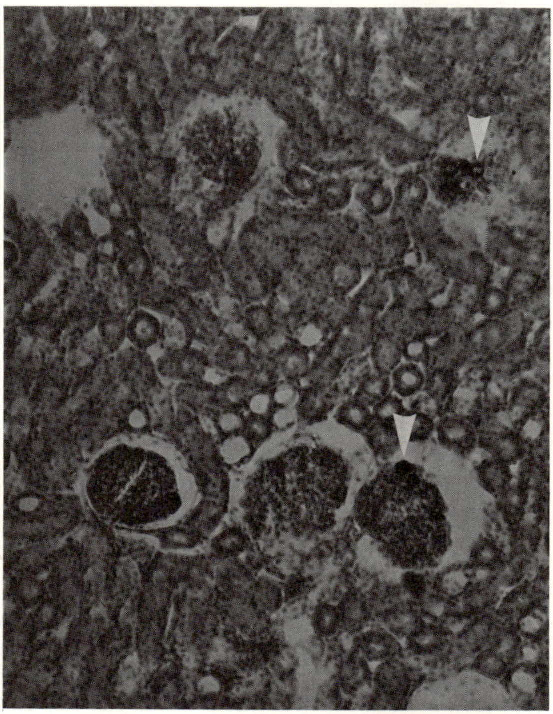

Fig. 2. Representative section of renal cortex after four serial injections of microspheres. Entrapment of microspheres along the periphery of glomeruli exclusively is indicated.

made during each experiment. Following the experiment the kidneys were removed and prepared for sectioning according to the methods of McNay *et al.* (1965) and Katz *et al.* (1971). Blocks of kidney tissue were mounted in a cryostat and serially cut from capsular cortex through papilla. A total of 20 or 21 sections were obtained from each block of kidney tissue, 13 of which were sections of cortex. Duplicate sections from each kidney were accurately weighed, placed in plastic tubes, and counted on a Baird-Atomic gamma-ray spectrometer system. The concentration of each isotopically labeled microsphere type in each section of each kidney was expressed as a count density (CD) (c.p.m./gm tissue). The CD of each isotope in all kidney sections were then graphically plotted in order to obtain a profile of cortical microsphere distribution.

Blood samples for renin assay were drawn from both renal veins simultaneously. Renal venous plasma renin activity was estimated using radio-immunoassay for angiotensin I (A_I). In addition, renin secretion rates were calculated using total RBF from each kidney at the time of blood sampling.

Dogs were given 250–300 mg/kg creatinine s.c. (as a 15% solution) at least 45 min prior to starting an experiment. Most dogs received 400–700 ml of isotonic saline in order to assure adequate urine flow. Urine losses were replaced with isotonic saline after each 5-min urine collection period in order to prevent renin secretion as a result of electrolyte or volume loss. A recovery time of at least 1 hr was allowed after finishing surgery for stabilization of all parameters prior to starting an experiment. Isotonic saline was infused (0.01 ml/kg/min IRA) in seven placebo experiments. Prostaglandin E_1 (PgE_1) was infused (0.05 γg/kg/min IRA for 10 min) in six dogs.

With this model bilateral renal function may be studied while administering an agent to a single kidney. In this way the contralateral kidney acts as a control since it is subject to the same environment as the infused kidney.

RESULTS

The responses of several parameters to unilateral saline or PgE_1 infusion will be briefly summarized. The experimental protocol consisted of three periods; a pre-infusion or control period of 15 min duration, a 10-min intrarenal arterial infusion period, and a post-infusion, or recovery, period of 15 min duration. All parameters were recorded continuously throughout the experiment and the mean response for the group is illustrated.

Mean blood pressure and heart rate remained essentially unchanged in both saline-infused and PgE_1-infused dogs (Fig. 3a,b). In these experiments a constant blood pressure was necessary in order to exclude juxtaglomerular baroreceptor stimulation as a provocator of renin secretion (Skinner *et al.*, 1964). It should be noted that the placebo-infused dogs were remarkably stable throughout the experimental period.

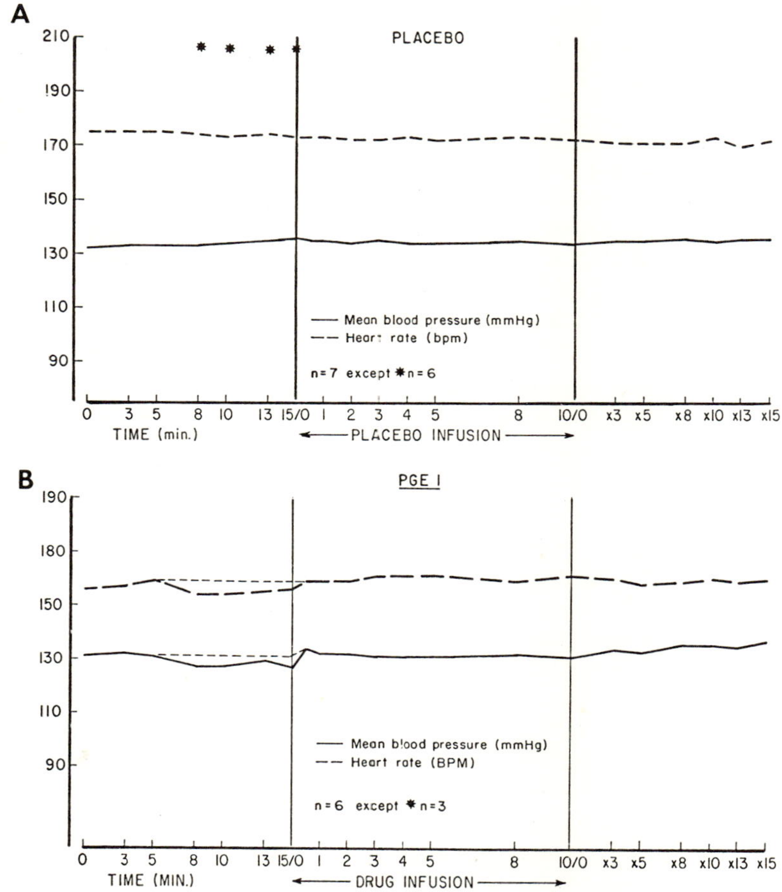

Fig. 3. Mean blood pressure (mm Hg) and heart rate (bpm) responses prior to, during, and after infusion of (a) isotonic saline, or (b) PgE_1 into the left renal artery.

Renal Blood Flow

In the saline-infused dogs, total RBF remained essentially constant for the duration of the experiment (Fig. 4a). Total blood flow in the left kidneys was consistently higher than in the right kidneys since the dogs lay on the right side causing some compression of the right kidney. During PgE_1 infusion, the total left RBF rose from 170 to 300 mg/min with essentially no change in right RBF (Fig. 4b). Following the infusion period, the left RBF rapidly returned to pre-infusion levels and remained constant for the remainder of the period.

Microsphere Distribution

In order to achieve consistent responses among all dogs within the groups, the count density (CD) of each isotope in each tissue section was plotted as a percentage of the section with maximal CD (Fig. 5). The initial subcapsular tissue section was aglomerular, and therefore contained few microspheres (Katz *et al.*, 1971). The inner cortical and outermost medullary sections have 10–20% of maximal CD. In the inner medulla and papilla the CD's are not representative of blood flow distribution since microspheres cannot gain access to these areas. The region of highest cortical CD during the pre-infusion period was generally 2 mm from the capsular surface. The general distribution BF pattern seen during control periods in these studies was in agreement with results reported by others using the microsphere technique (Bovee and Webster, 1972; Katz *et al.*, 1971; Slotkoff *et al.*, 1971; Stein *et al.*, 1971).

In the placebo-infused dogs there were no apparent changes in the relative distribution of microspheres in either kidney during or after saline infusion

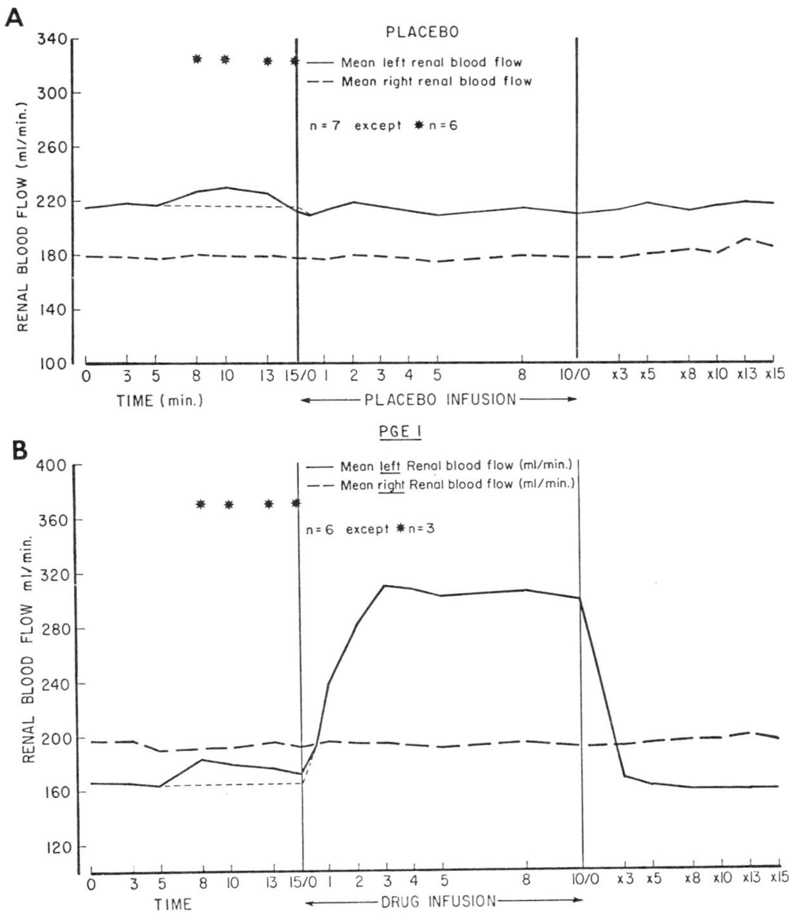

Fig. 4. Bilateral total RBF recordings (ml/min) prior to, during, and after infusion of (a) isotonic saline, or (b) PgE_1 into the left renal artery.

(Fig. 5a). The pre-infusion distribution in PgE_1 experiments was similar to the control distribution pattern on placebo dogs (Fig. 5b). After 4 and 8 min of constant PgE_1 infusion, the highest CD's were still found in the outermost cortex. In the mid and inner cortex, however, the CD's were approximately 70% of maximal CD, indicating a preferential increase in inner cortical blood flow during vasodilation. A similar occurrence has been previously reported (Vander, 1968; Jirakulsonchok and Moore, 1971). Following PgE_1 infusion, CD returned to pre-infusion levels throughout the cortex.

Relative microsphere distribution may be expressed also as a ratio of the CD's in mated left and right kidney sections, respectively. In the placebo infusion experiments left to right *cortical* CD ratios all fell very close to the unity line, indicating that the relative distribution of blood flow at comparable cortical depths is essentially equivalent in both kidneys (Fig. 6a). Again, CD ratios obtained from inner medullary and papillary areas are not legitimate estimates of normal blood flow distribution in these areas.

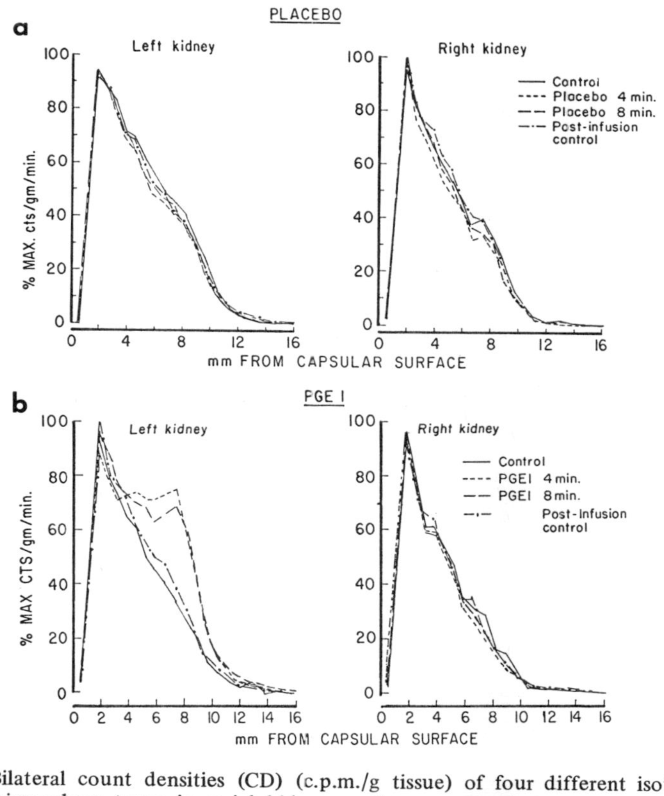

Fig. 5. Bilateral count densities (CD) (c.p.m./g tissue) of four different isotopically labeled microsphere types in serial kidney sections expressed as a percentage of the section with highest CD. Microspheres were injected prior to, during, and after infusion of (a) isotonic saline, or (b) PgE_1 into the left renal artery.

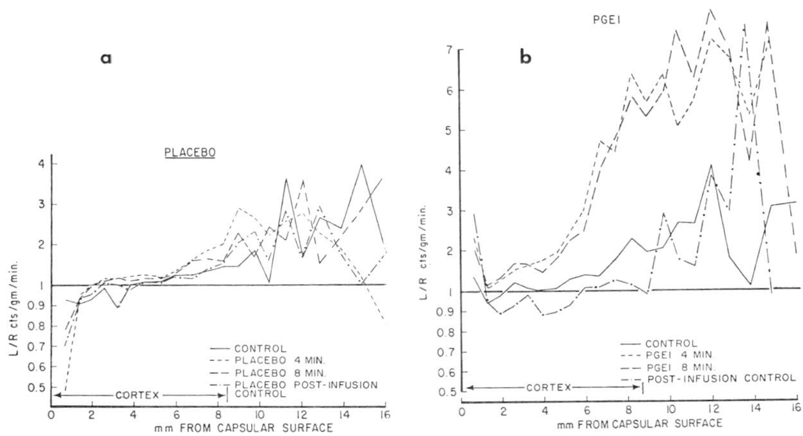

Fig. 6. Left to right renal CD ratios (left/right c.p.m./g tissue) of four different isotopically labeled microsphere types in serial sections from both kidneys. The CD of each isotope in each section from the left (infused) kidney is compared with a 'mated section' from the right kidney. Microspheres were injected prior to, during, and after infusion of (a) isotonic saline, or (b) PgE_1 into the left renal artery.

In PgE_1 infusion experiments the pre-infusion cortical CD ratios fell close to the unity line as in placebo experiments (Fig. 6b). During unilateral intrarenal infusion of PgE_1, cortical CD ratios were consistently higher than in the pre-infusion period. Since the same tissue sections were used to determine CD ratios prior to, during, and after PgE_1 infusion, increases or decreases in these ratios represent actual increases or decreases, respectively, in blood flow to these regions of the renal cortex. Although highest CD ratios are found in the inner cortex and outer medulla during infusion of PgE_1, absolute blood flow is increased *throughout the cortical mass.*

The microsphere data indicate that PgE_1 infusion increases blood flow throughout the cortex, but that the increases in inner cortical flow are proportionally greater than in outer cortical flow. In addition, contralateral blood flow and blood flow distribution were unaltered even during the period when the total left RBF is highest. The left RBF distribution returned to the pre-infusion condition soon after stopping the infusion.

Renal Electrolyte Excretion

Bilateral sodium, potassium, and chloride excretion rates and total kidney GFR remained constant throughout the experimental period in dogs receiving intrarenal infusion of saline (Fig. 7a). During PgE_1 infusion there were significant, unilateral increases in excretion of urinary electrolytes and in GFR (Johnston, Herzog, and Lauler, 1967; Lee, 1967; Lipson and Sharp, 1971; Martinez-Maldonado *et al.,* 1972). These saluretic, kaliuretic, and diuretic responses to PgE_1 infusion were completely reversible within 15 min of ending the intrarenal infusion of PgE_1 (Fig. 6b).

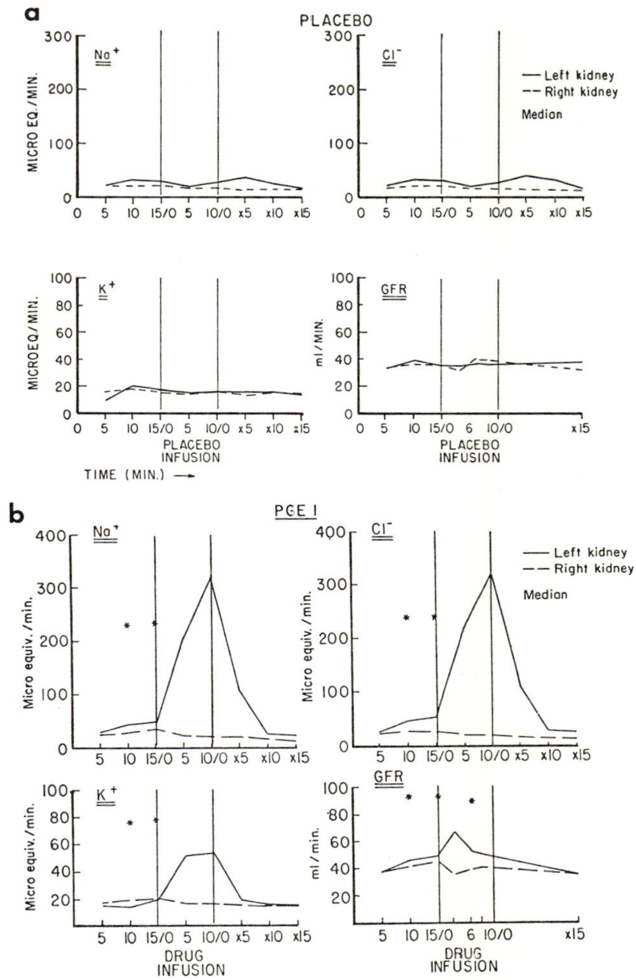

Fig. 7. Bilateral renal sodium, potassium and chloride excretion rates (μeq/min) and GFR (ml/min) prior to, during and after infusion of (a) isotonic saline, or (b) PgE_1 into the left renal artery.

Renin Secretion

Renal venous plasma renin activity values in anesthetized, surgically traumatized dogs are known to be highly variable and difficult to predict (Assaykeen and Ganong, 1971; Granger, unpublished thesis, Dept. of Investigative Medicine, McGill Univ., Montreal; Granger, Boucher, and Genest, 1970; Johnston, *et al.*, 1968; MacKenzie, Ryan, and Lee, 1967; Robertson and Michelakis, 1972). Because of this variability in RVPRA among anesthetized dogs we elected to study the changes in *renin secretion rate* in response to vasodilata-

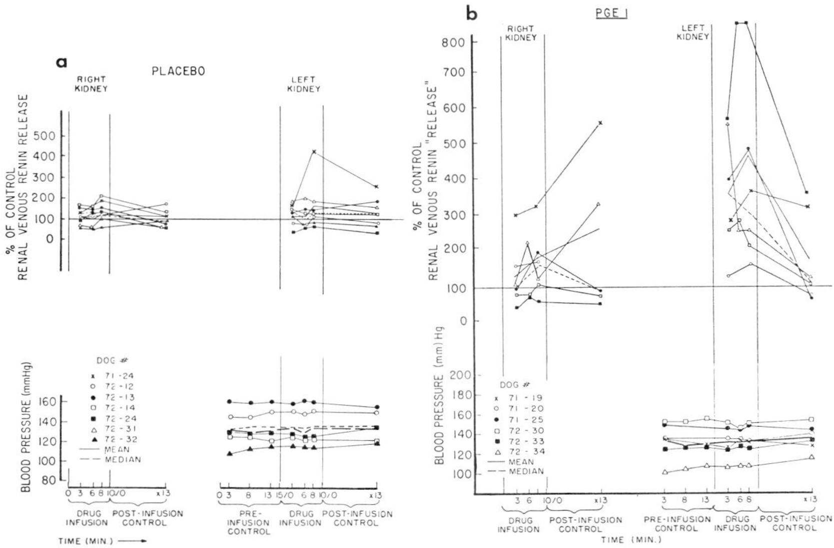

Fig. 8. Bilateral percentage changes in the rate of renal venous renin secretion in individual dogs from pre-infusion rates during and after infusion of (a) isotonic saline, or (b) PgE_1 into the left renal artery. Mean blood pressure responses in these same dogs are shown.

tion. Renin secretion combines the effects of changes in RVPRA and in renal plasma flow and in these studies demonstrates the contribution of each to changes in peripheral PRA.

In the placebo (saline)-infused dogs bilateral renal venous renin secretion rates, in all but one instance, changed very little (Fig. 8a). Changes in renal venous renin secretion of ±50% were not considered significant under circumstances of extreme renin lability. As noted previously, mean blood pressure remained stable in all dogs throughout the experiment.

In the PgE_1-infused kidneys renal venous renin secretion was stimulated in every case (Fig. 8b). Values were generally 2- to 4-fold higher during PgE_1 infusion than during the pre-infusion period. During the post-infusion period renin secretion gradually returned toward pre-infusion levels. In these dogs *left RVPRA* was also elevated during the infusion period. Renin secretion rates by the contralateral kidney were generally within the same limits as in placebo studies. Again, mean blood pressure was stable during and after PgE_1 infusion.

DISCUSSION

We have demonstrated that the dog model reported here is uniquely capable of assessing changes in a large number of intrarenal and systemic factors within a single animal. Further justification of the microsphere method for determining small changes in zonal cortical blood flow has been presented. In addition, some potential criticisms of the microsphere method have been allayed.

First, since the microsphere distribution represents particulate flow, rather than plasma flow, there is the potential for plasma streaming of spheres, especially in the intralobular arteries, and thus the possibility of an inappropriate distribution of spheres to the outer cortex (as proposed by Papenheimer *et al.,* 1956, for red blood cells). Under these circumstances, microsphere distribution would not accurately represent plasma flow. However, when normal cortical count density is plotted against glomerular density, it is evident that microsphere distribution is very closely correlated with glomerular distribution (Horiuchi *et al.*, 1971) (Fig. 9). In addition, intrarenal dilators should exaggerate any plasma streaming effects and produce an even greater artifact of sphere distribution toward the *outer* cortex. As noted in Fig. 6b, however, the outer cortical CD ratios do increase during PgE_1 infusion, but there is a proportionally greater increase in CD ratios in mid and inner cortex indicating that the microspheres do not stream to a significant extent.

A second criticism is that spheres may enter a glomerulus in such a way as totally to occlude flow and therefore decrease the number of active nephrons. Most investigators report no vascular damage as a result of intraglomerular residence of one or more 15γ-diameter microspheres (Katz *et al.,* 1971; Stein *et al.,* 1971). In these studies histological examination has revealed no microsphere-induced glomerular trauma after four serial injections of spheres, even in cases where more than one sphere resides in a glomerulus (Fig. 2). In

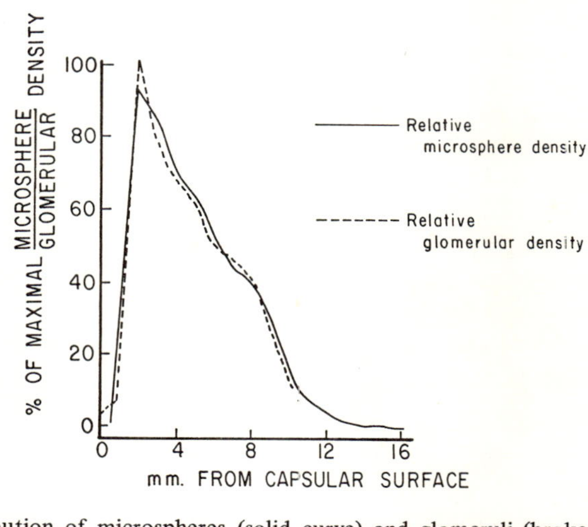

Fig. 9. Distribution of microspheres (solid curve) and glomeruli (broken curve) in the renal cortex. Microsphere distribution in proportion to the regional glomerular population is indicated. See text.

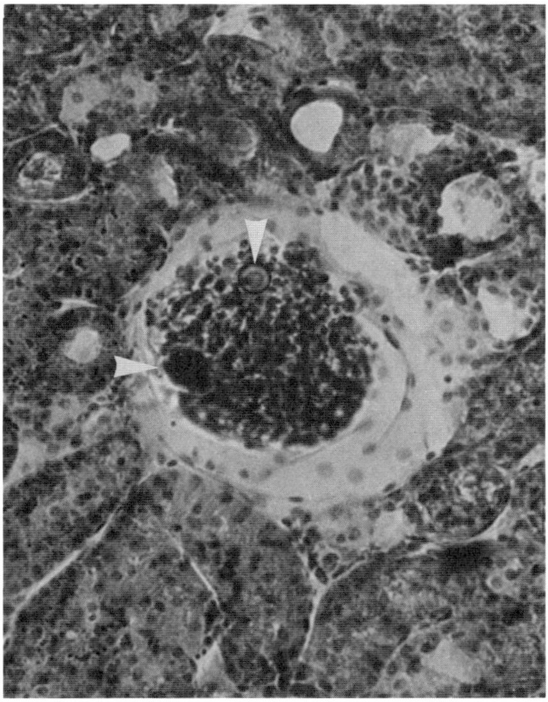

Fig. 10. Single glomerulus showing entrapment of two microspheres injected at different times. Continued glomerular perfusion despite the presence of one or more microspheres is indicated.

addition, the presence of one sphere does not preclude flow within a glomerulus. Figure 10 demonstrates the presence of two spheres in a single glomerulus, one black and one amber. These two types of spheres were injected at different times during the experiment, and thus one had to enter the glomerulus while the other was already *in situ.* The explanation of blood-flow maintenance in these glomeruli is that the afferent arteriole initially divides to form several capillaries which perfuse the periphery of the gomerular tuft. A sphere may lodge in one of these capillary units without occluding flow through the remainder of the capillaries.

Although the method described cannot permit a final evaluation of the mechanisms of vasodilator-induced renin secretion, it does provide abundant data from individual dogs and allows statistical correlations to be made with greater efficiency and confidence. The same procedure, with modification (i.e., denervations, nonfiltering kidneys, dietary electrolyte control, receptor blockade, etc.), can also be used to investigate further the elements associated with renin secretion. In addition the reliability of the method precludes the necessity of using large numbers of test animals in order to secure sufficient data for analysis of renal function.

REFERENCES

Assaykeen, T.A., and W.F. Ganong. 1971. The sympathetic nervous system and renin secretion. *In* L. Martini and W.F. Ganong (eds.), Frontiers in Neuroendocrinology, Oxford University Press, New York, pp. 62–102.

Ayers, C.R., R.H. Harris, and L.E. Lefer. 1969. Control of renin release in experimental hypertension. Circulation Res. 24 & 25(1): 103–112.

Bovee, K.C., and G.D. Webster. 1972. Values for intrarenal distribution of blood flow using Xe^{133} in the anesthetized dog. Am. J. Vet. Res. 33: 501–510.

Goldblatt, H., J. Lynch, R.E. Hanzal, and W.W. Summerville. 1934. The production of persistent elevation of systolic blood pressure by means of renal ischemia. J. Exp. Med. 59: 347–479.

Granger, P., R. Boucher, and J. Genest. 1970. A method for determination of renin in dog's plasma and renal tissue. Can. J. Physiol. Pharm. 48: 457–462.

Gutmann, F.D., H. Tagawa, E. Haber, and A.C. Barger. 1973. Renal arterial pressure, renin secretion and blood pressure control in trained dogs. Am. J. Physiol. 224: 66–72.

Horiuchi, K., H. Tanaka, K. Yamamoto, and J. Ueda. 1971. Distribution of renin in the dog kidney. Life Sci. 10(1): 727–734.

Jirakulsonchok, D., and W.W. Moore. 1971. Effect of PgE_1 on renal function and the distribution of renal blood flow. Physiologist 14: 168 (abstr.).

Johnston, C.I., J.O. Davis, C.A. Robb, and J.W. MacKenzie. 1968. Plasma renin in chronic experimental heart failure and during renal sodium 'escape' from mineralcorticoids. Circulation Res. 22: 113–125.

Johnston, H.H., J.P. Herzog, and D.P. Lauler. 1967. Effect of PgE_1 on renal hemodynamics, sodium and water excretion. Am. J. Physiol. 312: 939–946.

Katz, M.A., R.C. Blantz, F.C. Rector, Jr., and D.W. Seldin. 1971. Measurement of intrarenal blood flow. I. Analysis of microsphere method. Am. J. Physiol. 220: 1903–1913.

Lee, J.B. 1967. Antihypertensive activity of the kidney: the renomedullary prostaglandins. New Engl. J. Med. 277: 1073–1079.

Lipson, L.C., and G.W.G. Sharp. 1971. Effect of PgE_1 on sodium transport and osmotic water flow in the toad bladder. Am. J. Physiol. 220: 1046–1052.

MacKenzie, J.H., J.W. Ryan, and M.R. Lee, 1967. Effect of laparotomy on plasma renin activity in the rabbit. Nature (Lond.) 215: 542–543.

Martinez-Maldonado, M., N. Tsaparas, G. Eknoyan, and W.N. Suki. 1972. Renal actions of prostaglandins: comparison with acetylcholine and volume expansion. Am. J. Physiol. 222: 1147–1152.

McNay, J.L., and Y. Abe. 1971. Redistribution of cortical blood flow during renal vasodilatation in dogs. Circulation Res. 27: 1023–1032.

McNay, J.L., R.H. McDonald, Jr., and L.I. Goldberg. 1965. Direct renal vasodilatation produced by dopamine in the dog. Circulation Res. 16: 510–517.

Pappenheimer, J.R., and W.B. Kinter, 1956. Hematocrit ratio of blood within mammalian kidney and its significance for renal hemodynamics. Am. J. Physiol. 185: 377.

Robertson, D., and A.M. Michelakis, 1972. Effects of anesthesia and surgery on plasma renin activity in man. J. Clin. Endocr. Metab. 34: 831–836.

Rudolph, A.M., and M.A. Heymann. 1967. Circulation of the fetus *in utero*. Circulation Res. 21: 163–190.

Selkurt, E.E. 1963. The renal circulation. *In* Handbook of Physiology. Circulation, sec. 2, vol. 2, chap. 43, American Physiological Society, Washington, D.C., pp. 1457–1516.

Skinner, S.L., J.W. McCubbin, and I.H. Page. 1964. Control of renin secretion. Circulation Res. 15: 64–76.

Slotkoff, L.M., A. Logan, P. Jose, J. D'Avella, and G.M. Eisner, 1971. Microsphere measurement of intrarenal circulation in the dog. Circulation Res. 28: 158–166.

Stein, J.H., T.F. Ferris, J.E. Huprich, T.C. Smith, and R.W. Osgood. 1971. Effect of renal vasodilatation on distribution of cortical blood flow in the kidney of the dog. J. Clin. Invest. 50: 1429–1438.

Vander, A.J., 1968. Direct effects of prostaglandins on renal function and renin release in anesthetized dog. Am. J. Physiol. 214: 218–221.

Alterations in Renal Function during Vasodilator Therapy

Gerald R. Zins
Cardiovascular Diseases Research
The Upjohn Company
Kalamazoo, Michigan

Minoxidil (2,6-diamino-4-piperidinopyrimidine-1-oxide) is a sustained action, peripheral vasodilator (DuCharme *et al.,* 1973) which is being investigated clinically as an antihypertensive drug. Its effectiveness in reducing elevated blood pressure, especially in severe drug-refractory cases, now has been documented on a number of occasions (Gilmore, Weil, and Chidsey, 1970; Gottlieb, Katz, and Chidsey, 1972; Limas and Fries, 1973). Side actions from this drug have not been numerous, although salt and water retention generally has occurred.

Salt and water retention has been a recognized property of most antihypertensive drugs for many years. For this reason occurrence of this phenomenon during the preclinical investigation of minoxidil was not entirely a surprise. However, while characterizing this effect in animals, renal hemodynamics were found not to be compromised and, therefore, it was impossible to explain the minoxidil-induced retention on the basis of this frequently invoked mechanism (Dollery, Emslie-Smith, and Milne 1960; Bayliss and Harvey-Smith, 1962; Lauler *et al.,* 1963; Smith, 1965). Subsequently, in man, renal hemodynamic changes were not found nor was enhanced elaboration of aldosterone demonstrable (Gilmore *et al.,* 1970; Gottlieb *et al.,* 1972). Hence it was necessary to seek an alternative explanation for this alteration in renal function.

MATERIALS AND METHODS

Renal Hemodynamics, Fluids, and Electrolytes

Adult female beagle dogs were force fed, daily by stomach tube, amounts of dog chow in slurry form which had been found in a preliminary balance study to be required for maintenance of body weight. Feeding preceded biological measurements by 18–24 hr. Polyethylene cannulas for i.v. infusion and for blood pressure recording were surgically implanted in the right heart and abdominal aorta, respectively, two weeks prior to pretreatment measurements. Up to 250 ml of blood was also collected in citrated containers at this time and was kept refrigerated until used to replace blood samples taken during the experiment. While measurements were being made, dogs were housed in cages fitted with water-tight swivel assemblies which enabled continuous i.v. infusion of indicator substances. Foley catheters were used to obtain urine samples and to rinse bladders.

Mean arterial blood pressure (MAP) was recorded directly from PE-20 cannulas during the equilibration interval for renal hemodynamic indicators. Glomerular filtration rate (GFR) and effective renal plasma flow (ERPF) were measured over a 40-min period using ^{14}COOH-labeled inulin (specific activity, ca. 1.5 μCi/mg) and p-aminohippurate (PAH) clearances, respectively. Plasma levels of ^{14}C and PAH were in the range of 500–1000 c.p.m./ml and 2–4 mg% for the respective indicators. The [^{14}COOH] inulin was analyzed by counting 0.5-ml volumes of urine and 5% trichloroacetic acid (TCA) filtrates of plasma, suspended in diatol (Herberg, 1960) by means of an equal volume of Cab-o-sil® (Packard Instrument Co.), using a liquid scintillation spectrometer. The PAH was analyzed by the method of Harvey and Brothers (1962).

Total body exchangeable sodium ($TBNa_e$), potassium (TBK_e) and water (TBH_2O) were measured by conventional isotope dilution techniques using ^{24}NaCl (10 μCi per dog), ^{42}KCl (50 μCi per dog), and tritiated water (6 μCi per dog), respectively. Radioactive sodium and potassium were given via the aortic cannula, immediately after stomach tube feeding, on the day prior to the intended measurement. Urine was collected subsequently and the radioactive residues of both isotopes were determined after a 24-hr equilibration. The specific activity of sodium (^{24}Na/^{23}Na) was then measured in a plasma sample and of potassium (^{42}K/^{40}K) in a urine sample by means of a two-channel gamma spectrometer and an internal standard flame photometer. Tritiated water was also administered into the aortic cannula but in this case, a 6-hr equilibration interval was employed. A blood sample was then taken and lyophilized, and the water was trapped and then counted in diatol to determine the specific activity applicable at the time of isotope administration.

Plasma volume (PV) and extracellular fluid volume (ECFV) were measured with Evans blue dye and [^{14}COOH] inulin, respectively. A carefully measured dose of dye was given i.v. and a jugular vein plasma sample was obtained 4 min later. Pre-injection background was routinely determined. Dye concentration was measured by the method of Jarnum (1959) and, on the basis of pilot studies which showed that 4-min samples consistently had dye concentrations which were 98% of zero time extrapolates, was corrected to estimate PV. A priming dose of 1.4–1.8 × 10^6 c.p.m. [^{14}COOH] inulin was given into the jugular vein cannula, and a similar quantity was given per hour as a continuously infused maintenance dose. Administered amounts were carefully measured and corrected for quantities appearing in the urine throughout the study. After a 2-hr equilibration plasma samples were obtained from the jugular vein, tritiated water was removed by lyophilization, protein in reconstituted samples was precipitated with 5% TCA, and 0.5 ml of filtrate was counted in 15 ml of diatol-Cab-o-sil® as described above. A sufficient interval between acquisition and counting was routinely allowed to permit total decay of the ^{24}Na and ^{42}K also present.

Renal Artery Infusion

Adult mongrel dogs of either sex were used. The animals were anesthetized with pentobarbital, a mid-line abdominal incision was made, and both ureters were cannulated. A 26 ga. needle, connected by means of polyethylene tubing to an infusion pump, was inserted into the left renal artery. Both renal veins were cannulated with PE-100 tubing. Approach to the renal vessels was via separate flank incisions. The dogs were primed initially with 0.9% NaCl (1 ml/min for 40 min), after which the rate of saline infusion was continually adjusted to be equivalent to the combined rate of urine flow from the two kidneys. The dogs were then primed and continuously infused with PAH and inulin, and equilibrated for an additional 40 min before beginning the pretreatment clearance periods. Minoxidil was dissolved in water by using appropriate amounts of HCl and was then incorporated into Krebs-Ringer-bicarbonate (K-R-B) buffer. This solution was infused into the left renal artery at a rate to produce a total body dose of 1 mg/kg within a 15-min period. The K-R-B, with HCl only, served as the infusion fluid in vehicle control runs.

The GFR and ERPF were monitored with inulin and PAH, respectively. Renal venous plasma was obtained simultaneously with carotid arterial plasma at the midpoint of clearance intervals in order to determine renal PAH extraction efficiency. Total renal plasma flow (TRPF) was then calculated by dividing ERPF by extraction efficiency. Flow not defined by PAH clearance was also calculated ($TRPF-C_{PAH}$). Renal blood flow resistance and filtration fraction were estimated by dividing MAP and GFR, respectively, by TRPF. The MAP was recorded from the carotid artery.

The data from each kidney were analyzed separately for statistically significant changes as a two-way classification (dogs and times). All data were transformed to logarithms for this analysis. The means for both the infusion and post-infusion periods were compared statistically with the mean of the three 10-min pretreatment periods. Differences were considered significant if $p \leqslant 0.05$. The data were also analyzed to estimate the rate of change during successive 5- or 10-min intervals for the responses in the infused and noninfused kidney. The model $R = Ae^{bt}$ was applied to the values for each kidney during the time of minoxidil infusion. This model is equivalent to the regression equation $\log_e R = \log_e A + bt$ which was calculated by methods given in Snedecor and Cochran (1967).

Tubular Site of Antinatriuretic Action

Adult female beagle dogs which weighed an average of 11.0 kg were used. Right heart (0.04-inch i.d. Dow-Corning silastic tubing inserted via the jugular vein) and abdominal aorta (PE-20 tubing inserted via the femoral artery) cannulas were surgically introduced at least one week before experimentation for the purpose of infusing fluids and recording blood pressures, respectively. After an overnight fast and 3 hr before the intravenous loading phase, dogs were given 50 ml/kg of water orally to insure constant hydration. With only a few exceptions this water load was totally excreted during the ensuing 3 hr. Dogs were then secured in supporting slings and indwelling catheters were introduced into the bladders. Pre-equilibration blood pressures were directly recorded at this time. Zero-time blood samples were then taken, and animals were primed with PAH (10 mg/kg) and inulin (80 mg/kg), and an infusion of 3% glucose in water at a rate of 2.5 ml/kg/min was begun with a variable-speed infusion pump. This infusion was continued for 20 min by which time a water load of 50 ml/kg had been administered. The urine collected during the second 10 min of this loading period was added to a reservoir containing 100 ml of 0.25% inulin and 0.04% PAH in 3% glucose from which infusion was continued during the ensuing 10 min at the prior rate of urine flow. This practice of maintaining the dogs' state of hydration and osmolal dilution by infusing previously excreted urine at the rate of its formation was continued for the remainder of the experiment.

A period of 40 min was allowed after the glucose load for equilibration and the disappearance of antidiuretic hormone (ADH). Reinfusion of urine was then supplemented with a modified air and carbon dioxide (95%–5%) gassed K-R-B buffer (in mEq/liter: Na^+, 114.7; K^+, 5.9; Ca^{2+}, 5.1; Mg^{2+}, 2.4; Cl^-, 99.6; $H_2PO_4^-$, 1.2; SO_4^{2-}, 2.4; HCO_3^-, 24.9; total cation, 128.1; total anion, 128.1) at a rate of 5.25 ml/min. Aliquots of the 10-min urine samples collected after equilibration were withdrawn for analysis and replaced before reinfusion with 0.5% inulin and 0.08% PAH in 3% glucose. Blood samples were drawn by individual jugular vein punctures at the midpoint of alternating or every third 10-min clearance period. Analytical results for these samples were interpolated to obtain plasma level data for all intervals.

Plasma and urinary osmolality were determined on the basis of freezing-point depression in 2-ml sample volumes using an Advanced Instruments osmometer. PAH and inulin were quantified with an autoanalyzer in dilutions of urine and Somogyi filtrates of plasma according to the methods of Harvey and Brothers (1962) and Roe *et al.* (1949), respectively. Plasma glucose concentrations were quantified with the automated technique of Hoffman (1937) and, along with the nonglucose background in plasma, were used to correct appropriately the measured plasma inulin levels (100 mg% glucose routinely appeared as 2.8–3.0 mg% inulin by the Roe procedure). Sodium and potassium in plasma and urine were quantified by lithium internal standard flame photometry using the autoanalyzer system. The $TBNa_e$ and PV were quantified as described earlier.

Renal clearances of sodium, potassium, inulin, PAH, and osmolality were calculated as UV/P where U represents the urinary concentration, V the rate of urine flow in ml/min and P the plasma concentration. Plasma sodium and potassium concentrations were multiplied by 0.95 to correct for the Donnan equilibrium. The rate of free-water clearance (CH_2O) was calculated as the rate of urine formation (V) minus the rate of osmolal clearance (C_{osm}). PAH clearance was used as an index of renal plasma flow (RPF) and inulin clearance as a measure of GFR. The rate of urine formation and of the various other clearances were expressed as ml/100 ml of GFR.

Renal Blood Flow Distribution

Adult beagle dogs of either sex were intubated with a PE-60 cannula in the abdominal aorta via a femoral artery and a PE-20 cannula in the left ventricle via the left carotid artery several days before blood flow was to be measured. Both cannulas exited through the skin between the shoulder blades; cannulas were filled with heparinized saline and plugged when not in use. Dogs were fasted overnight before experimentation. Minoxidil was administered orally in capsule 4 hr before measurements were made.

Fifteen-micrometer (±5) diameter microspheres (3M Co.), labeled with either ^{85}Sr or ^{141}Ce and suspended in 20% dextran containing Tween-80, were diluted 10-fold with 10% dextran (minimal amount of Tween-80 added) by vigorous agitation with a Teflon stirring bar followed by vortex mixing. Aggregates were totally dispersed by this procedure and the resulting suspension was stable for several minutes. A volume containing sufficient spheres to provide a dose of 10^5 spheres/kg was then drawn into a plastic syringe fitted with a blunt 26 ga. needle. The actual dose was quantified by weighing the syringe before and after injection. Injection was made manually into the ventricular cannula over a period of 1 min. The cannula was then quickly rinsed with 3 ml of saline. Calibration of tissue blood flow in respect to radioactivity content was accomplished by counting a known volume of a blood sample withdrawn from the abdominal aorta by pump at a constant rate during a carefully timed interval starting 15 sec before and continuing for 1 min after microsphere injection and cannula rinse. This sample was kept from clotting during acquisition by administering i.v. 200 units/kg of heparin no more than 5 min earlier.

Dogs were unanesthetized and suspended in slings during these procedures. No evidence of intolerance to microsphere injections was obtained. Blood pressure was monitored from the abdominal aorta cannula until it was used for sample withdrawal. Animals were eventually sacrificed by i.v. administration of saturated aqueous KCl. Both kidneys were excised and dissected sagittally to produce equal halves. One half from each kidney was further subdivided to enable introduction into vials, weighing, and finally counting to determine whole kidney blood flow. Thin (2–3 mm) sagittal sections of the remaining halves were also prepared and dissected manually into 4 equi-thick zones of cortex (1–4, outer to inner), and outer and inner medulla. Corresponding zones were pooled (at least 200 mg tissue in each) and introduced into separate vials to quantify zonal blood flow. Counting was done with a gamma spectrometer (Nuclear of Chicago). Blood flow rate was expressed as ml/g wet tissue wt/min and blood flow resistance was calculated from the following formula:

resistance = arterial blood pressure/blood flow rate.

RESULTS AND DISCUSSION

Effects of Minoxidil on Fluids, Electrolytes, and Renal Hemodynamics

The effects of minoxidil, administered once daily by mouth, on MAP and renal hemodynamics in normal unanesthetized beagle dogs are shown in

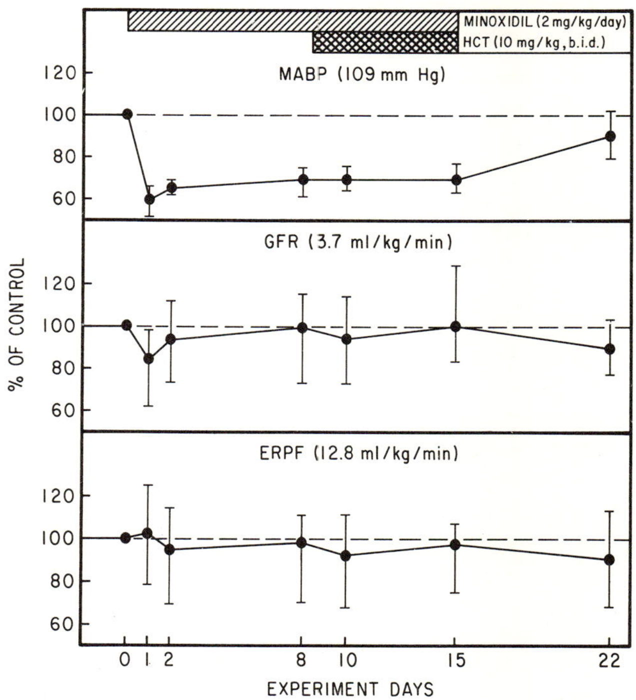

Fig. 1. The MABP, GFR, and ERPF in beagle dogs treated orally once daily with minoxidil. Numbers in parentheses represent the mean value for control measurements made before drug treatment began. Points on the graph represent the mean and range for six animals. Treatment measurements were made 4 hr after minoxidil administration.

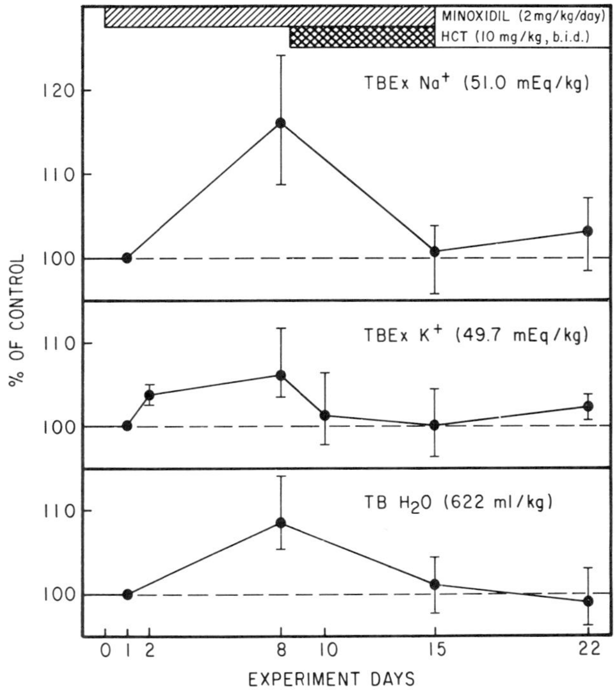

Fig. 2. Total body exchangeable sodium (TBEx Na^+) and potassium (TBEx K^+) and total body water (TBH_2O) in beagle dogs treated orally, once daily with minoxidil. Numbers in parentheses represent the mean value for control measurements made before drug treatment began. Points represent the mean and range for six animals. Treatment measurements were made 4 hr after minoxidil administration.

Fig. 1. The MAP was consistently reduced when minoxidil alone was given. Nevertheless, GFR and ERPF were preserved within normal limits in the face of this marked reduction in perfusion pressure. The addition of hydrochlorothiazide to the regimen after the first week of treatment was not evidenced by further changes in any of these parameters.

In spite of the persistence of normal renal hemodynamics, minoxidil treatment resulted in a dramatic retention of electrolytes and fluid in these animals (Fig. 2). Thus, on the eighth day of treatment, $TBNa_e$ was increased approximately 80 mEq, TBK_e approximately 25 mEq, and TBH_2O approximately 600 ml. Simultaneous measurement of PV and interstitial fluid volume (ISFV) disclosed a 30% increase in both compartments which precisely accounted for the 600 ml increase in TBH_2O. Body weight changes also reflected this increment in body water in that an average gain of 0.6 kg occurred. (Fig. 3). The retention process was not progressive, however, since balance in terms of body weight, and presumably body water and electrolyte, was restored at a now elevated extracellular fluid volume on the fourth day of treatment. Introduction of hydrochlorothiazide on the eighth day of treat-

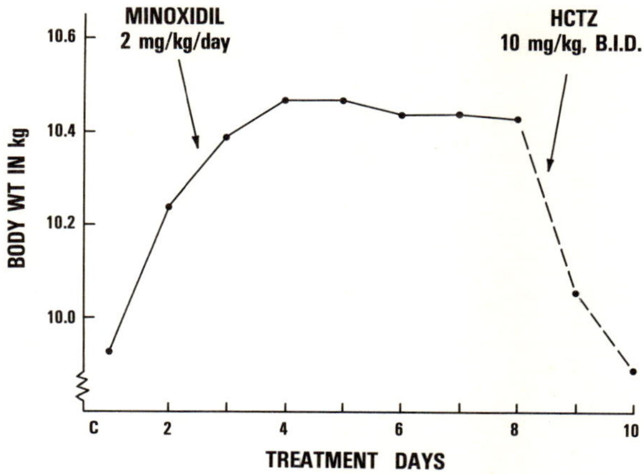

Fig. 3. The effect of orally administered minoxidil, alone and combined with hydrochlorothiazide (HCTZ), on body weight in beagle dogs (n=6).

ment resulted in a prompt increase in salt and water excretion and, on the basis of changes in body weight, pretreatment conditions were again approached within a single day. Continued treatment with this combination regimen saw complete restoration of normal body fluid and electrolyte levels after another week.

Direct Effect of Minoxidil on Renal Sodium Excretion

In view of the marked salt and water retention evoked by minoxidil in the absence of renal hemodynamic dysfunction, it seemed possible that renal electrolyte reabsorption might have been directly stimulated by the drug. In order to address this question, minoxidil was directly infused into the left renal artery of pentobarbital-anesthetized dogs and functions of the two kidneys were compared. These results appear in Table 1.

Tubular rejection of sodium (TRF–Na) by the infused kidney was actually enhanced during drug administration in contrast to reduced sodium excretion on the opposite side. Both kidneys retained sodium when the infusion was terminated. Control experiments in which vehicle was infused in place of the minoxidil solution showed negligible changes (less than 10%) in TRF-Na for either kidney in relation to control. Inspection of the hemodynamic findings in the infused kidney during the natriuretic response provides little insight as to the mechanism of this effect, since none of the measured parameters was appreciably altered. However, when the rates of change in these various endpoints during the 15-min infusion period were calculated, first-order kinetics could be applied to the increase in TRF-Na and to the decrease in filtration fraction and renal vascular resistance. This kinetic similarity is considered presumptive evidence of a mechanistic relationship, and, therefore, suggests that diminished colloidal osmotic pressure and/or

Table 1. Effect of renal artery infusion of minoxidil (1 mg/kg) on sodium excretion and renal hemodynamics in dogs

	Infused kidney			Noninfused kidney		
	30 min control	15 min infusion	30 min post-infusion	30 min control	15 min infusion	30 min post-infusion
TRF for Na^+ (% of GFR)	4.31	6.07[a]	3.25[a]	3.93	2.65[a]	1.24[a]
C_{PAH} (ml/min)	101	104	95	98	87[a]	76[a]
TRPF − C_{PAH} (ml/min)	40	47	39	40	35	32[a]
FF (GFR/TRPF)	0.29	0.27	0.27	0.30	0.30	0.29
RVR (MAP/TRPF)	0.89	0.82	0.82	0.93	1.05	1.03
GFR (ml/min)	42	42	38	41	37	35[a]
MAP (mmHg)	130	126	111[a]			

Abbreviations: TRF, tubular rejection fraction; C_{PAH}, PAH clearance; TRPF, total renal plasma flow; FF, filtration fraction; RVR, renal resistance; GFR, glomerular filtration rate; MAP, mean arterial pressure.

Values represent means for six dogs; infused kidney and noninfused kidney data obtained from the same animals.

[a]Different from control ($P < 0.05$).

increased hydrostatic pressure in peritubular capillaries contributed to the minoxidil induced natriuresis.

In terms of the sodium retention, the decrease in TRF-Na during both periods in the noninfused kidney and post-infusion in the infused kidney also conformed to first-order kinetics. However, no relationship could be established with any of the hemodynamic parameters. Thus it must be concluded that the salt-retaining action of minoxidil, while associated with peripheral vasodilatation and a decline in systemic blood pressure, cannot be explained in terms of measurable hemodynamic changes on a whole kidney basis and, furthermore, is not the result of a direct action of minoxidil on the kidney.

Tubular Site of the Antinatriuretic Effect of Minoxidil

The approach to assessing the renal tubular site of the enhanced electrolyte reabsorption following minoxidil treatment was to produce a state of maximal water diuresis in unanesthetized dogs and utilize urine volume as a measure of delivery of filtrate out of the proximal tubule and free-water clearance (C_{H_2O}) as an indicator of sodium reabsorption by the distal tubule (Seldin *et al.*, 1966). Four treatments were employed and dogs were studied twice at an interval of 1 week in a pretreatment - treatment sequence. Treatments were as follows: (1) control, no drug; (2) acute minoxidil, 1 mg/kg p.o. 4 hr before the treatment measurement; (3) chronic minoxidil, 1 mg/kg/day p.o. for 4 days, the last dose 4 hr before treatment measurement; (4) chronic minoxidil + HCTZ-minoxidil, 1 mg/kg/day p.o. for 4 days, the last dose 4 hr before treatment measurement, plus hydrochlorothiazide, 10 mg/kg p.o., twice on day 3, the last dose 20 hr before treatment measurement. These treatments were arrived at on the basis of the data in Fig. 3. They depict the following renal sodium reabsorption conditions: (1) normal; (2) avid minoxidil-induced sodium retention; (3) restoration of sodium balance during minoxidil treatment at elevated $TBNa_e$, i.e., 'minoxidil escape;' (4) analogous to 'minoxidil escape' in time but with a normal $TBNa_e$.

An indication of the extent and consistency of the water diuresis state in these animals appears in Table 2. Plasma osmolalities before 3% glucose loading were relatively constant within and among groups. The loading procedure, in turn, produced a uniform post-equilibration reduction in P_{osm} of 14–21 mOsm/kg (10-min values) and these levels were maintained throughout the 3-hr expansion phase (170 min). This constancy is important in ensuring the absence of ADH secretion and stems from the practice of continuously reinfusing the voided urine.

Several indicators of effects or the absence of effects of drug treatment in these four groups of dogs appear in Table 3. The various volume and electrolyte measurements were made before the 3% glucose loading period in both the pretreatment and treatment phase of the experiment but only changes from pretreatment are presented. As would be expected, plasma volume and $TBNa_e$ did not change in the control and acute minoxidil groups. On the other hand, dogs treated chronically with minoxidil showed increases

Table 2. Plasma osmolality during hypotonic volume expansion in minoxidil treated dogs

Treatment	Experiment phase	Preload (mOsm/kg)	Δ mOsm/kg during expansion	
			10 min	170 min
Control	Pretreatment	285 ± 4	−16 ± 3	−17 ± 2
	Treatment	290 ± 1	−15 ± 2	−18 ± 2
Acute minoxidil	Pretreatment	286 ± 4	−21 ± 3	−18 ± 2
	Treatment	280 ± 3	−21 ± 1	−21 ± 2
Chronic minoxidil	Pretreatment	284 ± 5	−18 ± 1	−18 ± 3
	Treatment	286 ± 5	−15 ± 2	−19 ± 2
Chronic + HCTZ	Pretreatment	285 ± 2	−18 ± 1	−18 ± 1
	Treatment	279 ± 4	−14 ± 1	−17 ± 3

Results given as mean ± s.d. for five dogs.

in PV and $TBNa_e$ comparable with similarly treated animals in Figs. 1–3. The effort to simulate chronic treatment conditions in all respects except for salt and water retention appeared successful, since the weight gain in the second chronic treatment group on day 3 was reversed by day 4 through administration of two doses of hydrochlorothiazide. The inulin and PAH clearances shown in this table are the mean values for the 3-hr hypotonic volume expansion period. They confirm the earlier finding that minoxidil fails to alter renal hemodynamic function under these treatment conditions.

Table 3. Pre-expansion plasma volume and body sodium, expansion renal hemodynamics, in minoxidil-treated dogs

Treatment	Δ from pretreatment				
	Plasma volume (ml)	$TBNa_e$ (mEq)	Body wt (kg)	C_{inulin} (ml/min)	C_{PAH} (ml/min)
Control	+6 ± 14	+15 ± 12		−1 ± 4	0 ± 23
Acute Minoxidyl	+24 ± 12	+6 ± 19		−1 ± 6	+23 ± 29
Chronic Minoxidyl	+142 ± 54[a]	+54 ± 16[a]		−1 ± 8	−21 ± 35
Chronic + HCTZ			(D3) +0.75±0.34[a] (D4) +0.15±0.35	−5 ± 10	+33 ± 61

Results given as mean ± s.d. for five days.
[a]Different from control ($P < 0.01$).
[b]Different from control ($P < 0.05$).

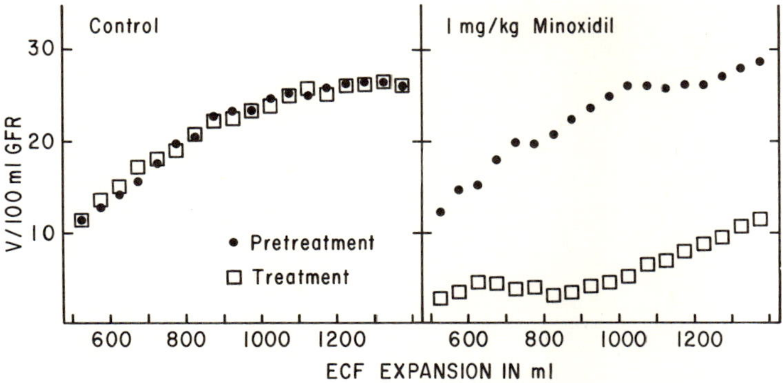

Fig. 4. Changes in fractional urine volume excretion (V/100 ml GFR) as a function of hypotonic ECF expansion in control and single-dose minoxidil-treated dogs. Pretreatment measurements preceded treatment measurements by 1 week. Treatment measurements were made during the 4–8 hr interval after oral dosing. Points represent mean values for five dogs.

The mean fractional urine volumes for the control and acute minoxidil groups, reflecting as they do the rate of delivery of isosmotic filtrate out of the proximal tubule, are plotted as a function of extracellular fluid (ECF) volume expansion in Fig. 4. Values were markedly reproducible during successive tests in untreated animals at an interval of one week and the well-known inhibition by ECF expansion of proximal tubular fluid reabsorption was clearly reflected by a progressive rise in urine volume. In contrast to controls, fractional V was markedly reduced (>80%) in animals given a single dose of minoxidil (all differences significant at $p<0.05$), although partial

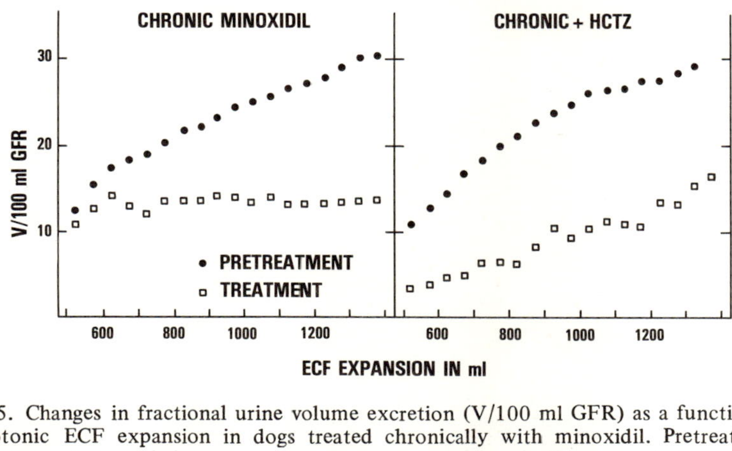

Fig. 5. Changes in fractional urine volume excretion (V/100 ml GFR) as a function of hypotonic ECF expansion in dogs treated chronically with minoxidil. Pretreatment measurements preceded treatment measurements by 1 week. Treatment measurements were made 4–8 hr after the fourth daily oral dose of minoxidil. Hydrochlorothiazide (HCTZ) was given twice daily by the oral route on the third day of minoxidil administration. Points represent mean values for five dogs.

reversal of this effect occurred when ECF expansion with K-R-B approached 500 ml. This responsiveness to volume loading takes on special significance in the light of the chronic treatment results in Fig. 5. Here fractional urine volume was indistinguishable from pretreatment during the early stages of supplemental ECF expansion in animals which were already expanded by minoxidil-induced retention of 54 mEq of sodium (Table 3). That this 'escape' by the proximal tubule from the influence of minoxidil on filtrate reabsorption was due to prior ECF expansion and not some other time-dependent adaptation is evident from the finding that avid reabsorption, similar to that seen in acutely treated animals, was restored during chronic treatment by reversing the sodium retention with a diuretic (Fig. 5). Although proximal tubular 'escape', mediated by ECF expansion, appears to have occurred during chronic minoxidil treatment, the function of this tubular segment remained abnormal since the usual increase in urine volume in response to further ECF expansion failed to occur. From the results it can be anticipated that the chronically treated dog, while essentially able to restore salt and water balance, would manifest delayed excretion of a large salt load.

The fractional free-water clearance and osmolal clearance values found in these experiments are presented in Figs. 6 and 7. Here they are plotted as a function of fractional urine volume which, in addition to representing the rate of delivery out of the proximal tubule, constitutes the distal tubular load. Again there is excellent agreement between measurements made at an interval of one week in control dogs. Furthermore, minoxidil, in either the acute or the two chronic treatment situations, failed to alter the well-defined relationship between solute reabsorption (C_{H_2O}) or solute excretion (C_{osm}) and the distal tubular load. These results do not permit evaluation of the possibility that minoxidil enhances electrolyte reabsorption in the distal tubule because sodium chloride, in our studies, is totally reabsorbed unless

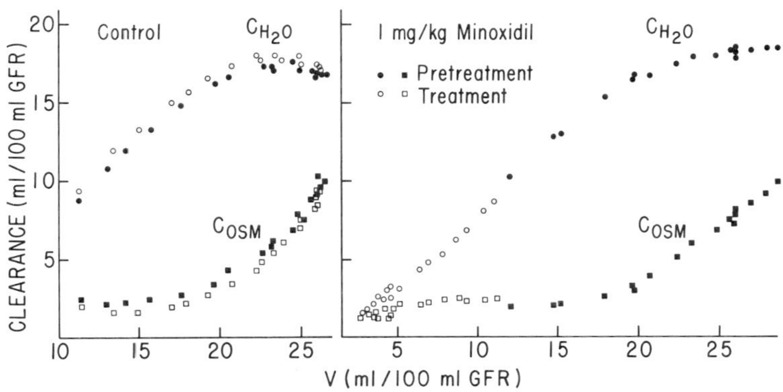

Fig. 6. Fractional (per 100 ml GFR), free-water (C_{H_2O}), and osmolal (C_{osm}) clearances as a function of distal tubular electrolyte load (V/100 ml GFR) in control and acute oral minoxidil-treated dogs. Pretreatment and treatment measurements were made one week apart. Points represent mean values for five dogs.

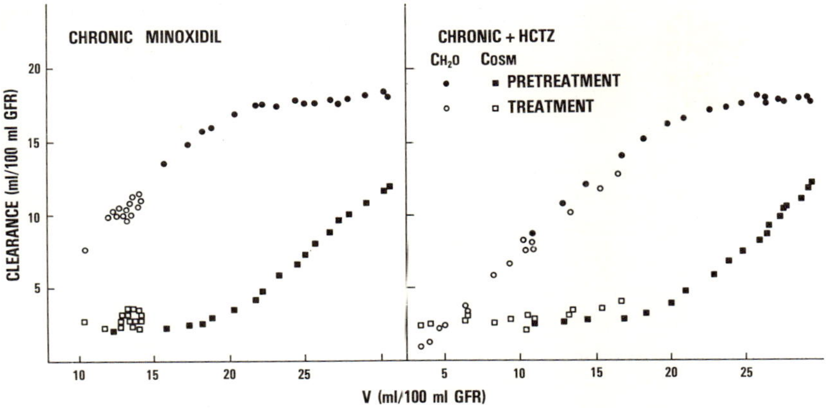

Fig. 7. Fractional (per 100 ml GFR), free-water (C_{H_2O}), and osmolal (C_{osm}) clearances as a function of distal tubular electrolyte load (V/100 ml GFR) in dogs treated chronically with minoxidil. Pretreatment and treatment measurements were made one week apart. Treatment measurements followed four daily oral doses of minoxidil. Hydrochlorothiazide (HCTZ) was given twice daily by the oral route on the third day of minoxidil administration. Points represent mean values for five dogs.

the quantity entering this segment exceeds the distal T_m. However, these results do help to eliminate the possibility that urine volume during water diuresis was reduced because of minoxidil-provoked ADH release, since, even after ECF expansion by 1400 ml, osmolal clearance was at the low level of 2–3% of GFR expected from delivery of small rather than large volumes of urine into the diluting segment.

In order to demonstrate further that the reduction in fractional urine volume produced by minoxidil in these studies was due to enhanced proximal tubular reabsorption and not ADH release, a study of the effect of ADH in the water diuresis model was conducted. Four dogs were loaded with 3% aqueous glucose, equilibrated, and then volume expanded in the usual manner for 3 hr. The ADH was then given i.v. at 10 mU/kg and maintained at 0.25 mU/kg/min for 20 min, after which an additional 23 mU/kg was given and the maintenance rate was increased 3.3-fold. From the results in Fig. 8 it is clear that ADH effected a reduction in C_{H_2O} in direct proportion to the reduction in urine volume, whereas osmolal and sodium clearances remained high and precisely consistent with the extent of ECF expansion. These findings contrast sharply with the low osmolal clearances in Figs. 6 and 7 and, therefore, support a proximal tubular site of enhanced electrolyte reabsorption with minoxidil.

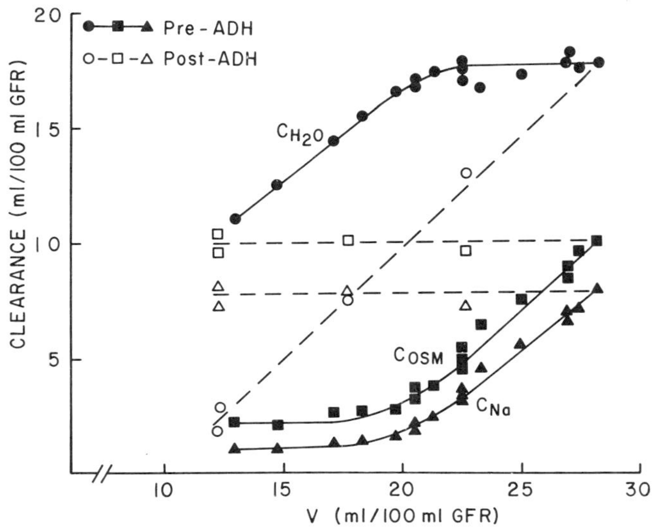

Fig. 8. The effect of vasopressin (ADH) infusion on fractional free-water (C_{H_2O}), osmolal (C_{osm}), and sodium (C_{Na}) clearances in maximal water diuresis dogs after a 1400 ml hypotonic volume expansion. Points represent mean values for four dogs.

Effect of Minoxidil on Blood Flow Distribution and Vascular Resistance in the Kidney

The lack of a direct action of minoxidil on renal tubular electrolyte transport coupled with the absence of change in hemodynamic parameters on a whole kidney basis left the possibility of redistribution of blood flow within the kidney as a means to explain the avid salt and water retention. Barger (1966) actually proposed this as a means to explain the absence of sodium excretion in congestive heart failure. This question was addressed by measuring total blood flow and its intra-organ distribution in the kidneys of control and acute minoxidil-treated, unanesthetized dogs and the findings appear in Table 4.

Consistent with earlier findings, whole kidney blood flow was not altered by minoxidil treatment in these animals. Of considerable interest, however, is the fact that treated animals manifested an appreciable redistribution of blood flow, i.e., zone 1 flow (outer cortex) was reduced 25% and zone 4 flow (juxtamedullary cortex) was approximately doubled. Redistributions of a remotely similar nature also have been described in conjunction with opposite changes in sodium excretion, i.e., natriuresis (Stein *et al.*, 1973), which raises a question about the relevance of such changes to the salt-retention phenomenon. However, it is important to recognize that only a relative reduction in outer cortical blood flow has been seen in conjunction with natriuresis, absolute flow to the outer cortex actually having increased in each of these cases. This is in distinct contrast to the data in Table 4 which show a true

Table 4. The effect of acute minoxidil (1 mg/kg p.o.) on renal blood flow distribution and renal vascular resistance in unanesthetized dogs

	No treatment (N=10)			Acute minoxidil (N=8)		
Anatomical locus	ml/min/g	Percentage total renal flow[a]	Resistance[b]	ml/min/g	Percentage total Renal flow[a]	Resistance[b]
Whole kidney	3.94 ± 0.20	100	29 ± 2	3.94 ± 0.34	100	22 ± 2[d]
Cortex[c]						
Zone 1	8.67 ± 0.71	53 ± 4	13 ± 1	6.40 ± 0.75[e]	39 ± 1[d]	14 ± 1
Zone 2	6.45 ± 0.69	31 ± 2	19 ± 3	6.96 ± 0.96	34 ± 1	13 ± 1
Zone 3	3.46 ± 0.46	12 ± 1	39 ± 7	4.77 ± 0.63	18 ± 2[d]	19 ± 2[d]
Zone 4	1.53 ± 0.24	4 ± 0	100 ± 26	2.93 ± 0.55[e]	8 ± 1[d]	36 ± 7[d]
Medulla						
Outer	0.22 ± 0.06	0 ± 0	1009 ± 26	0.41 ± 0.11	1 ± 0[e]	562 ± 307
Inner	0.10 ± 0.02	0 ± 0		0.09 ± 0.03	0 ± 0	

[a]Flow rates in ml/min/g are adjusted with the fraction of total kidney mass that a given zone represents (McNay and Abe, 1970) and values are expressed as percentage of total renal flow.
[b]Resistance is calculated in arbitrary units (mmHg min g/ml) with the equation resistance=MAP/flow.
[c]Ascending zone numbers for cortex correspond to outer to inner cortex.
[d]Significantly different from no treatment ($P < 0.01$).
[e]Significantly different from no treatment ($P < 0.05$).

redistribution of blood flow in the minoxidil-treated dogs with flow through the outer cortex being reduced and through the inner cortex increased.

The mechanism for this redistribution of renal blood flow is not entirely defined by the present data. The resistance to blood flow in the outer cortex was actually unchanged, flow being reduced entirely on the basis of a lowered blood pressure, and it is only on the assumption that resistance vessels in this part of the cortex should have been dilated by minoxidil as they appeared to be in the inner two regions (50% and 64% reduction in resistance) that it can be speculated that some active vasoconstrictor stimulus was imposed here. If, indeed, minoxidil is uniformly capable of dilating renal resistance vessels, thereby necessitating an antagonizing vasoconstriction in the outer cortex, such constriction was probably due to enhanced sympathetic nerve activity and/or intrarenal generation of angiotensin II. In this respect, minoxidil treatment may simulate thoracic inferior or superior vena cava constriction which likewise induces sodium retention by activating the sympathetic nervous system (Schrier, Humphreys, and Ufferman, 1971). The possibility that angiotensin II is the final link in this sequence of events is raised principally by the fact that it selectively constricts efferent arterioles in contrast to the afferent action of norepinephrine (Regoli and Gauthier, 1971; Finberg and Peart, 1972). An effect on the efferent arteriole would greatly enhance colloidal osmotic pressure as well as reduce hydrostatic pressure in peritubular capillaries associated with proximal tubules and, at the same time, these proximal tubules would be receiving sufficient filtrate such that enhanced reabsorption secondary to these physical factor changes would be of consequence. For that matter the possibility also exists that norepinephrine (Gill and Casper, 1972) or angiotensin II (Munday, Parsons, and Poat, 1972) stimulate proximal tubular reabsorption directly rather than through alteration of Starling forces.

It cannot be concluded with certainty that the reduced resistance in the inner cortical segments was entirely attributable to minoxidil vasodilatation since an autoregulatory mechanism, possibly involving renal prostaglandin synthesis, also may have been triggered by either the reduced blood pressure and/or a prior compensatory vasoconstriction. In any case, it seems reasonable to speculate that the reduced outer cortical blood flow was an important element in the mechanism for salt retention and apparently could not be antagonized in terms of effects on sodium excretion by opposite changes in flow in more inner cortical regions.

Tubular Site of the Antinatriuretic Action of Other Hypotensive Agents

Four additional hypotensive drugs were studied in dogs employing the water diuresis system. Three of these, hydralazine, diazoxide, and guancydine, produce peripheral vasodilatation as does minoxidil, while the fourth, guanethidine, blocks norepinephrine release at sympathetic nerve terminals. The treatment regimens and the effects of these drugs on renal hemodynamics

Table 5. Renal hemodynamics following hypotensive drug administration

Drug and dose	n	C_{inulin} (ml/min)	C_{PAH} (ml/min)
Control	4	70	232
Hydralazine HCl 2 mg/kg i.v. + 0.5 mg/kg/hr	3	76	298
Diazoxide 10 mg/kg i.v. + 2.5 mg/kg/hr	4	64	119[a]
Guancydine 50 mg/kg p.o. (1.5 hr)	3	71	206
Guanethidine SO_4 10 mg/kg i.v. (24 hr)	4	65	291

[a]Different from control ($P < 0.05$).

during the 3-hr expansion period are reported in Table 5. Because of a short duration of action, hydralazine and diazoxide were administered continuously by infusion after an initial priming dose. Guancydine, with which it is difficult to lower blood pressure in the dog (Cummings *et al.,* 1968), was given in a large dose shortly before the 3% glucose loading interval. In order to avoid the early pressor action of guanethidine secondary to catecholamine release, guanethidine was administered 24 hr before the study. None of these agents significantly altered GFR during the ECF expansion period and only diazoxide, which probably competes for PAH secretion, affected ERPF.

The effects of these compounds on blood pressure are shown in Fig. 9. The effect of minoxidil, obtained under identical conditions, is shown for comparison. Blood pressure reduction with diazoxide and guanethidine was comparable through the first half of the expansion period and the activity of hydralazine, guancydine, and minoxidil was similar throughout. Not surprisingly, blood pressure rose as a result of ECF expansion in control dogs.

The effects of these various hypotensive agents on fractional urine volume in relation to hypotonic ECF expansion are described in Fig. 10. Each of the vasodilators produced a 90% or greater initial reduction in apparent delivery from the proximal tubule and differences from control animals were statistically significant ($p<0.05$) throughout the expansion period. However, as with minoxidil, the effect on urine volume was also partially reversed by continued ECF expansion in every instance. Guanethidine, while appearing modestly to reduce urine volume, did not, in fact, exert a statistically significant effect. Thus, while the degree of hypotension induced by guanethidine and diazoxide was comparable through most of the observation period, their effects on proximal tubular reabsorption were markedly different.

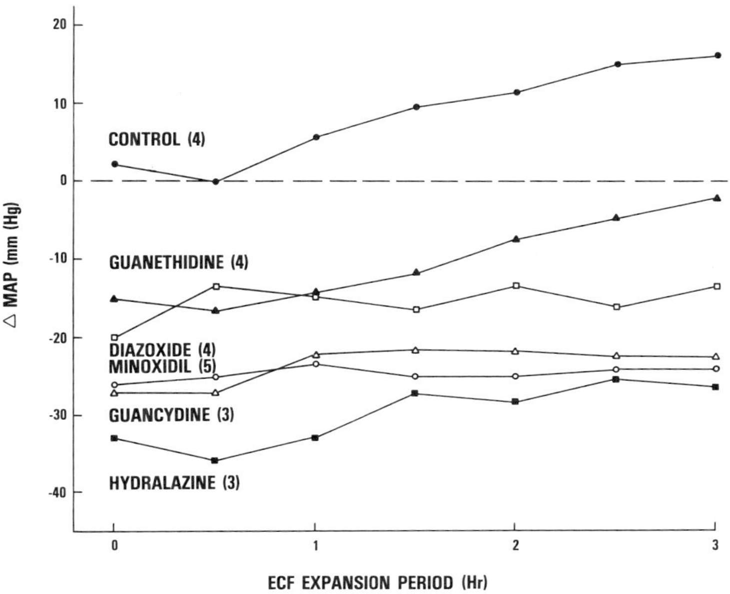

Fig. 9. Changes from pretreatment in MAP during hypotonic ECF expansion in antihypertensive drug-treated dogs. The number of animals per group is given in parentheses.

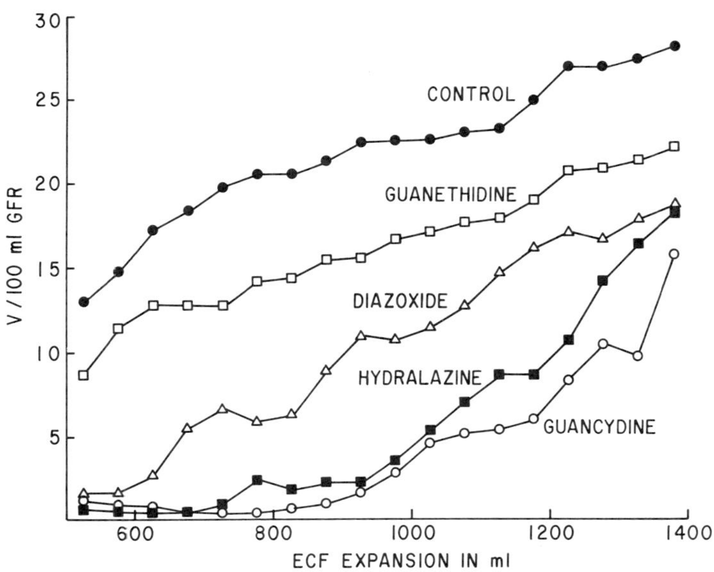

Fig. 10. Changes in fractional urine volume excretion (V/100 ml GFR) as a function of ECF expansion in dogs treated with various antihypertensive agents.

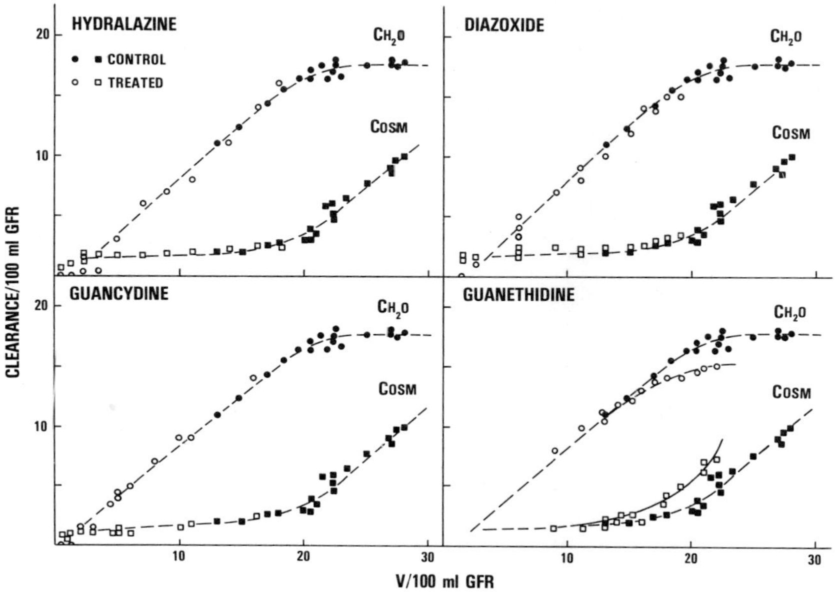

Fig. 11. Free-water (C_{H_2O}) and osmolal (C_{osm}) clearances as a function of distal tubular electrolyte load (V/100 ml GFR) in dogs treated with various antihypertensive agents.

The relationships between the free-water and osmolal clearances and fractional urine volume with these four drugs are plotted in Fig. 11. The results with the three vasodilators resemble closely those obtained with minoxidil, and suggest essentially normal diluting segment solute reabsorptive function relative to load and a definite enhancement of solute reabsorption by the proximal tubule. In the case of guanethidine C_{H_2O} was reduced from normal to about the same extent that fractional urine volume was decreased which, in conjunction with somewhat elevated osmolal clearance rates, suggests the elaboration of some ADH. Thus it is concluded that guanethidine was totally devoid of the propensity to promote proximal tubular electrolyte reabsorption, in contrast to the marked capability in this regard of drugs which lower blood pressure by a direct vasodilator mechanism. Other investigators likewise have concluded that diazoxide (Silver, Argy, and Schreiner, 1971) and guancydine (Gussin *et al.*, 1970) affect the retention of salt and water at least in part by promoting proximal tubular reabsorption.

CONCLUSIONS

Minoxidil, along with a number of other peripheral vasodilator drugs, produced marked salt and water retention in dogs in the total absence of reduced whole kidney renal hemodynamic function. The site of increased tubular fluid reabsorption was localized in the proximal tubule and the extent of the effect, amounting to at least an 80% reduction in delivery from this segment, was entirely adequate to account for the reduction in electrolyte excretion. Extracellular volume expansion was capable of reversing the augmented proximal tubular reabsorption and, since such expansion accompanies the administration of these drugs, salt and water retention with them becomes a self-limited process.

The mechanism for the increase in proximal tubular reabsorption was only partially defined. The inability of the nonvasodilator hypotensive drug, guanethidine, to evoke this response dissociated the effect from simply a reduction in blood pressure. Minoxidil reduced blood flow to the outer portion of the renal cortex and, at the same time, normal blood flow through the kidney as a whole was maintained by increased flow through the juxtamedullary cortex. No evidence was obtained for heightened resistance to blood flow in the outer renal cortex. However, if minoxidil relaxed resistance vessels here as it did in the inner cortex, the absence of reduced resistance implies an antagonistic active vasoconstriction. Such a change conceivably could have altered Starling forces in peritubular capillaries associated with proximal tubules such that salt and water reabsorption in this segment was facilitated.

ACKNOWLEDGMENTS

The author is deeply indebted to Mr. Stephen J. Humphrey for his collaboration in carrying out these studies and to Dr. John R. Schultz for performing statistical evaluations.

REFERENCES

Barger, A. C. 1966. Renal hemodynamic factors in congestive heart failure. Ann. N. Y. Acad. Sci. 139: 276–284.

Bayliss, R. I. S., and E. A. Harvey-Smith. 1962. Methyldopa in the treatment of hypertension. Lancet 1: 763–768.

Cummings, J. R., A. N. Welter, J. L. Grace, and L. M. Lipchuck. 1968. Cardiovascular actions of guancydine in normotensive and hypertensive animals. J. Pharmac. Exp. Ther. 161: 88–97.

Dollery, C. T., D. Emslie-Smith, and M. D. Milne. 1960. Guanethidine in the treatment of hypertension. Lancet 2: 381–387.

DuCharme, D. W., W. A. Freyburger, B. E. Graham, and R. G. Carlson. 1973. Pharmacologic properties of minoxidil: a new hypotensive agent. J. Pharmac. Exp. Ther. 184: 662–670.

Finberg, J. P. M., and W. S. Peart. 1972. The effect of angiotensin, noradrenaline and vasopressin on blood flow distribution in the rat kidney. J. Physiol. 220: 229–242.

Gill, J. R., Jr., and A. G. T. Casper. 1972. Effect of renal alpha-adrenergic stimulation on proximal tubular sodium reabsorption. Am. J. Physiol. 223: 1201–1205.

Gilmore, E., J. Weil, and C. Chidsey. 1970. Treatment of essential hypertension with a new vasodilator in combination with beta-adrenergic blockade. N. Engl. J. Med. 282: 521–527.

Gottlieb, T. B., F. H. Katz, and C. A. Chidsey, III. 1972. Combined therapy with vasodilator drugs and beta-adrenergic blockade in hypertension. Circulation 45: 571–582.

Gussin, R. Z., E. H. Stokey, M. A. Ronsberg, L. C. Malone, and J. R. Cummings. 1970. Mechanisms of antihypertensive-induced fluid retention. Clin. Res. 18: 500 (abstr.).

Harvey, R. B., and A. J. Brothers. 1962. Renal extraction of paraaminohippurate and creatinine measured by continuous *in vivo* sampling of arterial and renal vein blood. Ann. N. Y. Acad. Sci. 102: 46–54.

Herberg, R. J. 1960. Determination of carbon-14 and tritium in blood and other whole tissues. Analyt. Chem. 32: 42–46.

Hoffman, W. S. 1937. Glucose determination in biological samples. J. Biol. Chem. 120: 51–63.

Jarnum, S. 1959. A modified extraction method for determination of evans blue. Scand. J. Clin. Lab. Invest. 11: 332–339.

Lauler, D. P., A. I. Vagnucci, R. B. Hickler, and G. W. Thorn. 1963. Clinical features of sodium retention induced by antihypertensive therapy. Circulation 28: 754–755.

Limas, C. J., and E. D. Fries. 1973. Minoxidil in severe hypertension with renal failure. Am. J. Cardiol. 31: 355–361.

McNay, J. L., and Y. Abe. 1970. Pressure dependent heterogeneity of renal cortical blood flow in dogs. Circulation Res. 27: 571–587.

Munday, K. A., B. J. Parsons, and J. A. Poat. 1972. Studies on the mechanism of action of angiotensin on ion transport by kidney cortex slices. J. Physiol. 224: 195–206.

Regoli, D., and R. Gauthier. 1971. Site of action of angiotensin and other vasoconstrictors on the kidney. Can. J. Physiol. Pharmac. 49: 608–612.

Roe, J. H., J. H. Epstein, and N. P. Goldstein. 1949. A photometric method for the determination of inulin in plasma and urine. J. Biol. Chem. 178: 839–845.

Schrier, R. W., M. H. Humphreys, and R. C. Ufferman. 1971. Role of cardiac output and the autonomic nervous system in the antinatriuretic response to acute constriction of the thoracic superior vena cava. Circulation Res. 29: 490–498.

Seldin, D. W., G. Eknoyan, W. N. Suki, and F. C. Rector, Jr. 1966. Localization of diuretic action from the pattern of water and electrolyte excretion. Ann. N. Y. Acad. Sci. 139(2): 328–343.

Silver, L. J., W. P. Argy, and G. E. Schreiner. 1971. Acute renal effects of diazoxide. Fed. Proc. 30(2): 338 (abstr.).

Smith, A. J. 1965. Fluid retention produced by guanethidine. Circulation 31: 490–496.

Snedecor, G. W., and W. G. Cochran. 1967. Statistical Methods, 6th edn, Iowa State University Press, Ames, Iowa, pp. 135–171.

Stein, J. H., S. Boonjarern, C. B. Wilson, and T. F. Ferris. 1973. Alterations in intrarenal blood flow distribution. Circulation Res. 32–33 (suppl. 1): 161–172.

Inherited Causes of Nephrogenic Diabetes Insipidus in Mice

Heinz Valtin
Department of Physiology
Dartmouth Medical School
Hanover, New Hampshire

Experiments have been carried out on four abnormal genotypes of mice in order to identify the mechanism(s) for the vasopressin (ADH)-resistant urinary concentrating defect in each. In VII Os/+ mice the concentrating defect appears to be due to a reduction in renal size and in the number of nephrons, chronic renal failure, and consequent osmotic diuresis per nephron. When the gene for oligosyndactyly, Os, is introduced into the DI strain of mice, i.e., DI OS/+ animals, a severe concentrating defect results, which is due not only to renal failure and an osmotic diuresis per nephron but also to deficient water permeability of the distal tubules and collecting ducts, and to a shortening of the short loops of Henle. The last abnormality presumably reduces the interstitial osmolality of the outer medulla. In DI +/+ nonsevere mice, a mild deficiency in the water permeability of distal tubules and collecting ducts may be responsible; this suggestion is based in part on the conclusion that deficient water permeability is the main or sole cause of severe diabetes insipidus in DI +/+ severe animals. In both DI +/+ nonsevere and DI +/+ severe mice activation of the enzyme adenylate cyclase in response to saturating doses of ADH is reduced by about 23% and 40% respectively; this suggests, but does not prove, that deficient production of cyclic AMP may be involved in these two genotypes.

The results of this study show that a multiplicity of mechanisms, acting singly or together, may be responsible for ADH-resistant defects in urinary concentration; specifically, such defects do not *necessarily* entail deficient water permeability of tubular membranes.

During the past several years we have conducted studies on mice with hereditary urinary concentrating defects which are resistant to vasopressin (antidiuretic hormone or ADH) (Naik and Valtin, 1969; Naik and Sokol, 1970; Stewart, 1971; Kettyle and Valtin, 1972). These mice were first described by Falconer, Latyszewski, and Isaacson (1964). In the course of our work we have identified a number of different abnormalities which, singly or in combination, lead to nephrogenic diabetes insipidus. This paper will focus attention on this multiplicity of causes; specifically, I wish to emphasize that an ADH-resistant urinary concentrating defect does not *necessarily* entail a defect in the water permeability of tubular membranes.

The genotypes we have investigated are listed in Fig. 1 (Naik and Valtin, 1969; Kettyle and Valtin, 1972). The VII +/+ mice are considered normal, and serve as the controls in our studies. When eating and drinking *ad lib.* (open column), their urine is concentrated to a mean value of about 2800 mOsm/kg H_2O. This value is not significantly elevated when the mice are treated with supramaximal doses of ADH (shaded column), presumably because water permeability of distal tubules and collecting ducts is already maximal even at normal plasma concentrations of ADH. Introduction of the autosomal semidominant gene Os into the VII strain of mice causes not only oligosyndactyly but also a mild defect in urinary concentration. The mean urine osmolality of VII Os/+ mice is nearly 1000 mOsm/kg lower than that of controls, and again the defect cannot be corrected through exogenous ADH. A similarly mild defect in urinary concentration, also resistant to ADH, is seen in a different strain of mice, called DI. Urine osmolality in these mice may range from as high as 2000 to as low as 100 mOsm/kg; the variation occurs in part as a function of age (Fig. 2) and is in part genetically determined. In the present study DI +/+ animals were selected on the basis of whether they excreted urine of a fairly high osmolality or a very low

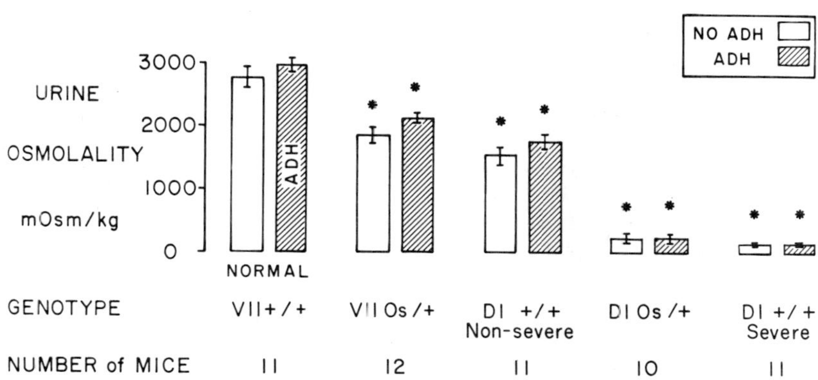

Fig. 1. Mean urine osmolalities, before and after treatment with vasopressin (ADH), in control mice and four abnormal genotypes, while eating and drinking *ad lib.* The striped columns represent the mean values after daily subcutaneous injections of ¼ unit Pitressin tannate in oil for three days. Asterisks denote values that are significantly different ($P<0.05$) from corresponding values in the normal VII +/+ genotype.

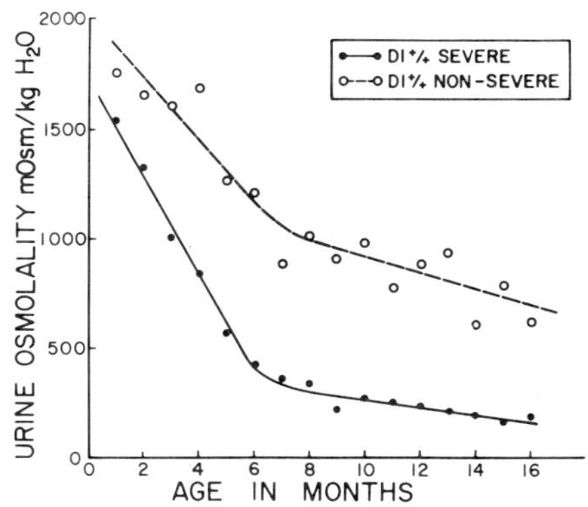

Fig. 2. Decline in urine osmolality with age, in the DI +/+ nonsevere and DI +/+ severe genotypes. The same mice were tested at different ages, although a single mouse was not necessarily examined over the entire age span, from 2–16 months. Each circle or dot represents the mean urine osmolality, while eating and drinking *ad lib,* of as many as 17 or as few as two mice (average 10) at any given age. (Data from Kettyle and Garrity, unpublished.)

osmolality; DI +/+ nonsevere mice had a mean urine osmolality, while eating and drinking *ad lib,* of about 1500 mOsm/kg, while DI +/+ severe mice excreted hypotonic urine with a mean concentration of about 150 mOsm/kg. Finally, when the Os gene is introduced into young DI +/+ animals, even of the nonsevere type, there results a much more severe concentrating defect than when the Os gene occurs in the VII strain (Stewart, 1971; Naik and Valtin, 1969). Again, the defect could not be corrected by giving ADH.

When dealing with ADH-resistant defects in urinary concentration, we try to distinguish between two general causes: (a) a deficiency in ADH-induced water permeability of the distal tubule and collecting duct; (b) a primary deficiency in building up the interstitial osmotic gradient from the cortico-medullary junction to the papillary tip. One can discriminate between these two causes by simultaneously analyzing the osmolality of the urine and that at the tip of the papilla. If the defect lies in water permeability, then the urine osmolality should be significantly lower than that at the papillary tip because osmotic equilibration between collecting-duct fluid and the surrounding interstitium could not occur. Conversely, if the primary defect is the build-up of the cortico-papillary osmotic gradient but water permeability is unimpaired, then the interstitial osmolality at the papillary tip and the urine osmolality will both be lower than normal but there will be no significant difference between the two. This experimental approach has been applied to each of the genotypes shown in Fig. 1 (Kettyle and Valtin, 1972).

Some of the results are shown in Fig. 3, in which the length of the renal countercurrent system, i.e., the distance from the cortico-medullary junction to the papillary tip, is plotted on the abscissa against osmolalities of the urine

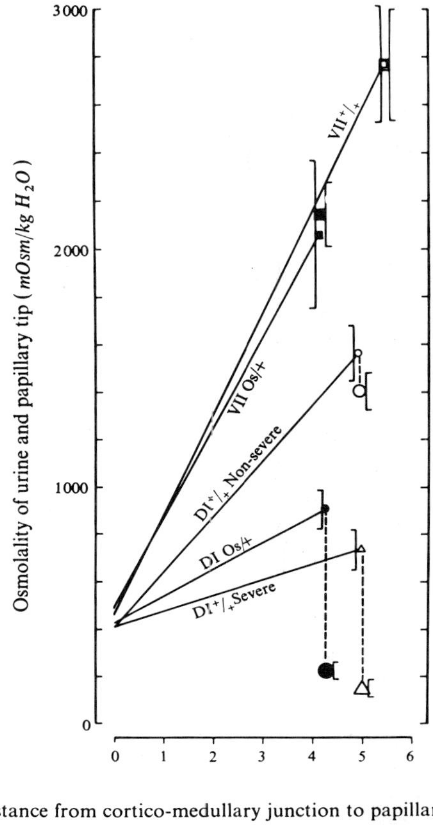

Fig. 3. Osmolalities of the urine (large symbols) and of the papillary tip (small symbols) in the genotypes of mice listed in Fig. 1. Osmolalities of cortical homogenates have been plotted at zero distance. Thus the graph indicates the approximate cortico-papillary osmotic gradient in each genotype; in this study the gradient was *assumed* to be linear. Each bracketed symbol represents the mean ±s.e.m. The difference between the mean papillary and urinary osmolality was not statistically significant for VII +/+, VII Os/+, and DI +/+ nonsevere mice, and had $P<0.001$ for DI +/+ severe and DI Os/+ animals. (From Kettyle and Valtin, 1972; published with permission of *Kidney International*.)

and papillary interstitium on the ordinate. In VII +/+ (normal) mice, the virtual identity of the urinary (large symbols) and papillary (small symbols) osmolalities presumably reflects high water permeability of the distal tubules and collecting ducts. The mean length of the countercurrent system in these mice is 5.41 mm, and the slope of the line between the cortico-medullary junction and the papillary tip gives the cortico-papillary osmotic gradient, which in this study was *assumed* to be linear (Kettyle and Valtin, 1972). The gradient had a value of 426 mOsm per kg tissue water per mm distance along the countercurrent system.

In VII Os/+ mice, the urine osmolality is also not significantly different from the osmolality at the papillary tip. Hence, in these mice, as in controls, there appears to be sufficient water permeability of distal tubules and collecting ducts to allow osmotic equilibration between tubular fluid and the surrounding interstitium. It should be noted, however, that the countercurrent system is foreshortened in these mice, being only 4.1 mm as opposed to 5.4 mm in the normal mice. This foreshortening is part of a general reduction in renal size, which is a pleiotropic effect of the Os gene. These mice have a reduced number of nephrons, and they are, in fact, in renal failure, manifesting significant nitrogen retention (Naik and Valtin, 1969; Stewart and Stewart, 1969). Like other individuals in chronic renal failure, these mice remain in solute and water balance on a normal diet. They therefore manifest an osmotic diuresis per nephron, which is the probable cause for the concentrating defect (Stewart, 1971). It is not yet known precisely how an osmotic diuresis leads to a reduction of the medullary interstitial osmolality, but it is likely that, in analogy with water diuresis, the phenomenon involves washout of solute particles by extra water which is reabsorbed from late portions of collecting ducts (Jamison, Buerkert, and Lacy, 1971) as well as decreased reabsorption of urea from these segments (Kettyle and Valtin, 1972; Stewart and Valtin, 1972).

Introduction of the Os gene into the DI strain of mice results in reduction of renal size, of number of nephrons, and of renal function roughly comparable with the changes seen in VII Os/+ animals (Naik and Valtin, 1969; Stewart, 1971), yet the defect in urinary concentration is much greater in DI Os/+ mice than in the VII Os/+ genotype. This suggests that chronic renal failure and osmotic diuresis per nephron is not the only mechanism contributing to their deficient urinary concentration. Two further factors have been identified. The first is a probable defect in the water permeability of the distal tubules and collecting ducts, as reflected in the osmotic disequilibration (Fig. 3) between the urine (222 mOsm/kg) and the papillary tip (911 mOsm/kg) (Kettyle and Valtin, 1972).

The second is a shortening of the short loops of Henle, illustrated diagrammatically in Fig. 4 (Stewart, 1971). Short loops, by definition (Peter, 1909; Kriz, Schnermann, and Dieterich, 1972), have their bends within the outer medulla, i.e., above the border between the outer and inner medulla. Since these loops, like long loops, presumably also act as countercurrent multipliers, curtailment of their length would be expected to lead to a reduction in the interstitial osmolality of the outer medulla, that reduction, in turn, would decrease the water that is reabsorbed from the early portion of collecting ducts and thereby diminish the ability to concentrate urine. It has been shown that the mean length of the short loops is 0.3 mm in DI Os/+ mice (Fig. 4), whereas it is about 1.0 mm in length when the Os gene is introduced into a control strain (Stewart, 1971). Although there is also a selective shortening of the pars recta in DI Os/+ mice (Fig. 4) only the

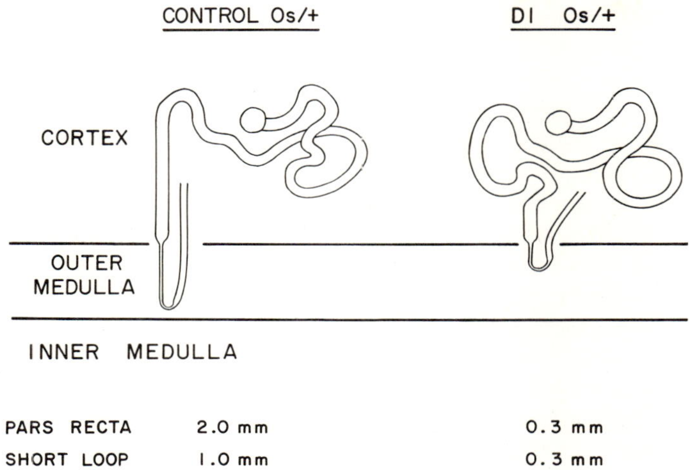

Fig. 4. Diagrammatic representation of the shortening of the short loops of Henle, which occurs when the gene for oligosyndactyly, Os, is introduced into the DI strain of mice (DI Os/+) but not when it occurs in control strains. There is concomitant shortening of partes rectae in DI Os/+ mice, but only the anatomical abnormality in the loops of Henle appears to contribute to the urinary concentrating defect. (Data from Stewart, 1971.)

anatomical abnormality of the short loops appears to be causally related to the defect in urinary concentration (Stewart, 1971).

Finally, what abnormalities appear to be responsible for the concentrating defect in DI +/+ mice? These animals, both nonsevere and severe, have kidneys of normal size with a normal complement of nephrons, and they are not in renal failure (Naik and Valtin, 1969; Stewart, 1971). In DI +/+ nonsevere mice, the small difference between urinary and papillary-tip osmolalities (Fig. 3) is not statistically significant ($P>0.2$). Nevertheless, in view of the conclusion to be drawn on DI +/+ severe mice (discussed below) and the worsening of the concentrating ability with age (Fig. 2), the small osmotic disequilibration between urine and papillary tip in DI +/+ nonsevere animals might reflect a mild defect in water permeability. The concomitant decrease in the cortico-papillary osmotic gradient might then well be secondary to a small deficiency of water permeability (Stewart and Valtin, 1972; also see next paragraph).

The large and highly significant ($P<0.001$) difference between the urinary and papillary osmolalities in DI +/+ severe mice (Fig. 3) almost certainly reflects impaired water permeability of the distal tubules and collecting ducts. The concomitant reduction in papillary interstitial osmolality is roughly the same as has been found by various techniques and in several species in the absence of ADH (Gottschalk, 1961; Levitin *et al.*, 1962; Valtin, 1966), or through computer simulation of water diuresis in which the only imposed change is a decrease in the water permeability of the distal tubules and collecting ducts (Stewart and Valtin, 1972). It seems likely, therefore, that no additional abnormality need be involked in order to explain the low papillary osmolality, but that it probably can be accounted for wholly as a consequence of the defective water permeability (Stewart and Valtin, 1972).

The conclusion that in DI +/+ mice the major or sole abnormality leading to diabetes insipidus may be a defect in ADH-induced water permeability has led to further experiments in these animals. The currently most popular scheme for the cellular mode of action of ADH (Orloff and Handler, 1967) is illustrated in Fig. 5. It is proposed that ADH activates the enzyme adenylate cyclase which converts ATP to the intracellular mediator cyclic AMP; this mediator, by a series of as yet undefined steps, is then thought to lead to increased water permeability of certain membranes, such as those lining the distal tubules and collecting ducts. We have investigated this reaction in normal and DI +/+ mice (Dousa and Valtin, 1973). The assay is performed *in vitro* on a cell-free particulate fraction of the renal medulla which contains the adenylate cyclase (Dousa *et al.,* 1971). Concentrations of ADH ranging from 10^{-9} to 10^{-5} M (about 40–400,000 μU/ml) is added to this preparation, and the conversion of ATP labeled with ^{32}P on the alpha phosphorus to labeled cyclic AMP is measured. The rate of this conversion is taken to reflect the activation of adenylate cyclase, which is maximal at an ADH concentration of 10^{-6} M.

The results are summarized in Fig. 6, in which maximal activation of adenylate cyclase (expressed as the maximal amount of cyclic AMP produced when supersaturating concentrations of ADH are added) is plotted against the mean urine osmolalities in the same animals. In DI +/+ severe animals maximal activation of adenylate cyclase is reduced by about 40% from the value found in VII +/+ (control) animals ($P<0.05$). Maximal activation is also lower than normal in DI +/+ nonsevere mice, but the reduction is not

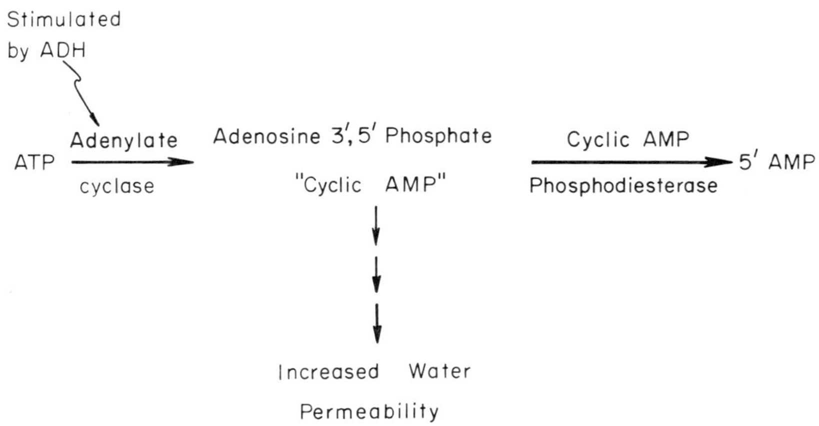

Fig. 5. Scheme for the cellular mode of action of vasopressin (ADH) which has been proposed by Orloff and Handler (1967).

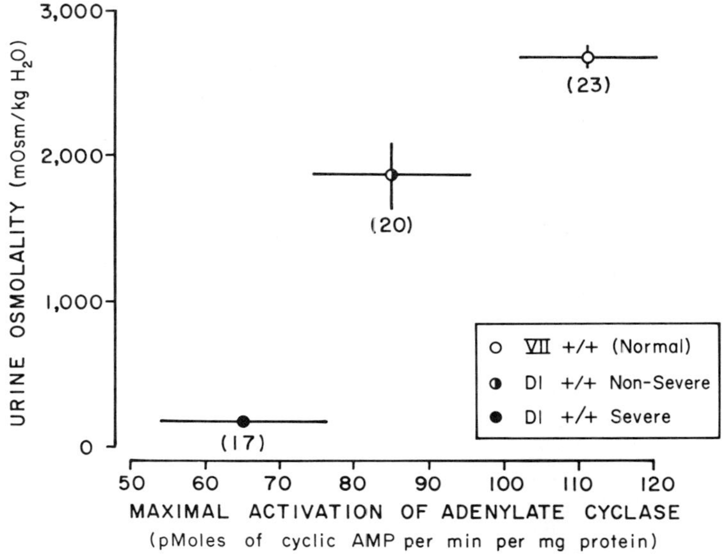

Fig. 6. Activation of adenylate cyclase by saturating doses (10^{-6}M) of ADH *in vitro,* in three genotypes of mice, plotted against mean urine osmolalities in the same mice while eating and drinking *ad lib.* Parentheses indicate ±s.e.m. The difference in urine osmolalities are all statistically significant, as is the difference in activation of adenylate cyclase between VII +/+ and DI +/+ severe mice ($P<0.05$). The difference in activation between VII +/+ and DI +/+ nonsevere animals has a $P>0.10$. (From Dousa and Valtin, 1973, and unpublished.)

statistically significant ($P>0.10$). These differences in the activation of adenylate cyclase are not seen in preparations of renal cortex from the same mice, nor in response to sodium fluoride, a nonspecific stimulator of the enzyme, nor in Brattleboro rats with hereditary hypothalamic diabetes insipidus [Schultz *et al.,* 1972], which, unlike the mice, can respond to exogenous ADH [Valtin, 1967]. Thus the findings illustrated in Fig. 6 *suggest,* but by no means prove, that a deficiency of ADH-induced activation of adenylate cyclase may lead to deficient water permeability in DI +/+ mice. A genetic experiment, which may support or disprove a causal relationship (Valtin and Kettyle, 1972), is now being done.

Preliminary experiments indicate that the activity of cyclic AMP phosphodiesterase (Fig. 5) as well as stimulation of protein kinase by cyclic AMP (possibly one essential step in the induction of water permeability denoted by the vertical arrows in Fig. 5) are the same in DI +/+ as in normal mice [Dousa and Valtin, 1973]. Beyond that, other aspects of the scheme shown in Fig. 5 will have to be studied before the cause for the concentrating defect in DI +/+ mice can be definitely established. Such studies are now in progress.

ACKNOWLEDGMENTS

This work was supported by the following grants from the U. S. Public Health Service: AM-08469-GM; AM-16105; HE-5322. Dr. Valtin is the recipient of U. S. Public Health Service Research Career Program Award 6-K3-GM 21,786 from The National Institute of General Medical Sciences. Mrs. Ethel B. Garrity gave able technical and clerical assistance in virtually all of these studies.

REFERENCES

Dousa, T., O. Hechter, I. L. Schwartz, and R. Walter. 1971. Neurohypophyseal hormone-responsive adenylate cyclase from mammalian kidney. Proc. Natl. Acad. Sci. 68: 1693–1697.

Dousa, T. P., and H. Valtin. 1973. Reduced activation of vasopressin (ADH)-sensitive adenylate cyclase in mice with hereditary nephrogenic diabetes insipidus. J. Clin. Invest. 52: 24a (abstr.).

Falconer, D. S., M. Latyszewski, and J. H. Isaacson. 1964. Diabetes insipidus associated with oligosyndactyly in the mouse. Genet. Res. 5: 473–488.

Gottschalk, C. W. 1961. Micropuncture studies of tubular function in the mammalian kidney. Physiologist 4: 35–55.

Jamison, R. L., J. Buerkert, and F. Lacy. 1971. A micropuncture study of collecting tubule function in rats with hereditary diabetes insipidus. J. Clin. Invest. 50: 2444–2452.

Kettyle, W. M., and H. Valtin. 1972. Chemical and dimensional characterization of the renal countercurrent system in mice. Kidney Internatl. 1: 135–144.

Kriz, W., J. Schnermann, and H. J. Dieterich. 1972. Differences in the morphology of descending limbs of short and long loops of Henle in the rat kidney, *In* H. Wirz and F. Spinelli (eds.), Recent Advances in Renal Physiology, S. Karger, Basel, pp. 140–144.

Levitin, H., A. Goodman, G. Pigeon, and F. H. Epstein. 1962. Composition of the renal medulla during water diuresis. J. Clin. Invest. 41: 1145–1151.

Naik, D. V., and H. W. Sokol. 1970. The hypothalamohypophyseal neurosecretory system in mice with vasopressin-resistant urinary concentrating defects. Gen. Comp. Endocr. 15: 59–69.

Naik, D. V., and H. Valtin. 1969. Hereditary vasopressin-resistant urinary concentrating defects in mice. Am. J. Physiol. 217: 1183–1190.

Orloff, J., and J. Handler. 1967. The role of adenosine 3′, 5′-phosphate in the action of antidiuretic hormone. Am. J. Med. 42: 757–768.

Peter, K. 1909. Untersuchungen über Bau und Entwickelung der Niere, Gustav Fischer, Jena.

Schultz, G., K. H. Jakobs, E. Böhme, and K. Schultz. 1972. Einfluss verschiedener Hormone auf die Bildung von Adenosine-3′:5′-monophosphat und Guanosin-3′:5′-monophosphat durch partikuläre Präparationen aus der Rattenniere. Europ. J. Biochem. 24: 520–529.

Stewart, A. D., and J. Stewart. 1969. Studies on the syndrome of diabetes insipidus associated with oligosyndactyly in mice. Am. J. Physiol. 217: 1191–1198.

Stewart, J. 1971. Renal concentrating ability in mice: a model for the use of genetic variation in elucidating relationships between structure and function. Pflügers Europa J. Physiol. 327: 1–15.

Stewart, J., and H. Valtin. 1972. Computer simulation of osmotic gradient without active transport in renal inner medulla. Kidney Internatl. 2: 264–270.

Valtin, H. 1966. Sequestration of urea and nonurea solutes in renal tissues of rats with hereditary hypothalamic diabetes insipidus: effect of vasopressin and dehydration on the countercurrent mechanism. J. Clin. Invest. 45: 337–345.

Valtin, H. 1967. Hereditary hypothalamic diabetes inispidus in rats (Brattleboro strain). A useful experimental model. Am. J. Med. 42: 814–827.

Valtin, H., and W. M. Kettyle. 1972. Mechanisms causing vasopressin-resistant urinary concentrating defects in mice. *In* H. Wirz and F. Spinelli (eds.), Recent Advances in Renal Physiology, S. Karger, Basel, pp. 172–183.

Renal Hormonal Interactions and Their Pharmacological Modification: Renin-angiotensin, Catecholamines, and Prostaglandins

Philip Needleman, Eugene M. Johnson, Jr., Sister Barbara Jakschik, James R. Douglas, Jr., and Garland R. Marshall

Departments of Pharmacology and of Physiology and Biophysics
Washington University Medical School
St. Louis, Missouri

1. The isolated perfused rabbit kidney releases prostaglandin (PG) when treated with angiotensin II (AII), angiotensin I (AI), epinephrine, or bradykinin.
2. The specific competitive angiotensin antagonist cysteine^8-angiotensin-II inhibits PG release by angiotensin but not by epinephrine or bradykinin.
3. Indomethacin blocks PG release induced both by AII and by epinephrine.
4. Epinephrine and norepinephrine are equipotent in the rabbit in producing renal vasoconstriction and PG release whereas the β-agonist isoproterenol does not cause renal PG release.
5. Catecholamine-induced PG release thus appears to be mediated by alpha-adrenergic receptor site stimulation, and this is confirmed by finding that blockade is achieved with phenoxybenzamine (α-blocker) but not propranolol (β-blocker). Phenoxybenzamine does not block PG release induced by AII.
6. Releasing a clamped renal pedical in rats results in the simultaneous appearance of AII in the blood and an elevated systemic blood pressure. Infusion of cysteine^8-AII immediately lowers the blood pressure and blocks the bioassayable circulating AII in the acute renal hypertensive rats.
7. Renal infusion of very low concentrations of angiotensin greatly enhances the vasoconstriction and catecholamine release produced by renal nerve stimulation, thereby indicating that circulating angiotensin can exert a positive

feedback on renal adrenergic nerve fibers. The augmented effect of adrenergic stimulation induced by angiotensin is inhibited by cysteine[8]-AII.

8. Inhibition of renal PG biosynthesis by indomethacin augments the renal vasoconstriction produced by nerve stimulation. Thus endogenous prostaglandins appear to plan a local renal regulatory role to modulate neural tone by a negative feedback mechanism.

Renal vascular tone is the result of a moment to moment interplay of a number of humoral substances. Neural control is exerted by catecholamines released by adrenergic innervation (Pitts, 1968; McKenna and Angelakos, 1968). The renal vascular bed is also exquisitely sensitive to angiotensin such that as little as 10 pg/ml blood can produce renal vasoconstriction (Hollenberg *et al.*, 1972). Prostaglandin-like substances (PLS), which also play a role in modulating renal vascular tone, have been identified in renal venous effluent from dog kidney (a) during nerve stimulation (Dunham and Zimmerman, 1970), (b) during renal ischemia (Jaffee *et al.*, 1972, McGiff *et al.*, 1970a), (c) upon infusion of norepinephrine (Dunham and Zimmerman, 1970), or (d) upon infusion of bradykinin (McGiff *et al.*, 1972b). The renal medulla has been demonstrated to be the site of PG biosynthesis both in rabbit kidney (Crowshaw, 1971) and in dog kidney (Crowshaw *et al.*, 1970).

Renal vascular smooth muscle can be directly constricted by either catecholamines or angiotensin, or can be dilated by prostaglandins (E type). However, the *in vivo* actions of these humoral substances on the kidney are not independent. Adrenergic stimulation will be shown to cause renal vasoconstriction, catecholamine release, prostaglandin release, and renin release. Exposure of the kidney to angiotensin results in renal vasoconstriction, enhanced adrenergic tone, and prostaglandin release. In fact, these substances (catecholamines, angiotensin, and prostaglandins) can simultaneously influence the kidney, and the vascular tone at any given time is the net result of their interaction. Furthermore, the current investigation will demonstrate the use of various pharmacological antagonists to elicit desired manipulations of renal adrenergic and vascular tone.

METHODS

Rabbit Kidney Perfusion

Some limitations to the previous experiments involving the measurements of PG in dog renal venous blood are as follows: (a) they required the use of the blood-bathed organ technique (Ferreira and Vane, 1967) which usually precluded the use of specific inhibitors; (b) they necessitated the use of large amounts of peptide agonists; (c) they made dose-response

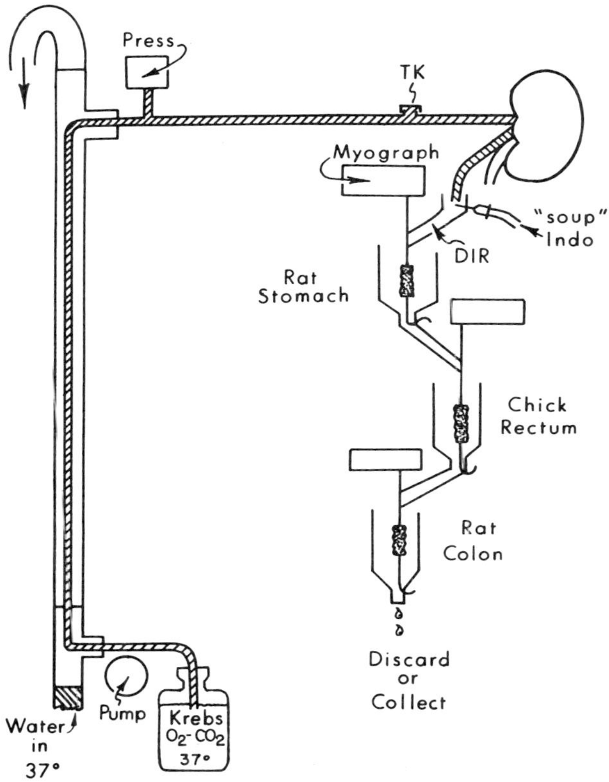

Fig. 1. Isolated rabbit kidney perfusion and superfused assay organs. TK designates injection of drug into the Krebs solution as it enters the renal artery. DIR indicates direct application of the agent across the assay organs. Soup (antagonist mixture) ingredients are described in the text.

and structure-activity studies exceedingly difficult. In the current investigation the isolated perfused rabbit kidney was found to release PG under all the conditions previously described for release from the kidney of the intact dog.

New Zealand rabbits (females) weighing 1.5–2 kg were anesthetized with pentobarbital sodium (30 mg/kg i.v.). After opening the abdominal cavity, the animal was heparinized (250 units/kg) and polyethylene catheters were tied into the renal artery (PE-160, Clay Adams), the renal vein (PE-205), and the ureter (PE-90). The kidney was placed in a warming jacket and perfused with oxygenated (95% O_2/5% CO_2) Krebs-Hensleit solution at 37°C at a constant flow rate (8 ml/min) (Fig. 1). Therefore changes in perfusion pressure were indicative of alterations in vascular resistance. Perfusion pressure was measured with a P-1000A linear core pressure transducer (Physiograph; Narco, Houston, Tex.).

Superfused Organ System

A series of isolated assay tissues, rabbit aorta, rat stomach strip, and chick rectum, were superfused by the venous effluent coming from the perfused kidney (Fig. 1) according to the procedure of Ferreira and Vane (1967). The rat stomach strip and chick rectum are particularly sensitive to prostaglandins. When the aorta was used it was the top strip of the superfused assay organs and was present for detection of catecholamines. A mixture of antagonists ('soup') was added to the superfusion fluid at 0.1 ml/min and rendered the assay tissues insensitive to catecholamines, acetylcholine, serotonin, and histamine. This antagonist reagent consisted of Krebs solution with 1 mg phenoxybenzamine, 20 mg propranolol, 1 mg hyoscine hydrobromide, 2 mg methysergide, and 1 mg diphenhydramine per 100 ml. Indomethacin (10 μg/min) was also perfused directly over the assay organs to eliminate the possibility that the assay organs might release PG and also to enhance the sensitivity of the assay organs to PG (Eckenfels and Vane, 1972). The mixture of inhibitors and indomethacin was injected below the aorta; thus the aorta responded to catecholamines, but the rat stomach and chick rectum were protected from catecholamines by specific antagonists.

Substances were tested (as a bolus injection) for their direct (DIR) effect on the assay organs by adding the agent to the perfusion fluid after it had passed through the kidney. The response of the perfused organ to the drug was determined by injecting the agent into the Krebs solution by way of an injection port just proximal to the arterial cannula (TK, through the kidney). Changes in smooth muscle tension were measured with F-50 microdisplacement myographs (Physiograph; Narco, Houston, Tex.)

RESULTS AND DISCUSSION

Angiotensin-Induced Renal Prostaglandin Release

The direct addition of AII to the assay organs resulted in contraction of the rat stomach strip and the rat colon but not of the chick rectum (Fig. 2). When AII was perfused into the kidney, the perfusion pressure increased and there was an immediate release of a PLS which was particularly apparent on the chick rectum. Epinephrine, when infused through the kidney, caused a marked increase in perfusion pressure which was accompanied by a distinct PLS release (Fig. 2). The ability of the perfused rabbit kidney to release prostaglandins following AII or epinephrine treatment is in agreement with the results obtained in dogs *in vivo* by McGiff *et al.* (1970a,b) and Aiken and Vane (1973).

Cysteine^8-AII has been shown to be a potent competitive antagonist of AII in isolated rat uterus strips and in rat blood pressure experiments

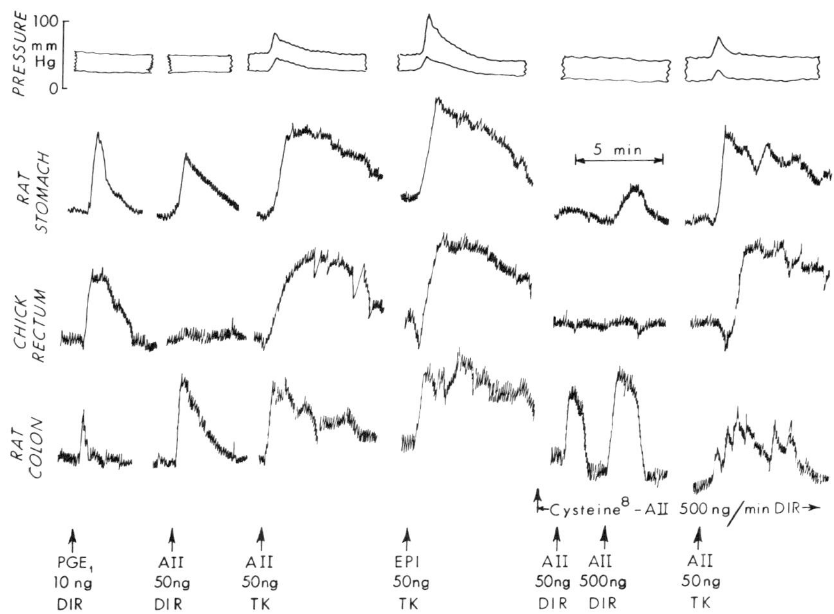

Fig. 2. Response of assay organs and the perfused rabbit kidney to AII and epinephrine (EPI) and the influence of infusion of cysteine^8-AII.

(Needleman *et al.,* 1972). Cysteine^8-AII was infused across the assay organs (DIR) and had no agonistic effect of its own, but it abolished the stomach contraction produced by 50 ng of AII (DIR) (Fig. 2). The competitive blockade was overcome by a very high dose of AII (500 ng, DIR). The AII (50 ng) was next injected into the kidney (TK) while cysteine^8-AII was being applied only to the assay organs (DIR, Fig. 2). The AII (TK) caused an increase in perfusion pressure (indicating renal vasoconstriction), and this was associated with a marked contraction of the chick rectum (normally unresponsive to AII) and the rat stomach (now unresponsive to AII because of the presence of the competitive antagonist), indicating PLS release. In contrast to this, when cysteine^8-AII was perfused through the kidney it completely blocked the increase in perfusion pressure and the PLS release induced by 50 ng of AII (TK) (Fig. 3). The inhibition was overcome by a 10 times higher dose of AII (500 ng, TK). The AII responsiveness returned within 15 min after stopping the cysteine^8-AII infusion (not shown). The specificity of the angiotensin antagonist was demonstrated by the fact that cysteine^8-AII did not alter the renal vasoconstriction and PG release induced by epinephrine (Fig. 3).

Indomethacin and aspirin-like drugs have been demonstrated by Vane (1971) to inhibit the biosynthesis of PG. Infusion of indomethacin

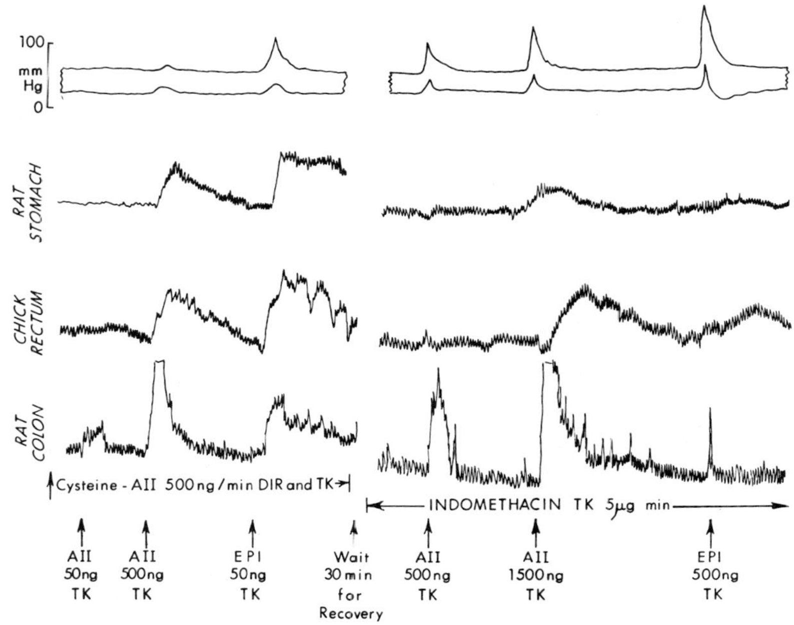

Fig. 3. Effect of cysteine⁸-AII or indomethacin infusion on renal prostaglandin release.

through the kidney abolished the release of PLS but not the increase in perfusion pressure by either AII or epinephrine (Fig. 3). However, very high doses of the agonists did break through the indomethacin blockade. The perfused kidney would appear to have a high capacity for destruction of AII, since 500 ng TK in the presence of indomethacin did not result in contraction of the rat stomach strip (Fig. 3) which could detect 5 ng of AII.

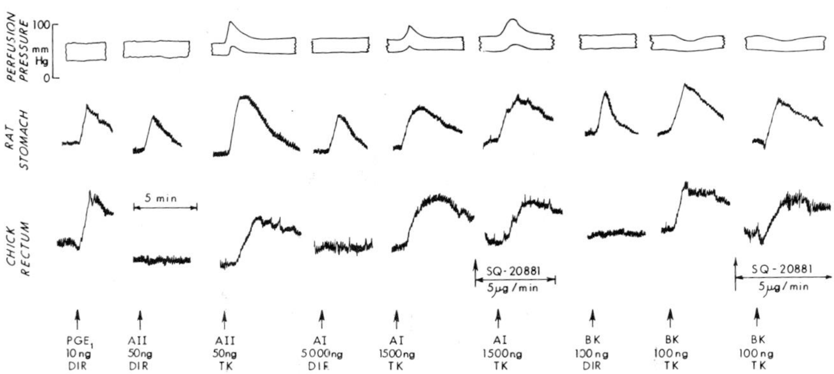

Fig. 4. Effect of angiotensin I and II and bradykinin directly on assay organs and on the perfused rabbit kidney and the influence of SQ-20881.

We compared AI and AII for their direct contractile action on rat stomach and their ability to release PLS (Fig. 4). The AI was found to possess only 1% of the activity of AII when tested directly on rat stomach, with 5000 ng of AI being required to produce a clearly detectable response. On the other hand, substantially less AI than this was required to produce a renal PG release (Fig. 4). Bradykinin potentiating factor (BPF) has been shown to inhibit the conversion of AI to AII. One such BPF, the nonapeptide SQ-20881, has been demonstrated to inhibit the enzyme(s) which converts AI to AII and it also blocks the degradation of bradykinin (Ferreira, 1965; Ferreira, Bartelt, and Green, 1970). Perfusion of SQ-20881 did not decrease the potency of AI in releasing PG (Fig. 4) nor did it enhance or prolong the action of bradykinin (Fig. 4). Bradykinin releases PG into the renal venous effluent even though it causes little change or a decrease in renal perfusion pressure (unlike AII or epinephrine). The AI, therefore, appears to induce renal PG release directly, without substantial conversion to the octapeptide, unless the rabbit kidney, unlike other tissues, contains a converting enzyme which is not susceptible to blockade by the nonapeptide.

Itskovitz and Odya (1971) bled dogs and found that the renal venous concentration of AI was 45 times that of AII. They noted a similar situation in blood from hypertensive patients with unilateral arterial abnormalities. The extreme preponderance of renal AI over AII, coupled with the demonstrated direct effects of AI on the kidney, support the hypothesis that the decapeptide rather than the octapeptide may be the major intrarenal vasoconstrictor. Escalante (unpublished data) has demonstrated high levels of AI by immunofluorescent localization in the kidneys of renal hypertensive rats.

Renal Prostaglandin Release by Catecholamines

Neural control of renal vascular tone is accomplished by the release of catecholamines from adrenergic nerve terminals. Infusion of epinephrine in the perfused rabbit kidney produced an immediate renal vasoconstriction and the renal venous effluent initiated an immediate contraction of the rabbit aorta (catecholamine sensitive) and of both of the PG sensitive organs, the rat stomach strip and chick rectum (Fig. 5). Norepinephrine was essentially equipotent with epinephrine as a vasoconstrictor and as a releaser of prostaglandin-like material. Indomethacin (10 μg/min through the kidney) blocked the contraction of the rat stomach and chick rectum which followed administration of epinephrine or norepinephrine, but did not inhibit renal vasoconstriction or aorta contraction (Fig. 3). The prostaglandin-like activity was shown to be PGE by radioimmunoassay (Douglas *et al.*, 1973). Dopamine had less than 0.1% of the vasoconstrictor and PG-releasing activity of epinephrine (Fig. 5). Dihydroxyphenylalamine (DOPA) was inactive at the high dosage tested. The beta-adrenergic agonist isoproterenol was entirely inactive in releasing PG from the kid-

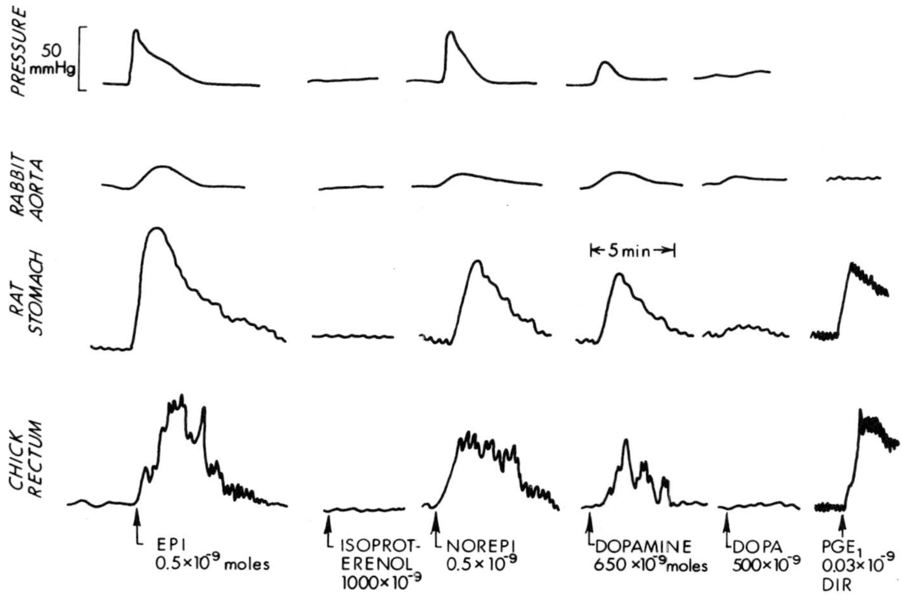

Fig. 5. Release of prostaglandins by isolated perfused rabbit kidney treated with exogenous catecholamines. All the drugs were injected as a bolus into the Krebs-Hensleit solution as it entered the renal artery, except the PGE_1 standard which was tested directly over the assay organs. Dosages are in moles. The results are traced from a typical experiment and the experiments were repeated in at least five rabbit kidney preparations with the same results.

ney (Fig. 5), nor did a constant infusion of isoproterenol alter norepinephrine-induced PG release (not shown). 3′5′-cyclic adenosine monophosphate, dibutyry-3′5′-cyclic adenosine monophosphate, and theophylline were inactive as inducers of renal PG release (not shown).

Effect of Adrenolytics on Catecholamine-Induced Renal Prostaglandin Release

Renal prostaglandin release appears to be the result of activation of alpha-adrenergic receptor sites. Consistent with the lack of effect of the beta agonist isoproterenol the beta-adrenergic blocking agent propranolol had no effect on epinephrine-induced renal PG release (Fig. 6). On the other hand, the alpha-adrenergic blocker phenoxybenzamine was a potent inhibitor of epinephrine-induced renal vasoconstriction and PG release. Phenoxybenzamine was acting as a specific adrenergic blocker since it was ineffective in inhibiting angiotensin-induced renal vasoconstriction and PG release (Fig. 6). Conversely, as shown above (Fig. 3), the specific angiotensin antagonist cysteine[8]-AII blocked angiotensin-induced PG release without blocking epinephrine-stimulated PG release.

Catecholamines and Renin Secretion

A primary endocrine function of the kidney is the elaboration of renin. Neural control is exerted on renin secretion by way of adrenergic nerve fibers. Enhanced adrenergic activity either evoked by renal nerve stimulation (Coote *et al.*, 1972; Loeffler, Stockigt, and Ganong, 1972; Vander, 1965) or by exogenous catecholamines (Bunag, Page, and McCubbin, 1966; Vander, 1965; Gutmann *et al.*, 1973; Winer, Chokshi, and Walkenhorst, 1971) leads to an enhanced renin secretion. Unlike renal PG release, which is mediated through alpha adrenergic receptor sites, the secretion of renin appears to be subserved to beta adrenergic receptors (Chokshi, Yeh, and Samet, 1972; Pettinger, Augusto, and Leon, 1972; Coote *et al.*, 1972; Loeffler *et al.*, 1972; Beck *et al.*, 1972; Winer *et al.*, 1971).

Enhanced adrenergic activity leads to renin secretion into the blood stream. Renin reacts with circulating renin substrate to produce the decapeptide AI which is cleaved to the octapeptide AII in the pulmonary circulation

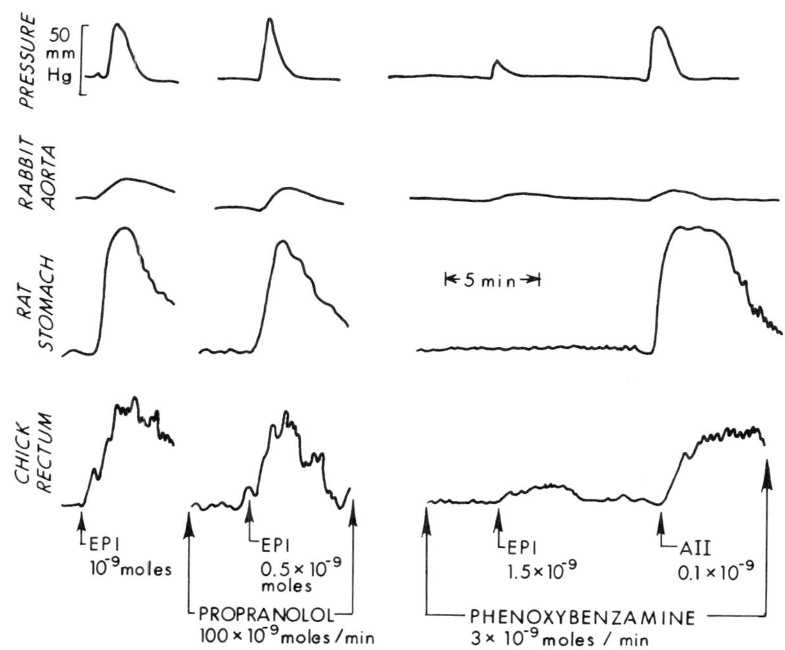

Fig. 6. Influence of adrenergic blocking agents on renal prostaglandin release induced by exogenous catecholamines. All drugs were administered into the kidney. The propranolol or phenoxybenzamine was infused through the kidney for 15 min before the kidney was challenged with some other agent. The response to AII was the same before and after infusion of the adrenergic blockers.

(Page and McCubbin, 1969). The resultant circulating AII amplifies adrenergic tone by stimulating catecholamine release from the adrenal medulla (Peach, Cline, and Watts, 1966) and by enhancing the release of catecholamines from sympathetic nerve terminals (Zimmerman and Gisslen, 1968; Schumann, Starke, and Werner, 1970; Peach *et al.,* 1970).

Angiotensin Antagonists in Renal Hypertension

The renin-angiotensin system can be selectively inhibited at a number of sites (Fig. 7). Renin reacts with angiotensinogen to form AI. Decapeptide AI is hydrolyzed to the octapeptide AII in the pulmonary circulation. The AI is usually less potent than AII but has been shown to act on the same receptor site (Needleman, 1972). The bradykinin-potentiating factors (BPF, e.g. SQ-20881) block the conversion of AI to AII. Decapeptide analogs (Ile^8-AI and Phe^4, Tyr^8-AI) were proved to compete with AI for converting enzyme as well as being specific antagonists for AI at its receptor sites (Needleman *et al.,* 1972). Finally, specific octapeptide angiotensin antagonists (such as $cysteine^8$-AII) are potent reliable inhibitors of both AI and AII (Fig. 7).

The effectiveness of a specific angiotensin antagonist in renal hypertension is demonstrated in Fig. 8. Acute renal hypertension was produced by unclamping the left renal pedicle after it had been occluded for 4 hr according to the method of Kreiger *et al.* (1971). The contralateral kidney was left intact. Upon removal of the clamp the elevation of arterial blood pressure was accompanied by appearance of a substance in carotid artery blood which contracts both the rat stomach and rat colon strips. These two strips are highly responsive to AII, and there appears to be an association between circulating angiotensin levels and the elevation in blood pressure. Arterial blood would be expected to contain high blood levels of AII and low levels of PG, since AI is converted into AII and PG is degraded in the pulmonary circulation. The presence of AII in the carotid blood, in temporal association with the hypertension, was confirmed by infusion of the specific antagonist $cysteine^8$-AII which concomitantly reduced the tone in the assay organs and lowered blood pressure (Fig. 8).

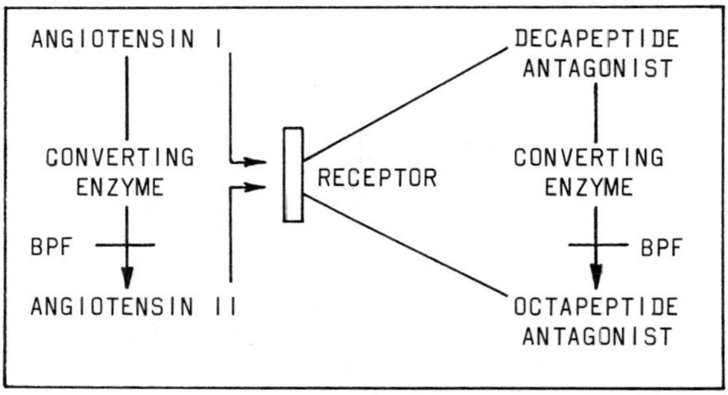

Fig. 7. Antagonists of the renin-angiotensin system.

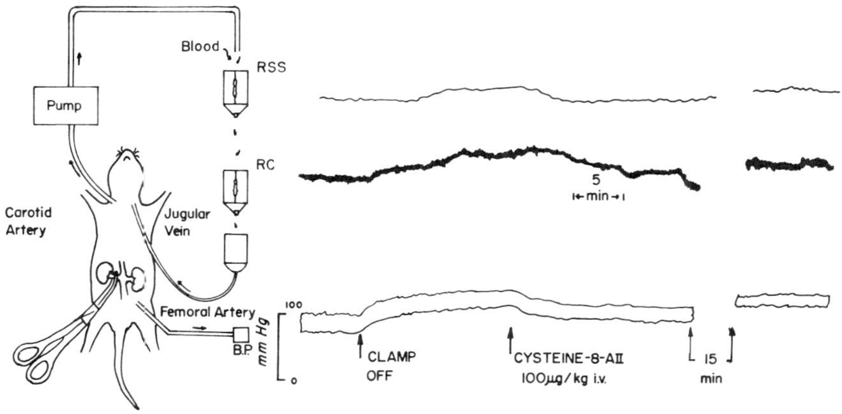

Fig. 8. Reversal of experimental acute renal hypertension in rats by infusion of cysteine^8-AII. Carotid artery blood was superfused at 5 ml/min across the assay organs and returned by way of the jugular vein. The reservoir for venous return was primed with 5 ml of blood from a donor rat. The blood superfusion was started 30 min before removal of the clamp.

When a converting enzyme inhibitor (BPF) was administered in renal hypertensive animals, there was an immediate drop in blood pressure, thereby indicating that AI cannot maintain the blood pressure (Kreiger *et al.,* 1971). Similarly, we have used decapeptide analogs Ile^8-AI and Phe^4, Tyr^8-AI of known angiotensin inhibitors, which are competitive antagonists of converting enzyme, and have been able to lower blood pressure in rats with acute renal hypertension (Needleman *et al.,* 1972). The quickness of the response to inhibition of either conversion of AI to AII or direct competitive inhibition of AII would imply that the conversion of AI is the rate-limiting step and that the concentration of AI must be very high.

The Influence of Angiotensin on Renal Adrenergic Stimulation

Stimulation of renal nerves was accomplished with an electrode placed around the renal artery of an isolated perfused rat kidney. The renal venous effluent superfused a rat aorta (present for catecholamine detection) and a rat stomach strip (present to detect prostaglandins) (Fig. 9). Stimulation (with fixed voltage) of the renal nerves resulted in a frequency-dependent increase in renal vasoconstriction with minimally detectable aorta contraction by the renal venous effluent following 6 and 12 c/sec and no apparent PG release. A bolus injection of norepinephrine into the kidney resulted in a characteristic renal PG release (equivalent to 10 ng of PGE_2). An extremely low concentration of angiotensin (150 pg/ml/min) was then infused into the kidney producing a mild renal vasoconstriction but no PG release. In the presence of angiotensin nerve stimulation resulted in enhanced renoconstriction associated with higher levels of catecholamines and PG in the renal venous

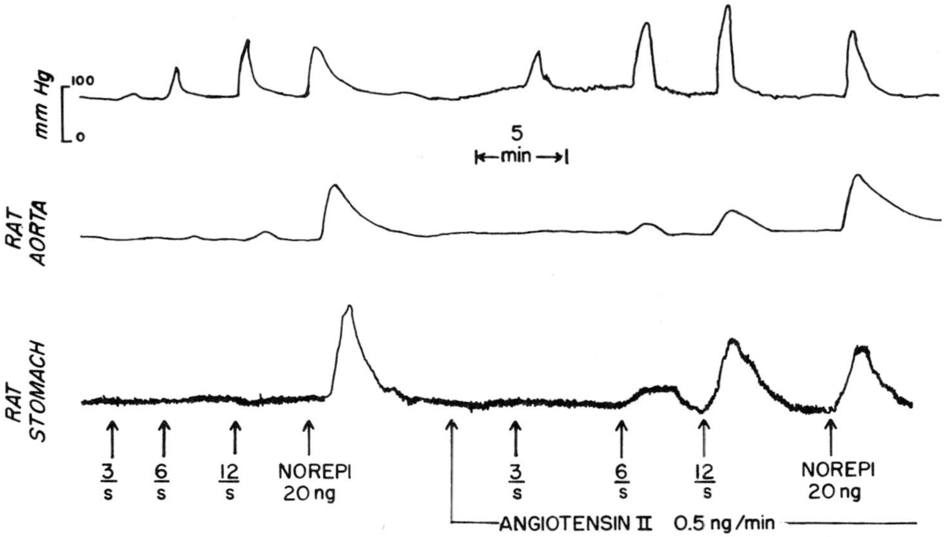

Fig. 9. Angiotensin enhancement of renal adrenergic stimulation. The rat kidney was perfused with Krebs-Hensleit media (95% O_2, 5% CO_2) at 3 ml/min. Stimulation was carried out by an electrode placed over the renal artery. A typical physiograph tracing of renal pressure changes is presented. The frequency (c/sec) of stimulation (indicated in figure) was carried out with a 15 V square wave stimulus for 30 sec.

effluent. The AII-induced enhancement appears to be presynaptic rather than postsynaptic since the renoconstriction produced by exogenous norepinephrine is not enhanced; in fact there appears to be some blunting of norepinephrine-induced renal PG release. The perfused rat kidney preparations deteriorate with time and the responsiveness to stimulation and AII

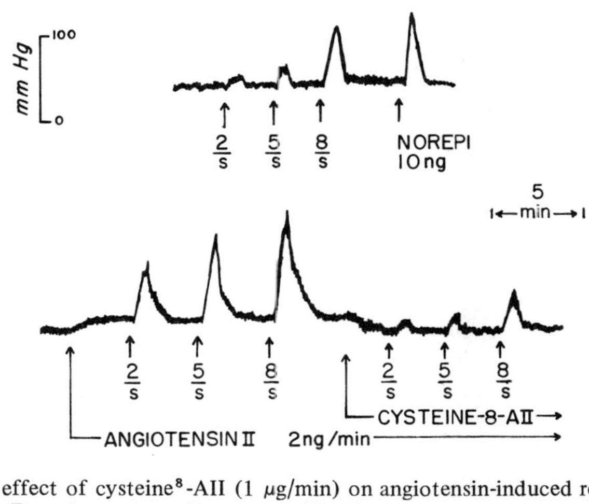

Fig. 10. The effect of cysteine[8]-AII (1 μg/min) on angiotensin-induced renal adrenergic enhancement. Experimental conditions as in Fig. 8.

enhancement are best in fresh preparations. The enhancement by AII of the responses to neural stimulation appears to be the result of action at specific angiotensin receptor sites, since the competitive antagonist cysteine^8-AII completely abolished the phenomenon (Fig. 10).

The vulnerability of the renal vascular bed to marked vasoconstriction is especially pronounced in shock. The profound hypotension leads to an increase in adrenergic tone with an associated elaboration of renin-angiotensin. The angiotensin itself is a potent renal vasoconstrictor but the peptide adds to the vicious cycle by enhancing adrenergic tone. It is our belief that angiotensin antagonists such as cysteine^8-AII have great therapeutic potential in such situations by helping to overcome vascular shutdown and enhancing renal perfusion. As shown, the antagonists can block both the direct effects of AII on renal vascular smooth muscle as well as the AII-induced enhancement of renal adrenergic tone.

Sympathetic Nerve Stimulation and Renal PG Release

Electrical stimulation of renal nerve fibers at high frequencies induced renal vasoconstriction (increased renal perfusion pressure), catecholamine release (contraction of rabbit aorta superfused by the renal venous effluent), and PG release (contraction of the rat stomach strips) (not shown). The PG release by electrical stimulation was blocked by indomethacin. On the other hand, phenoxybenzamine blocked both the vasoconstriction and the PG release caused by renal nerve stimulation, but propranolol was ineffective (not shown).

Dunham and Zimmerman (1970) demonstrated the release of prostaglandin-like material of the E type from autoperfused canine kidney by renal nerve stimulation and by infusion of norepinephrine. McGiff *et al.* (1970c; 1972a,b) found that renal infusion of norepinephrine was associated with increased levels of PGE-like material in the renal venous effluent, but when they stimulated renal nerves there was no PG release. The differences between these two investigations is unclear. Recently, Davis and Horton (1972) demonstrated that electrical stimulation of rabbit renal nerves increased the concentration of prostaglandins in renal venous blood and that indomethacin pretreatment prevented the renal PG release.

Modulating Effect of Prostaglandins on Renal Adrenergic Tone

At this point it appears that humoral influences on the kidney could result in a vicious cycle in which adrenergic stimulation causes renal vascular constriction and renin release. The resultant angiotensin, besides being a potent direct-acting vascular spasmogen, also causes a positive feedback which enhances adrenergic nerve stimulation. A possible endogenous mechanism for blunting the hormone-induced vasoconstriction may be provided by the prostaglandins shown to be generated in the vicinity of the neurons at the time of stimulation. Previous studies have demonstrated that prostaglandins (especially of the E type) can cause feedback inhibition of adrenergic nerve

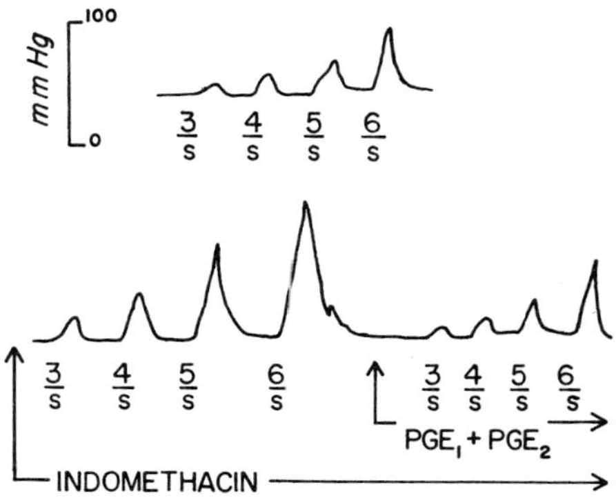

Fig. 11. The effect of indomethacin and prostaglandins on renal adrenergic stimulation. Rat kidneys were infused with indomethacin (10 μg/min) for 10 min prior to nerve stimulation. PGE_1 and PGE_2 was infused as a mixture at 2 ng/min.

stimulation in isolated vas deferens preparations and in isolated perfused hearts (Hedqvist, 1970; Stjarne, 1973). We have obtained results that indicate the prostaglandins must be exerting a negative feedback in the kidney as well. Indomethacin (which inhibits PG biosynthesis), when infused into isolated perfused rat kidneys, was found markedly to increase the renal pressor response to nerve stimulation (Fig. 11). The subsequent renal infusion of a mixture of PGE_1 and PGE_2 partially blocked the renal constriction. The results of Junstad and Wennmalm (1972), who placed rats in a cold room to increase total adrenergic activity and noted that treatment of such animals with indomethacin markedly increased the urinary excretion of norepinephrine, are in partial support of these findings.

When indomethacin was infused into the kidney at the start of the perfusion, at a time when neither basal nor stimulated renal PG release was observed, it had no clear effect on stimulation. However, when basal or stimulated PG release had increased indomethacin markedly exhanced the response to renal nerve stimulation. Completely analogous results were obtained by Ferreira, Moncada, and Vane (1973) in isolated perfused spleen preparations. Indomethacin enhanced the response to adrenergic stimulation only after 2–3 hr perfusion when basal PG release was apparent. They further noted that indomethacin treatment also augments the splenic vasoconstriction produced by angiotensin or norepinephrine.

Renal Hormonal Interactions and Their Modification

A more rational approach to the modulation of renal vascular tone as well as to renal hypertension or shock therapy should emerge when we achieve a clearer understanding of the renal interactions of catecholamines, renin-angiotensin, and prostaglandins (Fig. 12).

Adrenergic stimulation of β-receptors leads to renin secretion (blocked by propranolol). Renin acts on angiotensinogen (renin substrate) to produce the decapeptide AI, which is converted to the octapeptide AII (conversion blocked by SQ-20881, or Ile^{8}-AI or Phe^{4}, Tyr^{8}-AI). The AI has weaker biological activity than AII, but AI and AII appear to react at the same receptor sites (Needleman *et al.*, 1972). The AII acts on a wide variety of receptor sites, causing such responses as enhanced release of catecholamines from adrenergic neurons or the adrenal medulla, as well as release of renal prostaglandins or direct smooth muscle contraction (all blocked by angiotensin antagonists such as cysteine^{8}-AII). Prostaglandins, especially of the E type, cause renal vasodilation and thereby tend to blunt the vasoconstriction produced by either angiotensin or α-adrenergic stimulation (also blocked by α-adrenolytics). In addition PGE has been shown to inhibit the release of norepinephrine (N.E.) during nerve stimulation. The endogenous PG biosynthesis is blocked by pretreatment with indomethacin.

Experimental success in lowering blood pressure in animal models with high renin renal hypertension has been accomplished with specific AII antagonists (Marshall, 1970; Marshall, Vine, and Needleman, 1970; Needleman *et al.*, 1972; Regoli and Park, 1972; Pals *et al.*, 1971; Turker *et al.*, 1971; Vine *et al.*, 1973), with AI antagonists (Needleman *et al.*, 1972), with inhibitors of AI converting enzymes, (Ferreira *et al.*, 1970), and with propranolol alone or in combination with phenoxybenzamine (Michelakis and McAllister, 1972). Finally, the use in this situation of aspirin-like drugs, which inhibit prostaglandin biosynthesis, should be approached with caution as they have the

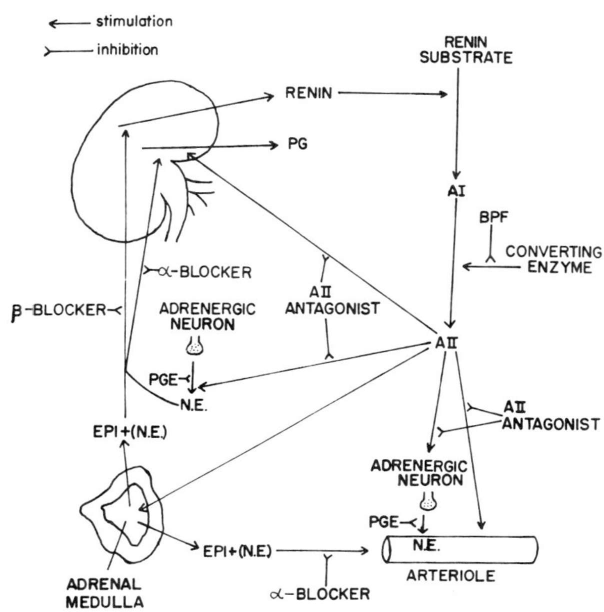

Fig. 12. Renal interactions and their modification.

potential of obliterating an important endogenous check on accelerated adrenergic tone.

ACKNOWLEDGMENTS

Technical assistance was provided by Mrs. Anne H. Kauffman, Mrs. Patricia B. Stoecklein, and Miss Janet Kourik. This research was supported by Established Investigatorships from the American Heart Association (68-115-P.N., 70-111-G.R.M.), and USPHS NIH grants HE-14397 and HE-14509, GM-02016 (Medical Scientist Training Program for J.R.D.), GM-00096-5-TO5, and GM 49033 (Predoctoral Fellowship for Sister Barbara J.) and American Heart Grant in Aid 70-672.

REFERENCES

Aiken, J. W., and J. R. Vane. 1973. Intrarenal prostaglandin release attenuates the renal vasoconstrictor activity of angiotensin. J. Pharmac. Exp. Ther. 184: 678–687.

Beck, N. P., S. W. Reed, H. V. Murdaugh, and B. B. Davis. 1972. Effects of catecholamines and their interaction with other hormones on cyclic 3′,5′-adenosine monophosphate of the kidney. J. Clin. Invest. 51: 939–944.

Bunag, R. D., I. H. Page, and J. R. McCubbin. 1966. Neural stimulation of release of renin. Circulation Res. 19: 851–858.

Chokshi, D. S., B. K. Yeh, and P. Samet. 1972. Effects of dopamine and isoproteranol on renin secretion in the dog. Proc. Soc. Exp. Biol. Med. 140: 54–57.

Coote, J. H., E. J. Johns, V. H. Macleod, and B. Singer. 1972. Effect of renal nerve stimulation, renal blood flow and adrenergic blockade on plasma renin activity in the cat. J. Physiol. 226: 15–36.

Crowshaw, K. 1971. Prostaglandin biosynthesis from endogenous precursors in rabbit kidney. Nature New Biol. 231: 240–241.

Crowshaw, K., J. C. McGiff, J. C. Strand, A. J. Lonigro, and N. A. Terragno. 1970. Prostaglandins in dog renal medulla. J. Pharm. Pharmac. 22: 302–303.

Davis, H. A., and E. W. Horton. 1972. Output of prostaglandins from the rabbit kidney, its increase on renal nerve stimulation and its inhibition by indomethacin. Brit. J. Pharmac. 46: 658–675.

Douglas, J. R., Jr., E. M. Johnson, Jr., G. R. Marshall, B. M. Jaffee, and P. Needleman. 1973. Stimulation of splenic prostaglandin release by angiotensin and specific inhibition by cysteine-8-AII. Prostaglandins 3: 67–74.

Dunham, E. W., and B. G. Zimmerman. 1970. Release of prostaglandin-like material from dog kidney during nerve stimulation. Am. J. Physiol. 219: 1279–1285.

Eckenfels, A., and J. R. Vane. 1972. Prostaglandins, oxygen tension and smooth muscle tone. Brit. J. Pharmac. 45: 451–462.

Ferreira, S. 1965. Bradykinin-potentiating factor (BPF) present in the venom of *Bothrops jararaca.* Brit. J. Pharmac. Chemother. 24: 163–169.

Ferreira, S. H., D. C. Bartelt, and L. J. Greene. 1970. Isolation of bradykinin-potentiating peptides from Bothrops jararaca venom. Biochemistry 9: 2583–2593.

Ferreira, S. H., L. J. Green, V. A. Alabaster, Y. S. Bakhle, and J. R. Vane.

1970. Activity of various fractions of bradykinin-potentiating factor against angiotensin converting enzyme. Nature (Lond.) 225: 379–380.
Ferreira, S. H., S. Moncada, and J. R. Vane. 1973. Some effects of inhibiting endogenous prostaglandin formation on the responses of the cat spleen. Brit. J. Pharmac. 47: 48–58.
Ferreira, S. H., and J. R. Vane. 1967. Prostaglandins: their disappearance from and release into the circulation. Nature (Lond.) 216: 868–873.
Gutman, F. D., H. Tagawa, E. Haber, and A. C. Barger. 1973. Renal arterial pressure, renin secretion, and blood pressure control in trained dogs. Am. J. Physiol. 224: 66–72.
Hedqvist, P. 1970. Studies on the effect of prostaglandins E_1 and E_2 on the sympathetic neuromuscular transmission in some animal tissues. Acta Physiol. Scand.79 (suppl. 345): 1–140.
Hollenberg, N. K., H. S. Solomon, D. F. Adams, H. L. Abrams, and J. P. Merrill. 1972. Renal vascular responses to angiotensin and norepinephrine in normal man. Circulation Res. 31: 750–757.
Itskovitz, H. D., and C. Odya. 1971. Intrarenal formation of angiotensin I. Science 174: 58.
Jaffee, B. M., C. W. Parker, G. R. Marshall, and P. Needleman. 1972. The renal concentrations of prostaglandin E in acute and chronic renal ischemia. Biochem. Biophys. Res. Comm. 49: 799–805.
Junstad, M., and A. Wennmalm. 1972. Increased renal excretion of noradrenaline in rats after treatment with prostaglandin synthesis inhibitor indomethacin. Acta Physiol. Scand. 85: 573–576.
Kreiger, E. M., H. C. Salgado, C. J. Assan, L. J. Green, and S. H. Ferreira. 1971. Potential screening test for detection of overactivity of renin-angiotensin system. Lancet 1: 269–271.
Loeffler, J. R., J. R. Stockigt, and W. F. Ganong. 1972. Effect of alpha- and beta-adrenergic blocking agents on the increase in renin secretion produced by stimulation of the renal nerves. Neuroendocrinology 10: 129–138.
Marshall, G. R., W. Vine, and P. Needleman. 1970. A specific competitive inhibitor of angiotensin II. Proc. Natl. Acad. Sci. 67: 1624–1630.
Marshall, G. R. 1970. Studies on the biologically-active conformations of angiotensin. Intra-Sci. Chem. Rep. 5: 305–316.
McGiff, J. C., K. Crowshaw, N. A. Terragno, A. J. Lonigro, J. C. Strand, M. A. Williamson, J. B. Lee, and K. K. F. Ng. 1970a. Prostaglandin-like substances appearing in canine renal venous blood during renal ischemia. Circulation Res. 27: 765–789.
McGiff, J. C., K. Crowshaw, N. A., Terragno, and A. J. Lonigro. 1970b. Release of prostaglandin-like substance into renal venous blood in response to angiotensin-II. Circulation Res. 26-27 (suppl. I): 1121–1130.
McGiff, J. C., K. Crowshaw, N. A. Terragno, and A. J. Lonigro. 1970c. Renal prostaglandins. Possible regulators of the renal actions of pressor hormones. Nature (Lond.) 227: 1255–1257.
McGiff, J. C., K. Crowshaw, N. A. Terragno, K. U. Malik, and A. J. Lonigro. 1972a. Differential effect of noradrenaline and renal nerve stimulation on vascular resistance in the dog kidney and the release of prostaglandin E-like substance. Clin. Sci. 42: 223–233.
McGiff, J. C., N. A. Terragno, K. U. Malik, and A. J. Lonigro. 1972b. Release of prostaglandin E-like substance from canine kidney by bradykinin. Circulation Res. 31: 36–43.
McKenna, O. C., and E. T. Angelakos. 1968. Adrenergic innervation of the canine kidney. Circulation Res. 22: 345–354.

Michelakis, A. M., and R. G. McAllister. 1972. The effect of chronic adrenergic receptor blockade on plasma renin activity in man. J. Clin. Endocr. 34: 386–391.

Needleman, P., E. M. Johnson, Jr., W. Vine, E. Flanigan, and G. R. Marshall. 1972. The pharmacology of antagonists of angiotensin I and II. Circulation Res. 31: 862–868.

Page, I. B., and J. W. McCubbin. 1969. Renal Hypertension, Year Book Medical Publishers, Chicago.

Pals, D. T., F. D. Masucci, F. Sipos, and G. S. Denning, Jr. 1971. A specific competitive antagonist of the vascular action of angiotensin II. Circulation Res. 29: 664–672.

Peach, M. J., W. H. Cline, Jr., D. Davila, and P. A. Khairallah. 1970. Angiotensin-catecholamine interactions in the rabbit. Eur. J. Pharmac. 11: 286–292.

Peach, M. J., W. H. Cline, Jr., and D. T. Watts. 1966. Release of adrenal catecholamines by angiotensin II. Circulation Res. 19: 571–575.

Pettinger, W. A., L. Augusto, and A. S. Leon. 1972. Alteration of renin release by stress and adrenergic receptor and related drugs in anesthetized rats. Adv. Exp. Med. Biol. 22: 105–117.

Pitts, R. F. 1968. Physiology of the Kidney and Body Fluids, 2nd edn, Year Book Medical Publishers, Chicago, p. 20.

Regoli, D., and W. K. Park. 1972. Pressor and myotropic effect and antagonist properties of several anglogs of angiotensin II. Can. J. Physiol. Pharmac. 50: 99–112.

Regoli, D., and J. R. Vane. 1964. A sensitive method for the assay of angiotensin. Brit. J. Pharmac. Chemother. 23: 351–359.

Schumann, H. J., K. Starke, and U. Werner. 1970. Interactions of inhibitors of noradrenaline uptake and angiotensin on the sympathetic nerves of the isolated rabbit heart. Brit. J. Pharmac. 39: 390–397.

Stjarne, L. 1973. Alpha-adrenoceptor mediated feedback control of sympathetic neurotransmitter secretion in guinea pig vas deferens. Nature New Biol. 241: 190–191.

Turker, R. K., M. Yamamoto, P. A. Khairallah, and F. M. Bumpus. 1971. Competitive antagonism of 8-ala-angiotensin II to angiotensin I and II on the isolated rabbit aorta and rat ascending colon. Eur. J. Pharmac. 15: 285–291.

Vander, A. J. 1965. Effect of catecholamines and the renal nerves on renin secretion in anesthetized dogs. Am. J. Physiol. 209: 659–662.

Vane, J. R. 1957. A sensitive method for the assay of 5-hydroxy-tryptamine. Brit. J. Pharmac. Chemother. 12: 344–349.

Vane, J. R. 1971. Inhibition of prostaglandin synthesis as a mechanism of action for aspirin-like drugs. Nature (New Biol.) 231: 232–235.

Vine, W. H., D. A. Brueckner, P. Needleman, and G. R. Marshall. 1973. The synthesis, biological activity, and ^{19}F NMR spectra of angiotensin II analogs containing fluorine. Biochem. J. 12: 1630–1637.

Winer, N., D. S. Chokshi, and W. G. Walkenhorst. 1971. Effects of cyclic AMP, sympathomimetic amines, and adrenergic receptor antagonists on renin secretion. Circulation Res. 29: 239–249.

Zimmerman, B. G., and J. Gisslen. 1968. Pattern of renal vasoconstriction and transmitter release during sympathetic stimulation in presence of angiotensin and cocaine. J. Pharmac. Exp. Ther. 163: 320–329.

Angiotensin II: Conformation and Interaction with the Receptor

Garland R. Marshall, Heinz E. Bosshard, William H. Vine, Jerry D. Glickson, and Philip Needleman

Departments of Physiology and Biophysics and of Pharmacology and
The Computer Systems Laboratory
Washington University
St. Louis, Missouri, and
Clinical Research and Training Center
University of Alabama School of Medicine
Birmingham, Alabama

The primary event of a hormone-induced physiological response[1] is that of recognition or binding. In order adequately to describe and understand this process, one must know the conformation(s) of the hormone in physiological solution and the conformation(s) when bound to the receptor, presumably on the cell surface. The structure and conformation(s) of the receptor with and without hormone must also be determined. This information would allow insight into the thermodynamics and kinetics of the hormone-receptor interaction and possibly into subsequent events leading to the physiological response.

Although recent efforts to purify and characterize hormone receptors may lead to the necessary information, only fragmentary data are presently available. We should like to consider the information available on the solution conformation of angiotensin II which has been gained by direct spectroscopic and other physical techniques. The data available on the receptor-bound conformation and that inferred for the receptor itself have been deduced from structure-activity studies of angiotensin analogs (Marshall, 1971; Marshall and Bosshard, 1972; Marshall, Eilers, and Vine, 1972c). While this approach is fraught with logical pitfalls and direct studies of the receptor

[1] A recent symposium on angiotensin has been published, *Chemistry and Biology of Peptides*, J. Meienhofer (ed.), Ann Arbor Science Publishing Co., Ann Arbor, Mich., which includes a review of the physiological actions of angiotensin.

itself would be more straightforward, the present state of the isolation of the receptor for angiotensin (Meyer *et al.*, 1972) is not yet developed sufficiently to offer a realistic alternative.

SOLUTION CONFORMATION

While the solution conformation(s) is amenable to examination by physical techniques, interpretation of results in terms of conformation is not unambiguous, and the results for angiotensin from different techniques have been interpreted in contradictory fashion. In particular, as physical measurements have been made models have been proposed which were ultimately rejected by further physical measurements. This process of model proposal, measurement, rejection, and new proposal leading hopefully to the correct model has been hindered by differences in conditions of the experiments which appear to be critical in the case of angiotensin.

A wide variety of physical and theoretical techniques have been used to study the solution conformation of angiotensin, including thin-film dialysis (Craig, Harfenist, and Paladini, 1964; Printz, Williams, and Craig, 1972b), titration (Paiva, Paiva, and Scheraga, 1963), hydrogen-tritium exchange (Paiva *et al.*, 1963; Printz *et al.*, 1972a), infrared and Raman spectroscopy (Fermandjian *et al.*, 1972a), electron spin resonance spectra of a free-radical analog (Weinkam and Jorgensen, 1971a), optical rotatory dispersion (Smeby *et al.*, 1962; Craig, 1968) and circular dichroism (Fermandjian, Morgat, and Fromageot, 1971a), potential energy calculations (Printz, Nemethy, and Bleich, 1972a), and nuclear magnetic resonance (see below).

Nuclear Magnetic Resonance

Studies by nuclear magnetic resonance (NMR) include proton NMR of [Asn^1, Val^5]-angiotensin II in deuterated dimethyl sulfoxide (Weinkam and Jorgensen, 1971b), proton NMR in D_2O of [des-Asp^1, Gly^2]-angiotensin II (Weinkam and Jorgensen, 1971b), proton NMR of [Asn^1, Val^5]-angiotensin II in D_2O and H_2O (Glickson, Cunningham, and Marshall, 1972a, 1973), hydrogen-deuterium exchange (Bleich, Galardy, and Printz, 1973), natural abundance ^{13}C NMR of [Asn^1, Val^5]-angiotensin II in water (Zimmer *et al.*, 1972), and ^{19}F NMR of [$pFPhe^4$]-angiotensin II and [$pFPhe^8$]-angiotensin II in water (Vine *et al.*, 1973).

Nuclear magnetic resonance offers the ability to identify and assign resonance signals to each nucleus of the angiotensin molecule under study and interpret the chemical shift, relative intensity, and splitting patterns of these resonance signals in terms of torsional rotations about bonds (coupling constants), proximity of different groups (ring current shifts, charged groups, and nuclear Overhauser effects), and rotational freedom about bonds (relaxation measurements). While the necessary experiments to propose and confirm a particular solution conformation of angiotensin are still being done, sufficient data is already at hand to rule out the models for angiotensin proposed to date and place strong constraints on future model building.

The assignment of specific resonances in the NMR spectra in D_2O as shown in Fig. 1 to specific hydrogens in [Asn^1, Val^5]-angiotensin II was accomplished (Glickson *et al.*, 1972a, 1973) by comparison with a spectrum computed for the component amino acids, by decoupling experiments, by chemical shift upon titration, and by synthesis. An example of each method of assignment will be given for illustration, using the two valine residues and phenylalanine. Because valine is the only amino acid residue in angiotensin with a single hydrogen on the β carbon, the two distinct doublets at 3.97 and 4.09 ppm in the α-proton region of the spectra must be assigned to valine-3 and valine-5. In order to distinguish between the two possible assignments, an analog of angiotensin with the valine in the 5 position replaced with a perdeuterated valine was synthesized (Marshall, 1970). This completely removed all signals arising from valine-5 and allowed unambiguous assignment of the remaining 3.97 ppm doublet to valine-3. By irradiating at 3.97 ppm and observing the β-proton portion of the spectra, a sharpening of the multiplet spectra at 1.92 ppm was observed, which was also seen when the valine methyl protons were similarly decoupled. This indicated a contribution by the Val-3 β-proton to the complex multiplet at 1.92 ppm. As the pH (pDc) was raised, one resonance in the α-proton region changed its position markedly with a pKa of 3.07±0.03. The agreement with the pKa value (3.34) obtained by direct titration of the C-terminal carboxyl group assigns this resonance directly to the α proton of the C-terminal phenylalanine residue.

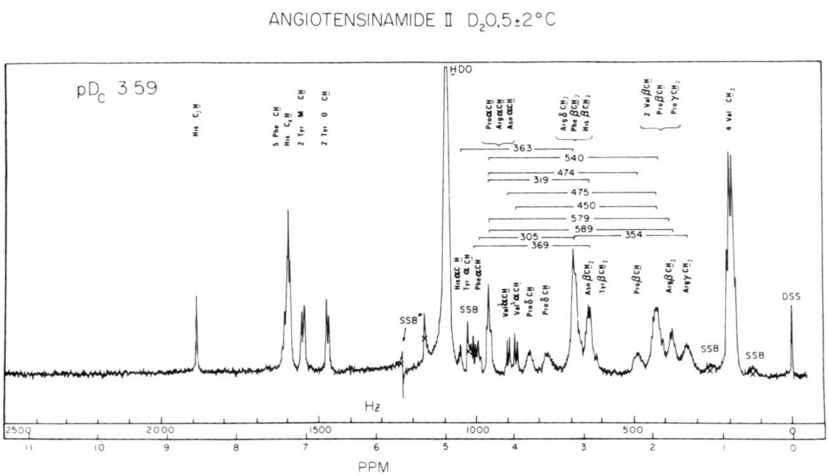

Fig. 1. 220 MHz NMR spectra of [Asn^1, Val^5]-angiotensin II in D_2O (pD_C 3.59, 5±2°C) with assigned resonances (Glickson *et al.*, 1972a, 1973).

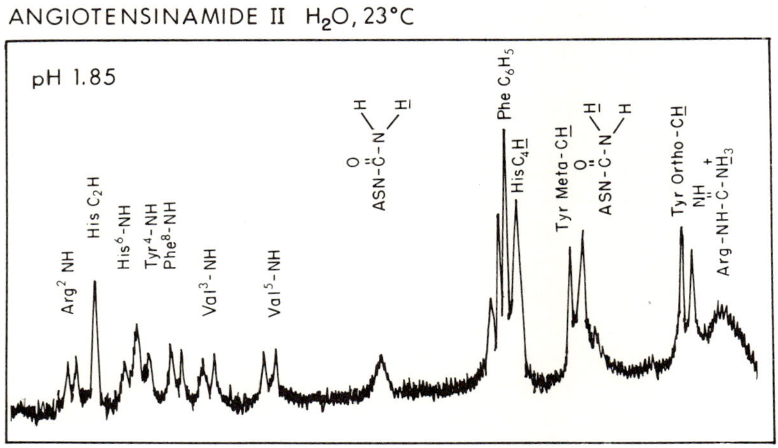

Fig. 2. Amide region of 220 MHz NMR spectra of [Asn^1, Val^5]-angiotensin II in H_2O (pH 1.85, 23°C) with assignments made by direct decoupling experiments (Glickson *et al.*, 1973).

By similar arguments and decoupling experiments, the entire spectrum in D_2O was assigned.

The situation in water presented additional difficulties. In D_2O, the resonance due to water is markedly diminished, but proton signals from exchangeable protons such as the amide protons are lost owing to their replacement by deuterium. This is unfortunate as the amide proton-carbon α-proton coupling constant provides critical information which places constraints on possible values of the torsional rotation ϕ about the amide-α carbon bond. By observing the spectra in water, one can measure the coupling constants of the amide protons (Fig. 2); the α-proton region is obscured, however, by the massive absorption due to water, and decoupling experiments to assign the amide resonances are extremely difficult on conventional spectrometers (Feeney *et al.*, 1971). By titration behavior in H_2O, the amide resonances belonging to arginine-2 and phenylalanine-8 could be assigned. Recently, Glickson, Dadok, and Marshall (1974) have been able to overcome the technical difficulties of decoupling the α protons in the presence of the water resonance using the spectrometer designed by Dadok *et al.* (1972b). This allowed unambiguous assignment of the amide resonances as shown in Fig. 2. Concurrent with these experiments, Bleich *et al.* (1973) have tentatively assigned the two valine resonances to two slowly exchanging protons, but could not distinguish between the two. Similar assignments were made for the other resonances, but no experimental details were given, and assignments based on the methods alluded to such as exchange rate for arginine-2 and pH profile for histidine-6 are not without pitfalls. Now that the assignments have been made by direct decoupling, the exchange data can be interpreted without fear of misassignment.

Interpretation of the coupling constants of the assigned amide protons is based on a correlation, the Karplus equation, between the peptide vicinal NH-C^{α}H coupling constant J and the dihedral angle θ, where θ is related to the torsion rotation ϕ as follows:

$$J_{NHCH} = A\cos^2\theta - B\sin\theta + C\sin^2\theta$$

and $\theta = | \phi - 60^\circ |$.

An initial difficulty concerns the choice of the constants A, B, and C. These are determined for a chemical class by examination of coupling constants for compounds of known conformation. Sets of values for A, B, and C have recently been proposed by Ramachandran, Chandrasekaran, and Kopple (1971) and by Bystrov *et al.* (1973) for the NH-CαH vicinal couplings. The possible values for the torsional rotation ϕ which are consistent with the observed NMR coupling constants J_{NHCH} have been calculated (Marshall *et al.*, 1973b) and are tabulated in Table 1. As is evident in several cases, there are four values (at most) of ϕ which will satisfy a given J_{NHCH}. An additional complication in interpretation arises from the fact that a measured J can be the average of those associated with sets of conformers whose interconversion is fast on the NMR time scale. In the ^{19}F NMR studies by Vine *et al.* (1973) of [pFPhe^8]-angiotensin II strong evidence was presented for conformers whose interconversion is slow on the NMR time scale as seen in Fig. 3. Since the angiotensin analog has only one fluorine per molecule, the increasing and reversible appearance of a second peak as the pH is increased is most readily interpreted in terms of two conformers with quite different environments of the C-terminal phenylalanine ring.

The pK of the transition seen with the fluorine analog is higher than a similar transition in the proton spectra, but sufficiently similar to be con-

Table 1. Constraints for the torsional rotation ϕ about the NH-C^{α}H bond based on measured coupling constants J_{NHCH}

Residue	Measured J_{NHCH} (Hz)	Calculated possible values	
		ϕ (degrees)[a]	ϕ (degrees)[b]
Arg-2	6.5±0.3	−159±3, −81±3, 60±10	−161±, −79±2, 30±2, 90±2
Val-3	7.9±0.3	−147±3, 93±3	−153±2, −87±2, 43±2, 77±3
Tyr-4	7.2±0.5	−153±4, −87±4	−157±3, −83±3, 36±5, 84±5
Val-5	8.0±0.4	−146±4, −94±4	−152±3, −88±3, 44±4, 76±4
His-6	6.0±0.5	−163±4, −77±4, 46±13, 74±13	−164±3, −76±3, 27±4, 93±4
Phe-8	7.3±0.3	−153±3, −87±3	−157±2, −83±2, 37±3, 83±3

[a]Data of Ramachandran *et al.*, 1971.
[b]Data of Bystrov *et al.*, 1973.

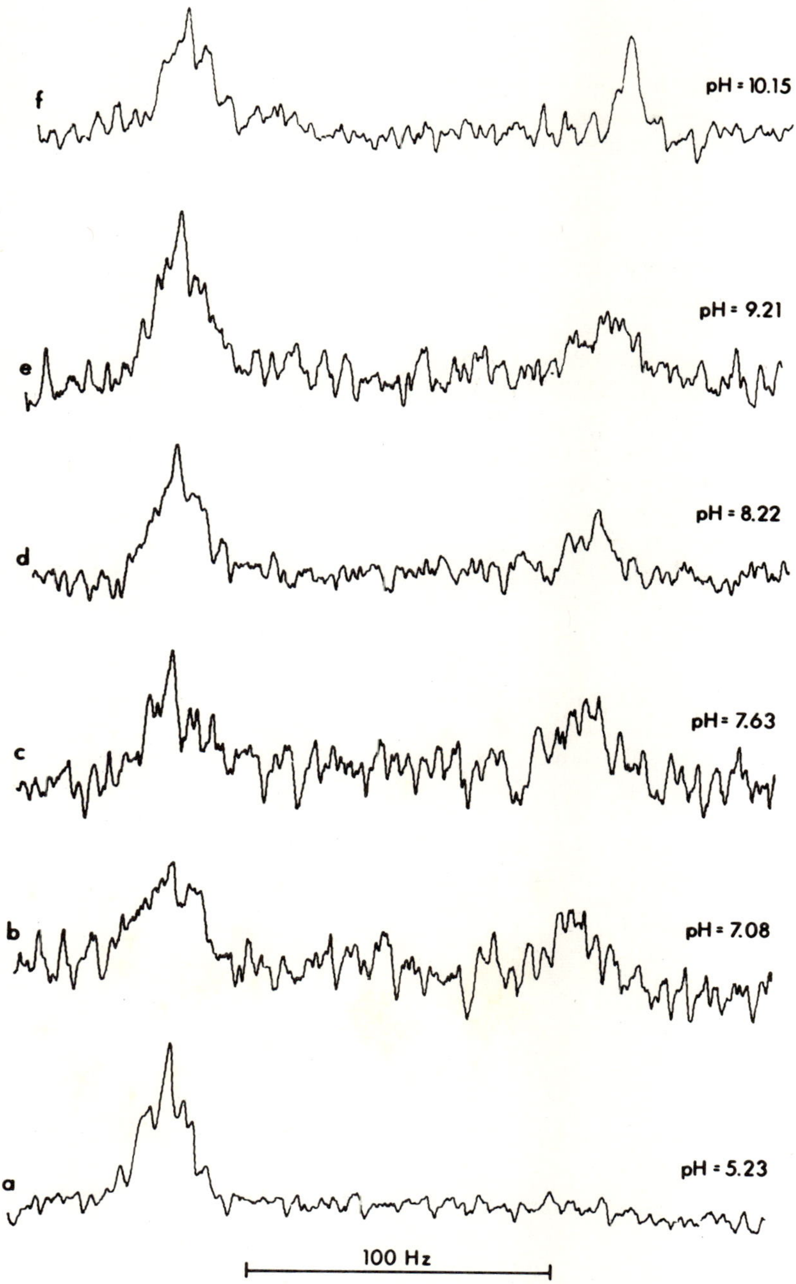

Fig. 3. Fluorine NMR spectra of [pFPhe[8]]-angiotensin II in H_2O as a function of pH (Vine *et al.*, 1973): (a) 64 scans, (b) 8 scans, (c) 8 scans, (d) 8 scans, (e) 8 scans, and (f) 32 scans.

sidered along with the evidence for a conformational transition of angiotensin near neutral pH. Changes in chemical shift of proton resonances as a function of pH can be due to ionization of groups and changes in electron density at adjacent protons, or to changes in the spatial orientation of groups with possible changes in chemical shift at groups removed from those undergoing primary ionization changes. In Fig. 4 both types of effects can be seen. For

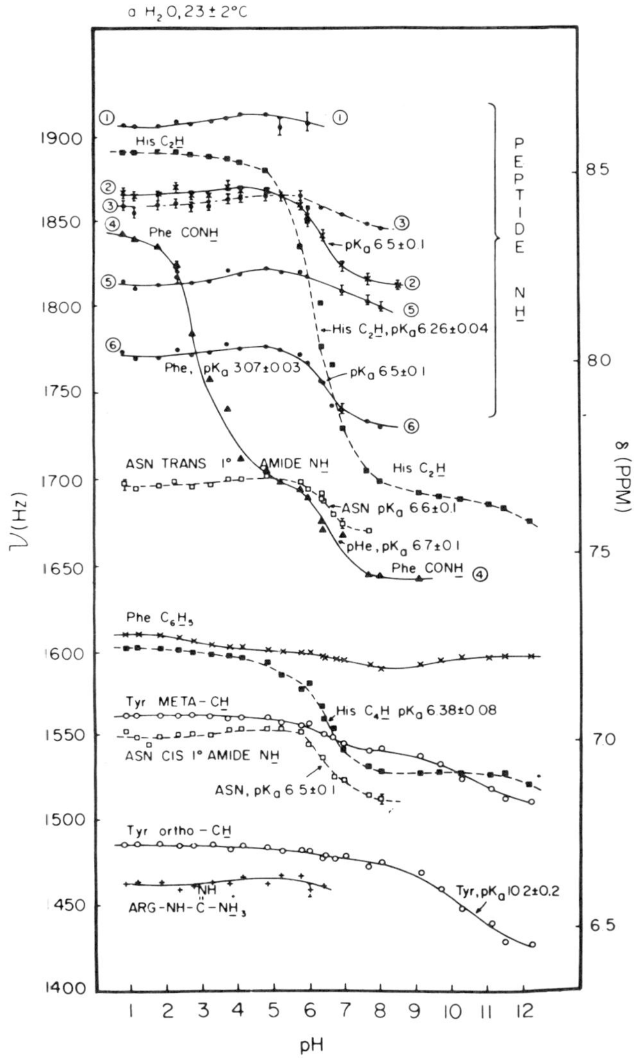

Fig. 4. Titration curves of proton resonances in [Asn[1], Val[5]]-angiotensin II at lower fields than H_2O adsorption. Amide resonances particularly show conformational changes.

example, changes in Phe-8 resonances as the carboxyl group is titrated, or His-6 resonances as the imidazole group is titrated, are direct ionization effects. Changes in the chemical shifts of the Tyr-4 α-proton (not shown), Asn-1 carboxamide protons, Tyr-4 meta protons, and five of the six amide protons (Val-3, Tyr-4, Val-5, His-6, and Phe-8) with a pK of approximately 6.6 indicate a major change in the solution conformation of [Asn^1, Val^5]-angiotensin II. This is substantiated by the absence of those effects attributed to conformation in the natural abundance ^{13}C NMR spectrum of angiotensin II, which shows only changes in chemical shifts of resonances of carbon atoms proximal to ionizing sites. This is due to the fact that ^{13}C spectra primarily reflect changes in charge density rather than conformational effect, i.e., through bond effects rather than through space effects. Indications of a similar conformational transition upon protonation of the tyrosine phenolic hydroxyl group are also seen in the titration data. Other evidence for such a conformational transition at pH 10 comes from thin-film dialysis and gel filtration studies (Franze de Fernandez, Delius, and Paladini, 1968; Ferreira, Hampe and Paiva, 1969).

Another possible indicator of side chain interactions is the pKa value of the ionizable groups. If these groups are involved strongly in intramolecular associations, this interaction should be reflected in their titration behavior. While the pKa's of [Asn^1, Val^5]-angiotensin II had been measured directly and spectrophotometrically (Paiva *et al.*, 1963), one must interpret a complex curve in order to determine the values for each ionizable group. Direct measurement of the titration behavior of individual ionizable groups is offered by NMR as seen in Fig. 4. A comparison between the values obtained by direct titration and by proton NMR (Glickson *et al.*, 1972a, 1973) and by

Table 2. Dissociation constants of angiotensin-II

Residue	Group	Method of Observation			
		PMR[a]		^{13}C NMR[b]	Direct titration[c]
		pK_a	pK_a^D	pK_a^D	pK_a
Phe^8	Carboxyl	3.07 ± 0.03		3.01 ± 0.1	3.34
His^6	Imidazole	6.26 ± 0.04	6.42 ± 0.02	6.54 ± 0.1	6.30
Asn^1	α-amino		6.58 ± 0.04		6.92
Tyr^4	Phenol	10.2 ± 0.2	10.1 ± 0.2	10.45 ± 0.1	10.04

[a]Data of Glickson *et al.*, 1973a. Carboxyl, imidazole, α-amino, and phenol titrations were monitored by displacement of Phe peptide N*H*, imidazole C_2H and C_4H, Asn α*CH*, and Tyr ortho-C*H* resonances, respectively. Measurements of pK_a's were made in H_2O at 23°C and of pK_a^D's in D_2O at 4°C and determined directly from pH meter readings.

[b]Data of Zimmer *et al.* (1972) in D_2O at 27°C.
[c]Data of Paiva *et al.* (1963) at 25°C in 0.1 M KCl.

Table 3. Comparison of ^{13}C NMR chemical shifts for proline carbons relative to tetramethylsilane

Compound	α Carbon	β Carbon	γ Carbon	δ Carbon
[Asn^1,Val^5]-angiotensin II[a]	61.6	30.15	25.25	48.88
PCA-His-Pro-NH_2,TRF(D_2O)[b]	61.5 (t)* – (c)*	30.56(t) 32.56(c)	25.56(t) 22.92(c)	48.90(t) 48.20(c)
PCA-His-Pro-NH_2 (DMSO)	61.59(t) – (c)	30.83(t) – c)	25.85(t) 23.45(c)	48.29(t) 47.69(c)
N-Acetyl-Pro-NH_2 (D_2O)[b]	62.66(t) 61.12(c)	31.36(t) 32.90(c)	25.45(t) 23.81(c)	49.69(t) 48.30(c)
N-Acetyl-Pro-NH_2 (DMSO)	61.88(t) 60.69(c)	31.10(t) 33.26(c)	25.71(t) 24.05(c)	48.98(t) 47.67(c)

Abbreviations: (b), *trans* orientation and (c), *cis* orientation of histidyl-proline amide bond; DMSO, dimethylsulfoxide.
[a]Data of Zimmer *et al.*, 1972. These data were reported relative to benzene and corrected according to Levy and Cargioli (1972).
[b]Data of Deslauriers *et al.*, 1972.

carbon NMR (Zimmer *et al.*, 1972) is shown in Table 2. These values fall within the normal range expected for solvated ionizable groups, including an apparently low pKa for the α-amino group which is associated with an N-terminal asparagine residue.

The chemical shift of proline resonances may be indicative of the orientation of the proline amide bond. Strong agreement exists between the chemical shift of the proline α proton (4.36 ppm) in angiotensin and that reported (Torchia and Bovey, 1971) for the α proton of poly-*L*-proline I (4.4 ppm) which exists in the *cis* orientation rather than the *trans* form (4.7 ppm) as was pointed out (Glickson *et al.*, 1973). The reliability of the chemical shift of the α proton of proline as an indicator of *cis* or *trans* conformation is highly questionable, as a survey of the literature indicates overlapping ranges of chemical shift for the *cis* and *trans* forms (Deber *et al.*, 1970). The suggestion of a *cis* orientation of the proline peptide bond was made originally by Fermandjian *et al.* (1971a) on the basis of circular dichroism studies. The natural abundance ^{13}C NMR spectra obtained by Zimmer *et al.* (1972) offer a less ambiguous criteria. Bovey (1972) has pointed out the advantages of ^{13}C spectra of proline residues in determining *cis* or *trans* orientations. Interpretation of the chemical shifts of Zimmer *et al.* (1972), which were measured against an external standard of benzene in terms of tetramethylsilane (TMS) (Levy and Cargioli, 1972), allows the comparison (Table 3) of the ^{13}C chemical shifts of the proline carbons with those of the thyrotropin releasing factor (TRF) (Deslauriers *et al.*, 1973) and oxytocin fragments

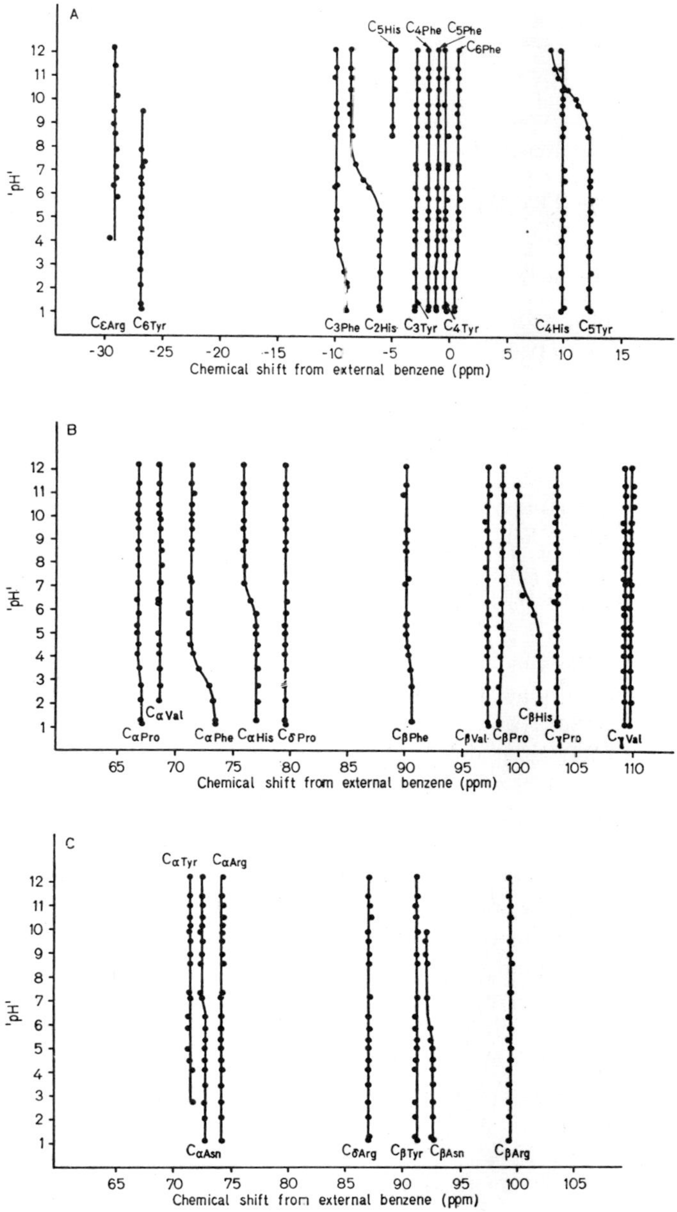

Fig. 5. Titration curves of ^{13}C NMR signals of [Asn^1, Val^5]-angiotensin II as reported by Zimmer *et al.* (1972): (a) aromatic ^{13}C resonances of angiotensin II; (b) aliphatic ^{13}C resonances of the four C-terminal residues of angiotensin II; (c) aliphatic ^{13}C resonances of Asn, Arg, and Tyr of angiotensin II.

Table 4. Amide exchange data[a] for [Asn[1], Val[5]]-angiotensin II at pH 2.3, 17°C

Residue	Half-life (min)
Arg-2	Fast
Val-3[b]	28.7 ± 1.2
Tyr-4	15.9 ± 0.6
Val-5[b]	30.2 ± 0.9
His-6	5.3 ± 0.5
Phe-8	5.8 ± 0.8

[a]From Bleich *et al.*, 1973.
[b]Correlated by Marshall *et al.* (1973a) based on the assignments by Glickson *et al.* (1974).

(Deslauriers, Walter, and Smith, 1972), in which both *cis* and *trans* orientations of proline are simultaneously observed. From the marked agreement of the angiotensin values for all the proline carbon chemical shifts with the *trans* orientations of TRF and N-acetyl-proline amide independent of solvent, one can conclude[2] that the proline amide bond has the *trans* orientation in aqueous solution regardless of the pH, as the chemical shifts for the proline carbons in angiotensin II are essentially independent of pH (Zimmer *et al.*, 1972) as seen in Fig. 5. It should be pointed out that TRF is a particularly good model for angiotensin II since it also contains a histidyl-proline bond.

Nuclear magnetic resonance has also been used to assign the different classes of exchangeable amide protons seen in hydrogen-tritium exchange studies (Printz *et al.*, 1972b). This was done directly (Bleich *et al.*, 1973) by measuring the rates of exchange, as shown in Table 4, of amide protons for deuterium by examination of the α-proton region upon dissolving [Asn[1], Val[5]]-angiotensin II in D_2O at pH 2.3, 17°C. As the amide protons exchange for deuterium, the coupling to the α proton is removed and the multiplet resonance simplifies. A different approach was used by Glickson *et al.* (1973) who measured line broadening of the NH resonances as a function of pH. This is based on the fact that the exchange rate increases with pH and that linewidth broadens when the exchange rate and the difference between the chemical shift of the exchanging protons becomes comparable. This means that conformational changes or changes in ionization must be consid-

[2]Independent ^{13}C NMR studies (Deslauriers, R., R. Walter, and I.C.P. Smith. Biochem. Biophys. Res. Comm. 53: 244, 1973.) have concluded that angiotensin II is predominantly in the *trans* configuration of proline in aqueous solution, and that the *cis* configuration, if present, represents less than 20% of the total population.

ered in this approach. The data obtained by Bleich *et al.* (1973) disagreed with that of Glickson *et al.* (1973) for the Phe-8 amide, which at pH 2.3 exchanged rapidly and yet was the most stable by the line-broadening approach. This is explained by the fact that the phenylalanine amide has a carboxyl adjacent with a pKa of 3.07 (Glickson *et al.*, 1972a). As the ionized carboxyl will destabilize the anion transition state for proton exchange on the adjacent amide by an inductive effect (Berger, Loewenstein, and Meiboom, 1959), the exchange behavior of the Phe-8 amide changes markedly with titration of the C-terminal carboxyl group. This does not imply that the Phe-8 amide proton is involved in hydrogen bonding or shielding from the solvent, which are probable explanations for such hindered exchange in the absence of an inductive effect. Stabilization of the amide anion transition state by an adjacent positively charged amino group explains the increased exchange rate seen by both methods for the Arg-2 amide. The fact that Glickson *et al.* (1973) failed to detect the slowly exchanging amides of Val-3, Val-5, and Tyr-4 probably reflects the large number of spectra at slightly different pH values which would be necessary to make the line-broadening approach as sensitive as the direct exchange rate measurements. It would be of considerable interest to determine if the same relative order of exchange rates for the amide protons, excluding Arg-2 and Phe-8, occur at other hydrogen ion concentrations.

The conformational lability of angiotensin II seen with pH can also be induced by solvent as suggested by the study of Weinkam and Jorgensen (1971b) on [des-Asp^1, Gly^2, Ile^5]-angiotensin in deuterated dimethylsulfoxide (DMSO). This shortened analog of angiotensin has coupling constants J_{NHCH} markedly different from those seen for [Asn^1, Val^5]-angiotensin II at acid pH. For example, both the Tyr-4 and His-6 amides in DMSO had a J_{NHCH} smaller than 3 Hz. In angiotensin itself in water the coupling constants are 7.2±0.5 and 6.0±0.5 Hz for Tyr-4 and His-6, respectively (Marshall *et al.*, 1973b). Similar conclusions relative to conformational changes as a function of condition have been reached with CD studies (Fermandjian *et al.*, 1971a). The presence of different conformations for oxytocin and lysine vasopressin in water *versus* DMSO has been shown directly by NMR (Feeney *et al.*, 1971; Glickson, Urry, and Walter, 1972b).

Other Techniques

Thin-film dialysis (Craig *et al.*, 1964; Printz *et al.*, 1972b) experiments were among the first to suggest a preferred solution conformation for angiotensin based on more rapid diffusion through a calibrated membrane than expected for a substance of that molecular weight. Examination under a variety of conditions also suggested a conformational transition to a more extended conformation at alkaline pH. This has been further studied by Franze de Fernandez *et al.* (1968) who found that the major expansion occurs between pH 9.3 and 10.7 and is associated with the ionization of the Tyr-4 phenolic hydroxyl group. It is interesting to note, however, that for [Asn^1, Val^5]-angiotensin II there appears to be increased diffusion between pH 5.05 and 7.60, which might also indicate a conformation transition. Urea addition also retarded the escape rate, a fact consistent with a compact conformation which expanded on addition of a known denaturant. Electrostatic effects were suggested as a complication in interpretation (Ferreira *et al.*, 1969) based on ionic strength effects on the slow-diffusing *versus* the rapid-diffusing component; this complication appears to have been overcome by the use of membranes treated to remove any charge (Printz *et al.*, 1972b).

Optical rotatory dispersion (ORD) measurements (Smeby *et al.*, 1962; Paiva *et al.*, 1963; Craig, 1968) also suggested a preferred time-averaged structure for angiotensin in that addition of urea modified the spectra (Smeby *et al.*, 1962) and a reversible change was seen upon changing the pH from 5.67 to 10.95 (Craig, 1968). Certainly a large part of the change seen at alkaline pH is due to tyrosine ionization and accompanying shifts in position and magnitude of the phenolic absorption bands. This is confirmed by the dispersion data for angiotensin which was not significantly altered by varying the pH between 2.5 and 8.5 (Paiva *et al.*, 1963). Also consistent with the importance of the tyrosine ionization in the observed ORD spectrum at alkaline pH is the observation (Franze de Fernandez *et al.*, 1968) that a similar ORD pattern is seen for [Val^5]-angiotensin II, [Asn^1, Val^5]-angiotensin II, and [Asn^1, Val^5]-angiotensin II amide, even though the change in retention time in thin-film dialysis is not seen for the latter peptide containing a C-terminal phenylalanine amide. This implies that the ORD changes observed signify primarily the changes in the tyrosine residue upon ionization and not those associated with the conformational transition seen by thin-film dialysis.

Circular dichroism (CD) studies (Fermandjian *et al.*, 1971a) showed four minima at 187, 203, 224, and 237.5 nm. Comparison with a mixture of free aromatic amino acids indicated that the amide transitions would be obscured. Comparison of the CD spectrum of [Phe^4]-angiotensin II with that of angiotensin, free tyrosine, and phenylalanine indicated that the tyrosine side chain behaves as if it were free of interactions limiting its rotation. This was confirmed by measurement of the fluorescence yield at 310 nm after excitation at 280 nm, which was identical for [Asn^1, Val^5]-angiotensin II and free tyrosine, and by measurements of the pK's of the phenolic hydroxyls of the two compounds, which were also identical (10.15). Increasing the temperature enhanced the two negative bands at 224 nm and 237 nm. Examination of the CD spectra in trifluoroethanol showed further enhancement of the peak at 224 nm. Fermandjian *et al.* (1971a) interpret these results to indicate that at pH 6 in aqueous solution the extent of ordered conformations was limited. Heating or organic solvents increased the stability and, thus, the concentration of the ordered structure represented by the band at 224 nm. The assignment of the negative band at 237 nm to the *cis* conformation of the proline-7 amide and the association of this conformational constraint with the ordered structure was also suggested. Films obtained by dessication from either trifluoroethanol or aqueous solution suggested a β structure owing to strong negative bands at 220 nm and strong positive bands at 195 and 198 nm. In view of the NMR evidence available, it would appear likely that temperature elevation at pH 6 might sufficiently alter the pK_a's of the ionizable groups to cause the conformational change seen by NMR with a pK of 6.6. The NMR data also makes it rather unlikely that the band at 237 nm indicates the *cis* orientation of the proline amide bond. The absence of strong bands in CD spectra assignable to regular structures such as α helix or β structures should not be interpreted as evidence for the absence of ordered structures or conformers. Regular structures allow the summation of amide transition bands of similar sign and position which may not occur in many other conformations which lack the regularity, but nevertheless have considerable order.

Infrared spectra were obtained on solid samples in KCl pellets, and Raman spectra were obtained on both solid samples and solutions varying in concentrations from 10 to 100 mM (Fermandjian *et al.*, 1972a). The data were reported to be consistent with an antiparallel β structure in the dry state or in concentrated aqueous solution. The ability to assign resonances and interpret results is limited at present to regular structures in infrared and Raman spectroscopy. Evidence from other techniques would indicate, however, that angiotensin does not have a regular structure in aqueous solution, but a conformation possessing considerable order.

Hydrogen exchange experiments were first done (Paiva *et al.*, 1963) by measuring the decrease in absorbancy at 1550 cm^{-1} after dissolving the peptide in D_2O. It was concluded that all the hydrogens exchanged at the same rate, which was the same order of magnitude as that for simple amides and peptides. Thus, a time-averaged preferred conformation with hydrogen bonding or steric shielding of an amide from the solvent was excluded. Using the more sensitive technique of automated tritium-hydrogen exchange, Printz *et al.* (1972b) indicated three classes of exchangeable protons at the pH of minimal exchange rate (pH = 2.5). Two hydrogens are in the slowest class with a half-life of 300 min, two of intermediate rate ($t_{1/2}$ = 80 min) and two exchange with a half-life of 8.7 min. While these values might be considered to agree qualitatively with those obtained by direct measurement (Bleich *et al.*, 1973), the absence of quantitative agreement and inability to identify the various groups of exchanging protons with individual amides indicates the clear superiority of NMR in this endeavor.

An interesting approach to the problem of the conformation of angiotensin was that of Weinkam and Jorgensen (1971a) who incorporated a spin-label analog of histidine, nitronylnitroxyalanine, into the C-terminal tripeptide of angiotensin II and studied its electron spin resonance spectra. On the basis of an inferred binding of the C-terminal phenylalanine carboxyl anion to the polar nitronyl nitroxide ring in the tripeptide, an ion-dipole bond between the C-terminal carboxyl group and the imidazole ring of His-6 was postulated. Glickson *et al.* (1972a, 1973) have pointed out that the absence of any perturbation in the C_2H or C_4H resonances of His-6 in the region of carboxyl titration clearly rule out this proposed interaction in aqueous solution for [Asn[1], Val[5]]-angiotensin II.

Proposed Models

As new experimental data has become available, old models of the solution conformation of angiotensin II have been discarded and new models proposed to take their place. It may be instructive to review the models, the information which led to their proposal, and the current data which leads to their demise.

α-Helix Model. This model was proposed by Smeby *et al.* (1962) in the midst of a great deal of enthusiasm for the α-helix conformation in proteins and particularly for the ability of ORD spectra to detect and quantitate helix content. The model proposed is shown in Fig. 6 and does accomodate some of the physical observations. It is as helical as can possibly be accomodated,

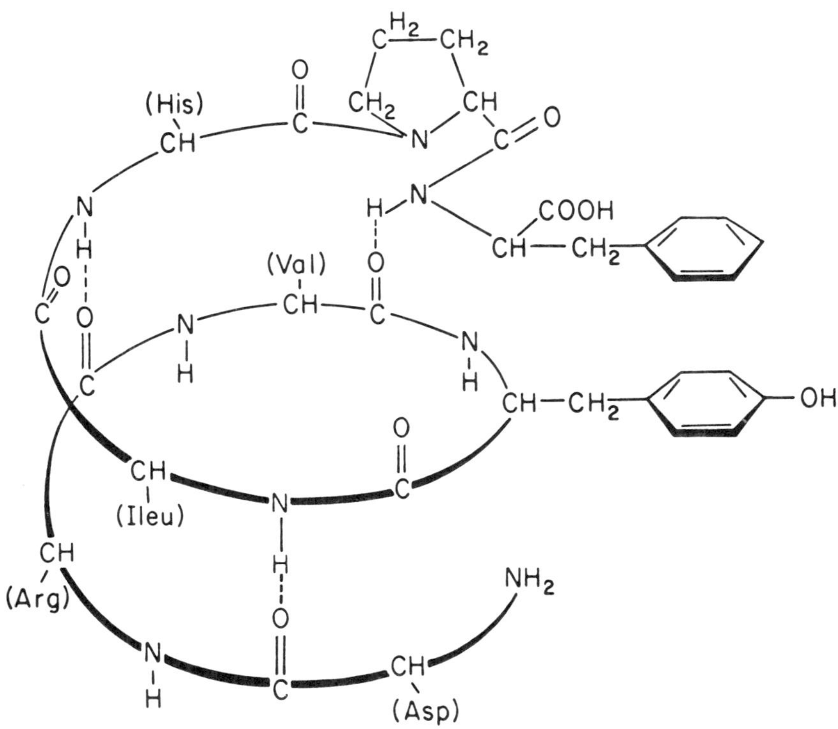

Fig. 6. First model proposed (Smeby *et al.*, 1962) for the solution conformation of angiotensin II.

with the assumption of hydrogen bonding of the Phe-8 amide proton to the Val-3 carbonyl as the Pro-7 amide does not have a proton to participate in the traditional α-helix bonding scheme. Other hydrogen bonds include the Val-5 amide proton to the Asn-1 carbonyl and the His-6 amide proton to the Arg-2 carbonyl. The Try-4 side chain is exposed to the solvent and does not participate in hydrogen bonding. While this model does accomodate some of the observed data, i.e. a hydrogen bond for the Val-5 amide and a free Tyr-4 hydroxyl, it is ruled out by other experiments. The hydrogen exchange data rule out participation of the His-6 amide in hydrogen bonding as well as the Phe-8 amide (at least at pH 2.5). Alpha helical angles ($\phi = -60°$) require J_{NHCH} to be approximately 3.3–3.8 Hz which is much lower than any of those observed in solution (Dadok, Glickson, and Marshall, 1974). In addition, the mean residue rotations for [Asn^1, Val^5]-angiotensin II calculated from the ORD spectra are at least an order of magnitude too low for significant helix content (Paiva *et al.*, 1963).

Random Conformation. Paiva *et al.* (1963) proposed that [Asn^1, Val^5]-angiotensin II exists in a random conformation in aqueous solution on the bases of hydrogen-deuterium exchange, titration, and ORD measurements. One assumes this to mean relatively free rotation about all the bonds in the molecule with no preferred time-averaged conformation but not simply equivalent to "neither α-helix nor β-pleated sheet." There is overwhelming physical data from NMR, hydrogen-tritium exchange, thin-film dialysis, circular dichroism, etc., that angiotensin exists in a preferred time-averaged conformation or sets of such conformers, the preponderant species depending on the conditions. How much rotational flexibility the molecule has remains to be determined, most likely by NMR relaxation measurements.

Nonhelix Model. Based on proposed helix-forming tendencies of each amino acid residue, Glauser *et al.* (1970) rejected the α-helix model and proposed an alternate "in accordance with the known behavior of polypeptides and proteins" which was described primarily by a series of photographs. Four major interactions were said to characterize this model: (1) hydrogen bonding between the side chains of Tyr-4 and His-6; (2) a hydrogen bond between the C-terminal carboxyl and the amide proton of Val-5; (3) an electrostatic interaction between the sidechains of Asp-1 and Arg-2; (4) hydrophobic bonding of the two valine and the phenylalanine sidechains. Nuclear magnetic resonance (Glickson *et al.*, 1973) effectively eliminates this model, since there is no effect on the Val-5 amide proton (amide 6) as the carboxylate is titrated and only slight reciprocal effects upon titration of either the tyrosine or histidine sidechains. Since there are observed conformational effects in the titration range of either His-6 or Tyr-4 and the pK's of the two groups are normal, the minor reciprocal perturbations are felt to be due to general conformational changes and not specific interactions.

Ion-Dipole Model. Weinkam and Jorgensen (1971b) proposed a preferred conformation for [des-Asp^1, Gly^2, Ile^5]-angiotensin II based on NMR measurements of the coupling constants in DMSO and ESR studies on a spin-labeled tripeptide analog of His-Pro-Phe (Weinkam and Jorgensen, 1971a). While this model may be relevant for the heptapeptide analog in DMSO, NMR spectra in aqueous solution for angiotensin show no perturbation of the histidine sidechain as the C-terminal carboxylate is titrated. Even more critical is the marked difference in coupling constants between water, J_{NHCH} (His-6) = 6.0 and J_{NHCH} (Tyr-4) = 7.2, and DMSO, J_{NHCH} (His-6) < 3 and J_{NHCH} (Tyr-4) < 3.

Beta-turn Model. Based on potential energy minimization techniques, Printz *et al.* (1972a) have proposed two specific conformations. The β-turn model has two hydrogen bonds, from the Val-3 NH to the His-6 carbonyl and from the His-6 NH to the Val-3 carbonyl. As Bleich *et al.* (1973) have pointed out, the exchange measurements rule out hydrogen bonding of the histidine NH. Marshall *et al.* (1973b) have also pointed out the inconsistency between coupling constants calculated from the model and those observed in solution.

Gamma-turn Model. The model preferred by Printz *et al.* (1972a) was the γ-turn model, which had the Val-3 NH hydrogen bonding to the Val-5 carbonyl and the Val-5 NH hydrogen bonding to the Val-3 carbonyl with a *cis* conformation of the proline amide bond. While the hydrogen-bond scheme fits the exchange data (Bleich *et al.*, 1973), the NMR data previously presented exclude the *cis* orientation for the proline peptide bond. In addition, Marshall *et al.* (1973b) have analyzed the coupling constants observed in NMR in terms of possible constraints on the torsional rotations about the NH-C*α*H bonds and find major discrepancies with those proposed for the γ-turn model. In particular, the γ-turn model leads to predicted values for coupling constants inconsistent with those observed. For example, the γ-turn model gives a predicted *J* of 2.5–3.2 Hz for the Val-3 amide and 4.5–4.7 Hz for the Phe-8 amide compared with the observed values of 7.9 Hz and 7.3 Hz respectively. The fact that the potential energy minimization procedure failed to predict a structure consistent with observed data can possibly be explained by the omission of solvent interactions from the calculations, overemphasis on the hydrogen-bond potential, or selection of local minima.

Cross β-Structure. Fermandjian *et al.* (1972b) have proposed a model based on their studies by circular dichroism, and infrared and Raman spectroscopy. It featured the *cis* orientation of the histidyl-proline peptide bond, hydrophobic interactions of the valine and phenylalanine sidechains, and a tyrosine sidechain free from interactions. In addition, hydrogen bonds between the Val-3 NH and His-6 carbonyl, and His-6 NH and Val-3 carbonyl are also shown. By virtue of its hydrogen-bonding scheme and *cis* orientation of the histidyl-proline bond, the model is excluded based on the exchange experiments of Bleich *et al.* (1973) and the analysis of the ^{13}C NMR presented previously which assigns the orientation of the histidyl-proline bond to the *trans* configuration.

Summary of Solution Studies

The combined results of the physical techniques used to study the solution conformation of [Asn^{1}, Val^{5}]-angiotensin II agree that this linear octapeptide, Asn-Arg-Val-Tyr-Val-His-Pro-Phe, has a time-averaged preferred solution conformation. In particular, the evidence from proton NMR indicates two conformational changes occurring as a function of pH, one with a pKa of 6.6 and the other with pKa of 10.2. The first conformational change would appear associated with the titration of either the N-terminal amino group (pKa = 6.98), or the imidazole of His-6 (pKa = 6.26), or more likely both. The second is associated with ionization of the phenolic hydroxyl of Tyr-4. Measurement and assignment of the NH-CαH vicinal coupling constants limit the possible values for the torsional rotations about the amide to α-carbon bond in [Asn^{1}, Val^{5}]-angiotensin II occurs in the *trans*-configuration. Exchange experiments indicate that the Val-3, Val-5, and possibly Tyr-4 amide protons are either involved in intramolecular hydrogen bonds or sterically protons are either involved in intramolecular hydrogen bonds or sterically shielded from the solvent. Studies of angiotensin analogs with a fluorine reporter group indicate that conformers whose rate of interchange is slow on the NMR time scale can occur in linear octapeptides. Combining these observations, it is possible to raise serious objections to all of the models proposed for the solution conformation of angiotensin II. Studies using a computer-based molecular modeling system (Barry *et al.*, 1972; Marshall *et al.*, 1972a) are underway to determine a model of angiotensin II consistent with the observations.

There is a wide variety of possible experiments which would offer insight and further constraints on the solution conformation of angiotensin II. An obvious approach would be the extension of the coupling-constant measurements to the α-β bond using the correlation recently proposed by Kopple, Wiley, and Tauke (1973) to determine the orientation of the amino acid sidechains. It has recently been proposed (Karplus and Karplus, 1972) to use the CαH-CN coupling constants to estimate the torsional rotation ψ about the α-carbon-carbonyl bond of the peptide backbone. While this would provide constraints for the second variable determining backbone conformation, it may require the introduction of ^{15}N into the amide group to be experimentally feasible. Perhaps the most critical experiments to be done are those measuring relaxation times for the various nuclei of the angiotensin molecule. This would allow an estimate of the rotational freedom around the various bonds in the molecule and shed new light on the problem of time-averaged conformation *versus* conformers whose interchange is slow. Lanthanide shift reagents may also be useful in determining the three-dimensional arrangement of groups in angiotensin II. Additional information of the proximity of sidechains can be obtained through nuclear Overhauser experiments and would place additional constraints on modeling.

RECEPTOR-BOUND CONFORMATION

While the solution conformation of angiotensin II is of interest in its own right and may shed important light on the interactions which determine conformation, the conformation assumed by angiotensin II while interacting with the receptor is of primary concern to those interested in the physiological and pathological roles of this hormone. Since the forces which determine the conformation are significantly different in the crystal, in solution, or when bound to the receptor (Marshall, 1970, 1971), it seemed appropriate to develop approaches which would allow one to infer constraints on the receptor-bound conformation based on structure-activity studies of peptide hormones (Marshall, 1970, 1971; Marshall and Bosshard, 1972; Marshall *et al.*, 1972b; Marshall *et al.*, 1973a). Our approach is somewhat analogous to the procedure used by Meister and co-workers (Glass and Meister, 1970; Meister, 1968) to determine the conformation at the active site of the substrate of glutamine synthetase. A report (Fermandjian *et al.*, 1971b) of small crystals of [Asn^1, Val^5]-angiotensin II from organic solvents may lead to the determination of the three-dimensional structure of the octapeptide in the crystalline environment. The progress in determining the solution conformation of angiotensin was summarized in the previous section. Determination of the receptor-bound conformation by solution techniques or even crystallography is theoretically feasible once the receptor is isolated in a homogenous state. Until then, indirect experiments using the biological response as an indicator of the correct orientation of function groups offer a method of determining constraints for the receptor-bound conformation.

Determination of Constraints

Systematic investigation (Marshall and Bosshard, 1972; Marshall *et al.*, 1972b) of the restrictions on conformational freedom[3] introduced by increasing the steric bulk of groups located on the peptide backbone was undertaken in order to reduce the inherent conformational flexibility available to a peptide hormone. In particular, the replacement of the hydrogen atoms of the peptide backbone by methyl groups, increasing the Van der Waals' radii from 1.2 to 1.85 Å has been investigated. The three categories of proton replacement examined were (1) the amide proton of the amino acid residue to give an N-methyl amino acid, (2) the α proton with a methyl group to give an α methyl amino acid, and (3) the amide proton of the subsequent amino acid, i.e., the effect of an N-methyl amino acid on a preceding residue. By assuming planarity of the amide bond due to its partial double-bond

[3]Conformational freedom is functionally defined and measured by referring to the area allowed on a plot of torsional rotation ϕ around the NH-CαH bond *versus* the torsional rotation ψ around the CαH-CO bond for a particular amino acid residue. This can be determined by calculations based on hard-sphere or other potential energy functions or by examination of large numbers of crystal structures.

character and spherical treatment of the methyl groups due to rapid rotation, the positions of all the atoms in space including the β carbon of the sidechain can be specified by torsional rotations about the NH-CαH (ϕ) and the CαH-CO (ψ) bonds of model compounds, N-acetyl-amino acid-methylamides.

In Figs. 7-10 are shown the results of calculations performed utilizing the Kitaigorodsky potential function (Venkatachalan and Ramachandran, 1967). These are similar to those obtained assuming a hard-sphere potential. The calculations for acetyl-L-alanine-methylamide (Fig. 7) show the agreement between the contours at 1 kcal/mole above the potential minimum and the values observed experimentally for 23 proteins (Marshall, Fritsch, and Bosshard, 1973c). The plot for N-acetyl-N-methyl-L-alanine methylamide (Fig. 8) is similar to that of the only common N-methyl amino acid found in proteins, proline. Because the torsional rotation ϕ about the NH-CαH bond in proline is required to be approximately $-60°$ by the cyclic imide (Balasubramanian *et al.*, 1971), all the values for proline should fall on a line where $\phi = -60°$. The scatter represents the error in the crystallographic determination, as proline would appear to serve as an internal standard. Proline values cluster in two regions: one at $\phi = -60°$, $\psi = -50°$ and the other at $\phi = -60°$, $\psi = 135°$. The plot for an amino acid preceding an N-methyl amino acid (Fig. 9) shows those experimental values for amino acids preceding proline. The allowed area is limited to positive values of ψ, except for a small area centered around the

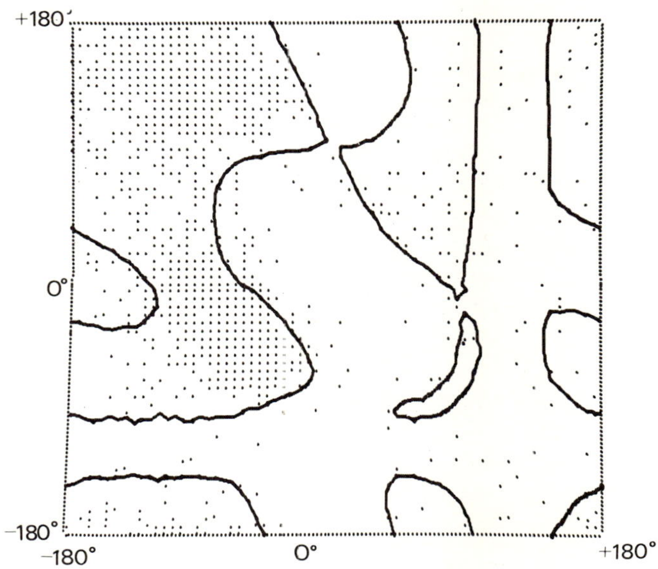

Fig. 7. Comparison of calculated allowed areas with values of ϕ and ψ observed in protein crystallography: plot for N-acetyl-L-alanine methylamide.

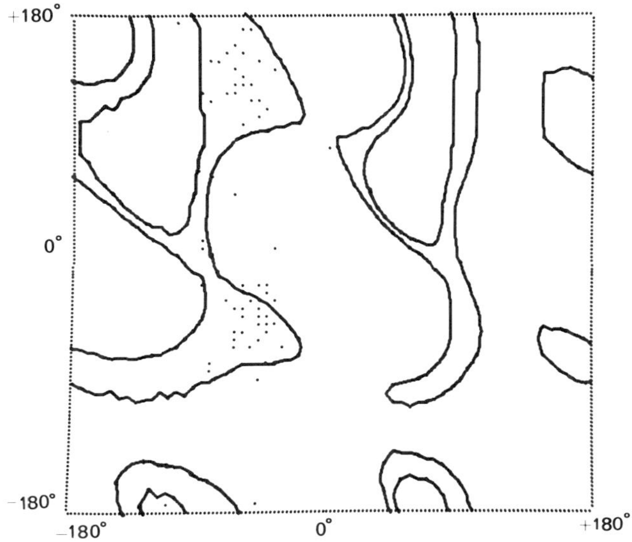

Fig. 8. Comparison of calculated allowed areas with values of ϕ and ψ observed in protein crystallography: plot for N-acetyl-N-methyl-L-alanine methyl-amide.

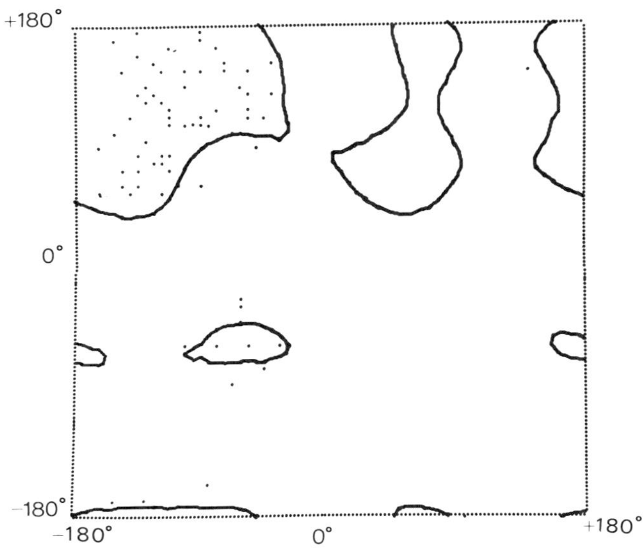

Fig. 9. Comparison of calculated allowed areas with values of ϕ and ψ observed in protein crystallography: plot for N-acetyl-L-alanine dimethylamide.

right-handed α-helix region ($\phi = -57°$, $\psi = -47°$). The plot for acetyl-amino-isobutyric methylamide (α-methylalanine) (Fig. 10) shows a marked restriction in conformational freedom with a decided preference for values associated with either a right-handed ($\phi = -57°$, $\psi = -47°$) or a left-handed ($\phi = 57°$, $\psi = 47°$) helical conformation.

The problem of interest is whether these calculated constraints apply to angiotensin when it binds to its receptor. Here the agreement with the observed values from protein crystallography offers some solace, as one would think that the range of interactions and potential distortions of the solution conformation which might occur on binding to the receptor had been adequately sampled by the interactions present in the folding of a large protein. In theory, a peptide would be expected to tolerate less distortion than a segment of a protein chain, as the end residues of the peptide can be moved without sacrificing a large number of energetically favorable interactions in order to relieve the local strain. Assuming these constraints are applicable to the angiotensin molecule and its analogs in association with the receptor, what information can we deduce with their use?

Examination of analogs of angiotensin in which chemical modification has introduced some of the constraints on conformational freedom has led to definite conclusions on the receptor-bound conformation. These conclusions depend strongly on one assumption which must be emphasized. Because the all-D analog of angiotensin is biologically inactive (von Vogler *et al.*, 1965), one can conclude that at least a three-point attachment to the receptor is

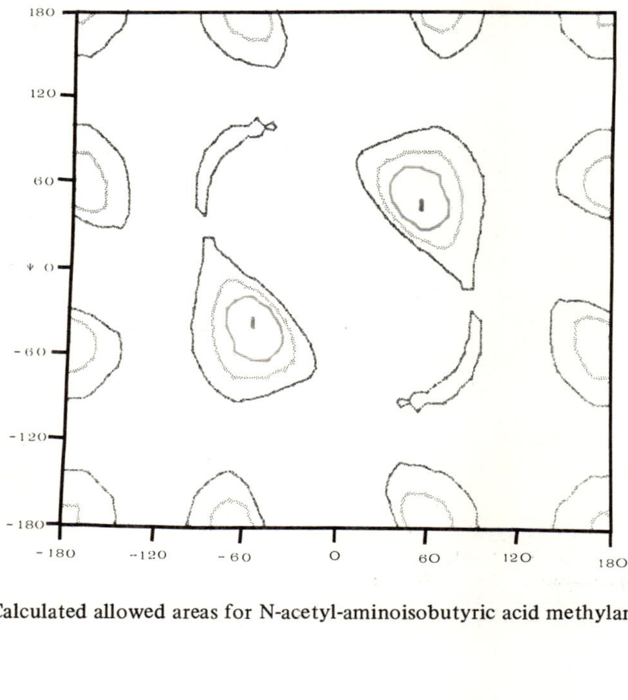

Fig. 10. Calculated allowed areas for N-acetyl-aminoisobutyric acid methylamide.

Table 5. Biological activity of angiotensin analogs with constraints on conformational freedom

Analog	Biological activity		Reference
	Rat pressor	Rat uterus	
[Asn^1, Val^5]-AII	100	100	
[Pro^3, Ile^5]-AII	40	80	Khosla *et al.*, 1968
[Aib^3, Val^5]-AII		1	Marshall *et al.*, 1972c
[Cle^3, Ile^5]-AII		1	Park *et al.*, 1972
[Leu^5]-AII	25		Schwyzer & Turrian, 1960
[Ala^5]-AII	5		Khosla *et al.*, 1968
[Pro^5]-AII	10		Jorgensen & Weinkam, 1973
[Aib^5]-AII	0.9		Marshall *et al.*, 1972c
[Cle^5]-AII	24		Jorgensen & Weinkam, 1973
[Cle^7]-AII		1	Park *et al.*, 1972
[Ala^7]-AII	0.83	1.4	Seu *et al.*, 1962
[Mal^7]-AII	22	4.3	Andreatta & Scheraga, 1971

Abbreviations: Aib, aminoisobutyric acid; Cle, 1-aminocyclopentane carboxylic acid; Mal, N-methyl-L-alanine; AII, angiotensin II.

necessary for activity. If the critical spatial orientation of the three or more groups can be accomplished by quite different backbone conformations, then the conclusions which follow are invalidated. It is assumed that the exquisite sensitivity and specificity associated with the interaction of angiotensin and its receptor preclude this possibility.

In Table 5 are listed several analogs of angiotensin II with their biological activity. The high activity associated with [Pro^3, Val^5]-angiotensin II of 40% and 80% in the two bioassays indicates that the constraint imposed by the cyclic imide ($\phi = -60°$) does not perturb the receptor-bound conformation to any degree. Since proline has only two possible conformational regions to occupy, substitution of an α-methyl residue which can occupy one of the two open to proline should prove instructive. Both [Aib^3, Val^5]-angiotensin II and [Cle^3, Ile^5]-angiotensin II show only 1% activity while complete omission of the Asp-Arg dipeptide only reduced the activity to 0.3% (Schattenkerk and Havinga, 1965). One is tempted to use the reduction of activity with an amino acid analog which can occupy only one of the two choices open to proline to eliminate the region common to both from consideration, i.e., $\psi_3 \simeq -135°$ for the active conformation. Reduction of activity could, however, occur from a variety of causes: increased degradation, steric interference of the α-methyl group with binding, etc. In any case, the high activity of the Pro-3 analog also makes it likely that the value of ψ_2 for Arg-2 is either positive, or $\phi_2 = -57°$, $\psi_2 = -47°$.

The substitution of proline for Val-5 also leads to relatively high activity (10%). Here substitution of cycloleucine, an α-methyl amino acid, retains

24% activity. Since the only region common to both substituted amino acids is that, associated with the right-handed α helix, the values for ϕ_3 and ψ_3 must be near −57° and −47° respectively at the receptor. The activity of the N-methyl residue at position 5 imposes constraints on position 4. Tyr-4 has either a positive value for ψ_4 or right-handed α-helical values. Position 7 is normally occupied by a proline. This imposes the N-methyl constraints on the preceding amino acid, His-6. The requirement for the N-methyl effect is substantiated somewhat by the higher activity of the N-methyl alanine analog compared with the alanine analog in position 7.

Comparison with Solution Conformation

Table 6 summarizes the conformational constraints which have been imposed on the receptor-bound conformation based on structure-activity studies. Marshall *et al.* (1973a) have compared these constraints with the possible values of ϕ for angiotensin based on the experimental coupling constants. It is particularly informative to compare the values for Val-3 and Val-5 by looking at the calculated coupling constants for the receptor-bound conformation. A torsional rotation of −60° would give 3.8 Hz by the formula of Ramachandran *et al.* (1971) and 3.3 Hz by that of Bystrov *et al.* (1973). This is considerably outside the range of 7.9 ± 0.3 Hz and 8.0 ± 0.4 Hz observed for Val-3 and Val-5 respectively. As there is no procedure available for preferring one of the four possible torsional rotations associated with a J_{NHCH}, the solution value for ϕ_3 could be −153°, −87°, 43°, or 77°, using the Bystrov *et al.* (1973) correlation since it gives values closest to those anticipated at the receptor. Assuming the value closest to that required for the Pro-3 analog of angiotensin, i.e., −87°, then a conformational change of 27° is still required to accomodate the solution conformation to that present at the receptor. Similar arguments give essentially the same value for the minimal change in ϕ_5. While it might be possible to ignore one of these required changes, the two together plus the likelihood that the conformational change might be much greater if the solution conformation actually prefers ϕ_3 = −153°, 43°, or 77°, requires only one possible conclusion. There is a conformational change of [Asn^1, Val^5]-angiotensin II from the time-averaged preferred

Table 6. Probable constraints on the receptor-bound conformation of angiotensin II

Residue	Amino acid	ϕ	ψ	Relevant analog
2	Arg		Positive	Pro^3
3	Val	−60°	+135°±45°	Pro^3; Ala^3; Aib^3; des-Asp^1, Arg^2
4	Tyr		Positive	Pro^5
5	Val	−60°±15°	−47°±15°	Aib^5; Cle^5; Pro^5
6	His		Positive	Mal^7, native
7	Pro	−60°		Native

solution conformation which is induced on binding to the receptor. Furthermore, solution studies indicate hydrogen bonding of the amide protons of Val-3 and Val-5 as contributing to the stabilization of the solution conformation. Substitution of proline at either position precludes the stabilization due to the hydrogen bond at that residue, as proline is an N-methyl amino acid and has no amide proton to contribute.

Considering the conformational lability of angiotensin II evident in solution studies, one should not be surprised that interaction with a receptor, which may include electrostatic, hydrogen-bonding, and hydrophobic interactions, effects the conformation of the peptide hormone. Evidence exists in another system that binding of a peptide to a protein induces a conformational change from that observed in solution. Finn, Dadok, and Bothner-By (1972) and Chaiken *et al.* (1973) have studied the binding of S-peptide to S-protein to form ribonuclease-S′. Upon binding of the peptide to the protein which generates enzymatic activity, a helical segment from residue 2-12, which is not present in a solution of the dissociated peptide, is induced in the peptide as seen in the crystal structure (Finn and Hofmann, 1973).

The implications of these findings are widespread. One of the factors encouraging the study of solution conformation of peptide hormones was the hope that this information would prove useful in understanding structure-activity relations. Unfortunately, the temptation to use models based on solution data to interpret analog activity and even project further to interrelations of the receptor has been too prevalent (Printz *et al.*, 1972a; Walter *et al.*, 1971).

RECEPTOR INTERACTION

The ultimate goal, of course, is to understand the interactions with the receptor which govern binding and activation of subsequent processes leading to the physiological response. Already the isolation of cell membranes enriched in binding sites for angiotensin has been reported (Meyer *et al.*, 1972). Further purification and characterization of these 'receptors' as well as their role in subsequent processes offers hope for the future. For the present and from the past, one can make some inferences from structure-activity studies.

Effects of pH.

The action of angiotensin could involve electrostatic binding of the peptide to charged groups in the receptor and, therefore, be influenced by the hydrogen ion concentration. Investigation of the effects of pH on the responsiveness of rat uterine strips to [Asn^1, Val^5]-angiotensin II showed a 100-fold shift of the dose-response curve with a change of pH from 6.8 to 8.6 (Needleman, Freer, and Marshall, 1972a) as shown in Fig. 11. A number of possibilities may be invoked to explain this increase in sensitivity with increasing pH: (a) pH affects the protonation of a group in angiotensin critically involved in an electrostatic interaction with the receptor; (b) pH affects the conforma-

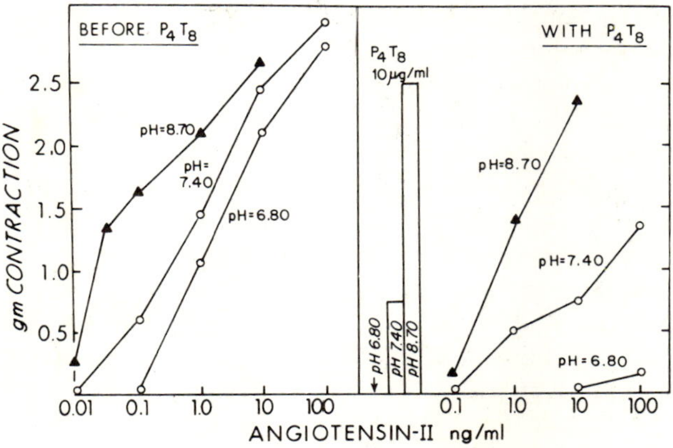

Fig. 11. Dose-response curve measuring uterine contraction induced by angiotensin II in the absence and presence of [Phe⁴, Tyr⁸]-angiotensin II at different pH's. The curves represent the angiotensin response and the bar graphs the response produced by [Phe⁴, Tyr⁸]-angiotensin II alone.

tion of angiotensin II increasing the more active conformation at high pH; (c) pH affects the ionization and/or conformation of the receptor in a critical way; (d) pH alters some necessary intermediary process involving ion permeability, etc.; (e) pH alters excitation-contraction coupling.

Since a conformational change occurs at approximately pH 6.6 and both the N-terminal amino group and imidazole of His-6 titrate in this range, some combination of the conformational or ionic change in the angiotensin molecule could explain these results. In order to exclude these possibilities, Needleman *et al.* (1972a) examined an analog of angiotensin prepared by Hofmann *et al.* (1968) in which His-6 was replaced by an isosteric analog, β-(3-pyrazolyl)-L-alanine, which has a pK_a of 2–3. In the range of 6.8–8.6 the degree of ionization of the histidine analog would not change significantly, while that of the histidine moiety of angiotensin II (pK_a = 6.26) would be modified considerably. The analog showed a similar increase in activity upon changing to the more alkaline conditions. Further studies (Needleman, Marshall, and Rivier, 1973b) using an analog, 3-methyl-histidine, which should increase the pK of the imidazole by approximately 0.5 pH units did not modify the increase in sensitivity with alkaline conditions. Needleman *et al.* (1973b) also prepared and tested the N-acetyl derivative of [Asn¹, Val⁵]-angiotensin II. The fact that this analog also showed increased sensitivity upon changing to more alkaline conditions excluded the possibility that changes in angiotensin itself, either ionic or conformational, were responsible for the observed changes in sensitivity.

This finding strongly supports the conclusions about a conformational transition in angiotensin II upon binding to the receptor. Since the amide coupling constants were determined at acid pH owing to line broadening at higher pH, it could have been argued that the conformational transition at pH 6.6 leads to a conformation identical to that which binds to the receptor. Because the binding constant could be greater, the resulting sensitivity would increase above pH 6.6. In other words, alkaline pH would cause the 'active' species to predominate in solution which could interact effectively at lower concentrations with the receptor. The fact that both modification of the amino group of Asn-1 and the imidazole groups of His-6 did not eliminate this pH-dependent sensitivity of the rat uterus indicates the improbable nature of the above interpretation.

Additional confirmation of the primary role of the receptor and/or subsequent processes in the pH effect comes from similar studies (Walaszek and Dyer, 1966) on the isolated guinea pig ileum, in which the sensitivity to angiotensin is relatively constant from pH 5–9 and shows a marked increase at pH 10. This is similar to the potentiation of the pressor effects of angiotensin by alkaline solution (pH 11) reported by Paladini, Delius, and Franze de Fernandez (1963). These studies imply that the properties of the receptor differ from tissue to tissue, and that the groups susceptible to pH modification of the medium are on the cell surface since the buffering capacity of the cell would be expected to keep the intracellular pH at a relatively constant value.

Inhibitors of Angiotensin II

While inhibitors of the renin-angiotensin system offer a unique tool for the study of the physiological, pharmacological, and pathological role of angiotensin (Marshall, Vine, and Needleman, 1970; Marshall, 1971; Pals *et al.*, 1971a,b; Brunner *et al.*, 1971; Needleman *et al.*, 1973a), the inhibitors also can contribute to our understanding of the hormone-receptor interaction. The fact that these compounds compete for binding to the receptor site without activating the subsequent processes leading to the physiological response indicates that some parts of the angiotensin molecule are primarily involved in binding while others are necessary for initiating the physiological response. As pointed out by Rudinger, Pliska, and Krejci (1972) for oxytocin analogs, the fact that a competitive inhibitor exists would appear to argue in favor of a 'participation' model of hormone action rather than a pure allosteric model. The evidence is not compelling, however. In an inhibitor the groups necessary for the physiological response would be missing or misaligned in the 'participation' model. The inhibitor would bind and yet fail to induce the conformational change in the allosteric model. One model on which the 'participation model' has been based (Finn and Hofmann, 1973) is the completion of the active site of ribonuclease S′ by the binding of the S-peptide to S-protein. One of the imidazole groups essential for activity in ribonuclease, His-12, is contributed by the peptide. In order for a peptide hormone to participate in a similar mechanism, one or more functional groups should be essential for the biological activity. The analogs of angio-

Table 7. Elimination of functional groups in angiotensin essential for biological activity

Group	Replaced Residue	Analog	Biological Activity (%)[a] Pressor	Oxytocic
α-Amino	Asp-1	Succinic acid	50	51
		Pyroglutamic acid	100	
		N-Acetyl-Asn	50	
β-Carboxyl	Asp-1	Asn	100	100
		Pyroglutamic acid	100	
		Gly	50	27
Guanidinum	Arg-2	Val	5	
		Orn	20	
		Arg (NO_2)	50	3
Phenol	Tyr-4	Phe	10	2.5
Imidazole	His-6	3-Pyrazolyl-L-alanine	79[b]	52[b]
		3-Methyl-L-His	5[c]	10[c]
C-Terminal Carboxyl	Phe-8	Phe-NH_2	3	
		Angiotensin I		
		Phe-OMe	10	

[a]Activities are taken from Page and McCubbin (1969) (unless otherwise indicated).
[b]Hofmann *et al.* 1968.
[c]Needleman *et al.*, 1973b.

tensin II listed in Table 7 indicate that all the groups which might be expected to contribute to an enzymatic active site have been eliminated individually while still maintaining significant activity. Participation of the carbonyl functions of the amide bonds in ion binding, as seen in ionophores such as valinomycin or enniatin, has not been eliminated, but neither has it been suggested on the basis of any experimental evidence. The evidence available would, therefore, support the allosteric model of hormone-receptor interaction for angiotensin II. Direct studies on the angiotensin-receptor interaction may be necessary to confirm this choice.

The first specific competitive inhibitor of angiotensin shown to be effective *in vitro* and *in vivo* was [Phe^4, Tyr^8]-angiotensin II (Marshall *et al.*, 1970). Khairallah, Toth, and Bumpus (1970) reported studies on [Ile^5, Ala^8]-angiotensin II which suggested that this compound showed cross-tachyphylaxis with angiotensin II on isolated guinea pig ileum, with 0.1% myotropic activity and 0.1% activity in the pressor assay. Turker *et al.* (1971) reported that further studies on [Ala^8]-angiotensin II demonstrated its action as a competitive antagonist on isolated rabbit aorta and rat ascending colon. Gagnon, Park, and Regoli (1971) also reported competitive antagonism for [Ala^8]-angiotensin II as well as for [D-Phe^8]-angiotensin II on the isolated rat colon assay. The peptide did not, however, antagonize the pressor and intestinal inhibitory effect of angiotensin when given intravenously to anesthetized cats (Turker *et al.*, 1971). In contrast, Pals *et al.* (1971b) showed that [Asn^1, Val^5, Ala^8]-angiotensin II was a competitive antagonist both *in vitro* with rabbit aorta strips and *in vivo* in the pressor assay on both conscious and pithed rats when infused. Park and Regoli (1971) confirmed the *in vivo* antagonism of [Phe^4, Tyr^8]-angiotensin II and [Ala^8]-angiotensin II, as well as reporting *in vivo* and *in vitro* antagonist data for analogs containing D-phenylalanine, cycloleucine (1-aminocyclopentanecarboxylic acid), or 1-aminocyclohexanecarboxylic acid substituted for Phe-8. Further improvements in potency and length of action of the inhibitors have been obtained by modification in positions 1 and 8 as shown in Table 8. Of possible pharmaceutical interest is the fact that substitution of sarcosine (N-methyl-glycine) in the one position increases both potency and duration of action (Pals *et al.*, 1971a; Turker *et al.*, 1972; Rioux, Park, and Regoli, 1973; Regoli, Park, and Rioux, 1973). Also of practical importance is the increased antagonist activity of [Ile^5, Ile^8]-angiotensin II (Khosla *et al.*, 1972a,b; Yamamoto *et al.*, 1972) and [Val^5, Cys^8]-angiotensin II (Needleman *et al.*, 1972b,c). Of particular interest to structure-activity studies is the inhibitory activity of [pFPhe^4, Val^5]-angiotensin II recently reported (Needleman *et al.*, 1972b,c; Vine *et al.*, 1973). This represents the first competitive antagonist of angiotensin in which the modification has been solely at the 4 position and implicates the 4 position as well as the 8 position in the activation process.

The implication of both Tyr-4 and Phe-8 sidechains in the activation process is consistent with the inhibitory activity of [Phe^4, Tyr^8]-angiotensin II. Single substitution of phenylalanine for tyrosine in [Phe^4]-angiotensin II or tyrosine for phenylalanine in [Tyr^8]-angiotensin II gives analogs with 10% and 83% activity and no antagonist activity. In other words, a compound with no phenolic hydroxyl groups, [Phe^4]-angiotensin II, or two phenolic hydroxyl groups, [Tyr^8]-angiotensin, has good intrinsic activity similar to that of the native hormone with one hydroxyl at the 4 position, while the competitive antagonist has a single phenolic hydroxyl at position 8. Insight into the unique inhibitory activity seen with [Phe^4, Tyr^8]-angiotensin II comes from the studies of Needleman *et al.* (1972a) which showed a striking reversal of the properties of the antagonist on isolated rat uterus by elevating the pH. At pH 8.6 [Phe^4, Tyr^8]-angiotensin II is a potent agonist with approximately the same concentration requirements for activity as for antagonism at pH 6.8 (Fig. 11). From these observations, it can be suggested that [Phe^4, Tyr^8]-angiotensin II may possess an intrinsic activity too low to activate fully the subsequent processes leading to contraction. An increase in

Table 8. Competitive inhibitors of angiotensin

Analog	Antagonist Activity[a]		Agonistic activity[a]	References
	In vitro	*In vivo*		
$[Phe^4, Tyr^8]$-AII	36:1(1)	+(5)	0.0025%(5)	Marshall *et al.*, 1970
	48:1(1)	+(5,8)		Needleman *et al.*, 1972b,c
	+(4,7)		0.1%(12)	Needleman *et al.*, 1973b
	5000:1(2)	50:1(5)		Park & Regoli, 1971
			+(5)	Regoli & Park, 1972
$[Ala^8]$-AII	125:1(3)		25/(9), 2%(5)	Peach *et al.*, 1969
	125:1(3)		0.1%(3), (5)	Khairallah *et al.*, 1970
	pA_2=8.3(11)	Negative(12)		Turker *et al.*, 1971
	+(2)			
	125:1(2)	50:1(5)		Park & Regoli, 1971
				Regoli & Park, 1972
	pA_2=6.8(11)	+(5)	+(5)	Pals·*et al.*, 1971[b]
	+(2)			Gagnon *et al.*, 1971
	pA_2=6.8(12)			Rioux *et al.*, 1971
	+(4)			Regoli, 1972
	+(4,7)			Needleman *et al.*, 1973a
$[D\text{-}Phe]^8$-AII	+(2)			Gagnon *et al.*, 1971
	500:1(2)	100:1(5)		Park & Regoli, 1972
				Regoli & Park, 1972
	pA_2=6.1(12)			Rioux *et al.*, 1971
	+(4)			Regoli, 1972

[Cle^8]=AII	250:1(2)	50:1(5)		Park & Regoli, 1971
	pA_2=5.7(12)			Rioux *et al.*, 1971
	+(4)			Regoli, 1972
[Ach^8]-AII	500:1(2)	100:1(5)		Park & Regoli, 1971
	pA_2=5.3(12)			Rioux *et al.*, 1971
	+(4)			Regoli, 1972
[Abu^8]-AII	pK_B=8.04(12)	+(5)		Regoli *et al.*, 1971
[Asn^1,Abu^8]-AII	pA_2=7.93(11)			Fessler *et al.*, 1972
[Leu^8]-AII	pK_B=9.03(12)	+(5)		Regoli *et al.*, 1971
	+(11)	+(5,12)	1.3%(5,13)	Khosla *et al.*, 1972a,b
[Asn^1,Leu^8]-AII	pA_2=8.26(11)			Fessler *et al.*, 1972
[Val^8]-AII	pK_B=7.94(12)	+(5)		Regoli *et al.*, 1971
	+(11)	+(5,12)	0.5%(5,13)	Khosla *et al.*, 1972a,b
[Asn^1,Val^8]=AII	pA_2=8.31(11)			Fessler *et al.*, 1972
[Ile^8]-AII	pA_2=9.21	+(5,13)	1	Khosla *et al.*, 1972a,b
	pK_2=8.86(1,11)			
	pK_2=9.47(11)	+(5,13)	0.33%(5,13)	Yamamoto *et al.*, 1972
	pK_B=8.36(12)	+(5)		Regoli *et al.*, 1971
	1:1(1)	3:1(5)		Needleman *et al.*, 1972b,c
	1:1(12)			Rioux *et al.*, 1972a
	+(4,7)			Needleman *et al.*, 1973a
[Asn^1,Gly^8]-AII	pA_2=6.54(11)			Fessler *et al.*, 1972
[Gly^8]-AII	pA_2=6.7(12)			Rioux *et al.*, 1973
[Asn^1,β-Ala^8] AII	pA_2=5.08(11)			Fessler *et al.*, 1972

Table 8 (continued)

Analog	Antagonist Activity[a] *In vitro*	Antagonist Activity[a] *In vivo*	Agonistic Activity[a]	References
[Cha^8]-AII	+(11)	+(5,12)	20%(11,5,12)	Khosla *et al.*, 1972a,b
[Phe^4,Ala^8]-AII	+(11)		0.001%(5,12) negligible(11)	Khosla *et al.*, 1972a,b
[Suc^1,Phe^4,Tyr^8]-AII		Negative(5)	0.19%(5)	Khosla *et al.*, 1972a,b
[Sar^1,Ile^8]-AII	+(11) pK_2=9.33(11)	+(13) 10X[Ile^8]-AII	+(13)	Turker *et al.*, 1972
			1%(5)	Khosla *et al.*, 1972a,b
[Sar^1,Ala^8]-AII	pA_2=8.61(11) 60X[Ala^8]-AII	+(5) 50X[Ala^8]-AII	+(5)	Pals *et al.*, 1971a
[Sar^1,Leu^8]-AII	pA_2=8.6(12) 1:1(12)			Rioux *et al.*, 1973
[$pFPhe^4$]-AII	100:1(1) +(7)	40:1(5) +(8)		Needleman *et al.*, 1972b,c Vine *et al.*, 1973
[Cys^8]-AII	1.2:1(1)	5:1(5) +(8)		Needleman *et al.*, 1972b,c
	+(4,7) +(6)			Needleman *et al.*, 1973a Douglas *et al.*, 1973
[Phe^4,Tyr^8]-AII	500:1(1)	+(8)		Needleman *et al.*, 1972b,c

[Ile^8]-AII	2000:1(1) +(4,7)	300:1(5),+(8)		Needleman *et al.*, 1972b,c
	pA_2=7.3(1) pA_2=7.9(3) pA_2=8.0(11)	+(5)		Paiva *et al.*, 1973
[Val^8]-AI	pA_2=7.3(1) pA_2=7.9(3) pA_2=8.0(11)	+(5)		Paiva *et al.*, 1973
[Chl^1]-AII	+(3) Up to 8 hr		20%(1),+(5)	Paiva *et al.*, 1972
Chl-AII	+(3) Up to 8 hr		20%(1),+(5)	Paiva *et al.*, 972
[Chl^1,Val^8]-AI	pA_2=7.4(1) pA_2=7.5(3) pA_2=7.6(11)	+(5)		Paiva *et al.*, 1973

Abbreviations: Cle, l-aminocyclopentanecarboxylic acid; Ach, l-aminocyclohexylcarboxylic acid; Abu, l-amino-*N*-butyric acid; Cha, β-cyclohexyl-L-alanine; Suc, succinic acid; Sar, N-methyl-glycine; pFPhe, *p*-fluorophenylalanine; Chl, chlorambucil; AI, angiotensin I; AII, angiotensin II.

[a]Assay systems: 1, isolated rat uterus; 2, isolated rat colon; 3, isolated guinea pig ileum; 4, perfusion pressure (isolated kidney); 5, rat pressor assay; 6, prostaglandin release (spleen); 7, prostaglandin release (kidney); 8, acute renal hypertensive model; 9, inhibition of norepinephrine uptake; 10, catecholanine release from isolated adrenals; 11, isolated rabbit aorta; 12, isolated rat stomach strip; 13, cat pressor assay.

pH either increases the intrinsic activity by forcing a realignment of certain groups, or decreases the stimulus threshold necessary for activity. The latter hypothesis is more plausible owing to the increased activity of angiotensin II at alkaline pH, a shift of approximately 100-fold in sensitivity (Needleman *et al.,* 1972a). Needleman *et al.* (1972c) reported similar conversion from antagonism to agonism by increasing the pH from 6.8 to 8.6 for [pFPhe^4]-angiotensin II and [Ile^8]-angiotensin I. Interestingly enough, [Ile^8]-angiotensin II and [Cys^8]-angiotensin II retained their antagonistic properties at pH 8.6 even though they were about 10-fold less potent as antagonists to angiotensin II at the elevated pH. This may indicate that there was a decrease in the threshold for initiation of contraction by angiotensin II sufficient to increase its sensitivity, but not sufficient to lower the threshold to allow the 8-substituted octapeptide analogs to exhibit agonist activity. The case for [Phe^4, Tyr^8]-angiotensin II, [pFPhe^4]-angiotensin II, and [Ile^8]-angiotensin I would imply that their intrinsic activity was greater than [Ile^8]-angiotensin II and [Cys^8]-angiotensin II and sufficient to cause contraction in view of the lowered threshold.

One possible explanation of a lowered threshold would be a higher intracellular concentration of calcium due to the reported higher influx of Ca^{2+} at elevated pH (van Breemen *et al.,* 1972). This might explain the increased sensitivity and spontaneous activity seen at pH 8.6. An alternate mechanism involves the spike-generating mechanism which appears to involve Ca^{2+} rather than Na^+ in smooth muscle (Nonomura, Hotta, and Ohashi, 1966) such as the taenia coli of the guinea pig, where tetrodotoxin, a known inhibitor of the Na^+ spike, was ineffective. Tetrodotoxin similarly does not affect the contractions of isolated rat uterus induced by angiotensin (Needleman and Marshall, unpublished). It is interesting that addition of Mg^{2+} to the assay solution at pH 8.6 returned the agonistic behavior of [Phe^4, Tyr^8]-angiotensin to that of an inhibitor (Needleman *et al.,* 1972a). In studies on tachyphylaxis at pH 6.8 associated with a positively charged residue at position six, Stewart and Freer (1972) reported that the tachyphylaxis could be reversed either by increasing the pH to 8.6 or increasing the Ca^{2+} concentration at pH 6.8. An anionic site near the receptor which could either bind tightly to the positively charged residue at position 6 to give tachyphylaxis or be neutralized by binding Ca^{2+} was proposed. An alternative explanation would be that the threshold was lowered either by increasing the pH or by increasing the Ca^{2+} concentration sufficiently that the added angiotensin could overcome the inhibition associated with the tachyphylaxis. It is hard to understand how the competition of Mg^{2+} for the anionic site binding Ca^{2+} would retain the tight association between the tachyphylactic peptide, or an inhibitor, and the anionic site. It seems more plausible that the Mg^{2+} is competing with Ca^{2+} for the intracellular pool or some other Ca^{2+} pool and preventing the lowering of the threshold associated with the increased Ca^{2+} influx. These findings are consistent with an interpretation based on receptor reserve and threshold (Krejci, Pliska, and Rudinger, 1970; Eggena, Schwartz and Walter, 1970).

Another interesting approach is that of affinity labels (Shaw, 1970) in which an activated group is incorporated into the peptide in hopes of forming a covalent bond with the receptor. This should lead to a specific long-acting antagonist exhibiting noncompetitive kinetics. This has proven to be the case *in vitro* with the bromoacetyl derivative of oxytocin (Walter *et al.*, 1972). Paiva *et al.* (1972) have incorporated *p*-[*N*, *N*-bis(2-chloroethyl)-amino]-phenylbutyric acid or chlorombucil (Chl), a nitrogen mustard derivative of phenylbutyric acid, as a terminating residue by reaction with the α-amino group of angiotensin II and C-terminal fragments of angiotensin. In the guinea pig assay the application of these derivatives gave long-acting inhibition, but it was not possible to obtain more than a 50% reduction in the maximal response. In addition, the compounds were agonistic, showing 20% activity in the rat uterus assay and a low order of activity in pressor assays which did not alter the subsequent response to angiotensin. This general approach, however, offers applications to receptor identification by specific labeling with a radioactive analog as well as the potential for organ-specific inhibition. Receptor differences have been suggested during the work on inhibitors; for example, the agonistic activity of [Ala^8]-angiotensin II in the assay for inhibition of norepinephrine uptake in sympathetic nerve endings in rabbit heart (Peach *et al.*, 1969) and in the release of catecholamine from perfused adrenals (Peach, 1971). While it may be possible to make use of these receptor differences to distinguish between some of the multitude of physiological and pharmacological activities of angiotensin I and II, the apparent similarity in receptor specificity in most assay systems would argue that the receptor in all tissues has some common biological precursor, and the structural features necessary for recognition and binding of angiotensin are shared. The evolutionary pressure to preserve the exquisite sensitivity and selectivity to angiotensin may preclude the possible development of competitive antagonists specific for each of the tissues responsive to angiotensin and hinder potential therapeutic applications. It would appear more reasonable to expect differences in functional groups adjacent to the binding site in the receptor as they have been less constrained by evolution. Thus, by placement of activated groups at various positions in the hormone molecule, one might expect tissue specificity of inhibition due to differences in nucleophilic or electrophilic groups adjacent to the receptor binding site.

Mechanism of Action

The basis of the pressor activity of angiotensin is the increase of peripheral resistance by smooth muscle contraction. Meyer and co-workers (d'Auriac, Baudouin, and Meyer, 1972; Baudouin *et al.*, 1972; Meyer *et al.*, 1972) have presented evidence for a proposed mechanism of action of angiotensin on smooth muscle. This mechanism involves inhibition of Ca^{2+} uptake by the sarcoplasmic reticulum which leads to an increased intracellular concentration of Ca^{2+} and contraction of the myofilaments. Since relaxation in smooth muscle has been associated with increases in cAMP (Triner *et al.*, 1970), it is postulated that angiotensin II reduces intracellular cAMP either by adenyl cyclase inhibition or by activation of phosphodiesterase. While this mechanism supplies many potential answers, many critical experiments remain before it can be accepted. In strong contrast to the uterus, the action of angiotensin to increase the production of aldosterone by the adrenal is not associated with a change in cAMP levels, while potassium and ACTH stimulation of aldosterone production are accompanied by elevated levels of cAMP (Saruta, Cook, and Kaplan, 1972).

CONCLUSION

Although the solution conformation of angiotensin has been under investigation for more than a decade, no model has yet been proposed which is consistent with the enormous number of observations which have been made by physical techniques. The observations are consistent with time-averaged preferred conformations which are sensitive to the environment, undergoing conformational transition with alterations in pH, solvent, or interaction with the receptor. This latter point is important owing to the tendency to postulate properties of the hormone-receptor interaction based on solution models.

The evidence predominates that the receptor in smooth muscle is located on the cell surface and that effects on Ca^{2+} transport either directly or indirectly via cAMP or other mechanisms underlie the action of angiotensin on this tissue. Recent discoveries of compounds with high affinities and low intrinsic activity have given the physiologist, pharmacologist, and, hopefully, the physician a useful tool in determining and modifying the ever expanding role of angiotensin in normal and pathological conditions.

ACKNOWLEDGMENTS

The authors acknowledge funding from the National Institutes of Health (AM13025, HE 14509, HE 14397, and RR 00396) as well as from the American Heart Association (68-722 and 70-672). In addition, Drs. Needleman and Marshall are Established Investigators of the American Heart Association. One of us (HEB) acknowledges a long-term fellowship from the European Molecular Biology Organization and another (WHV) a graduate fellowship in the Medical Scientist Training Program (NIH GM0-2016). In addition, the encouragement and discussions of Dan Urry, Charles Molnar, and many others are gratefully acknowledged.

REFERENCES

Andreatta, R.H., and H.A. Scheraga. 1971. Synthesis of [5-valine, 7-N-methylalanine]-angiotensin II, a hypertensive peptide. J. Med. Chem. 14: 489.

Balasubramanian, R., A. V. Lakshminarayanan, M. N. Sabesan, G. Tegoni, K. Venkatesan, and G.N. Ramachandran, 1971. Studies on the conformation of amino acids. VI. Conformation of the proline ring as observed in crystal structures of amino acids and peptides. Int. J. Protein Res. 3: 25.

Barry, C.D., R.A. Ellis, S.M. Graesser, and G.R. Marshall. 1972. CHEMAST: A computer program for modelling molecular structures. *In* Information Processing 71, North-Holland, Amsterdam, pp. 1552–1557.

Baudouin, M., P. Meyer, S. Fermandjian, and J.-L. Morgat. 1972. Calcium release induced by interaction of angiotensin with its receptors in smooth muscle cell microsomes. Nature (Lond.) 235:336.

Berger, A., A. Loewenstein, and S. Meiboom. 1959. Nuclear magnetic resonance study of the protolysis and ionization of N-methylacetamide. J. Am. Chem. Soc. 81:62.

Bleich, H.E., R.E. Galardy, and M.P. Printz. 1973. Conformation of angiotensin II in aqueous solution. Evidence for the γ-turn model. J. Am. Chem. Soc. 95:2041.

Bovey, F.A. 1972. NMR in the conformational analysis of polypeptides, especially cyclic polypeptides. *In* J. Meienhofer (ed.), Chemistry and Biology of Peptides, Proceedings of 3rd American Peptide Symposium, Ann Arbor Science Publishing Co., Ann Arbor, Michigan, pp. 3–28.

Brunner, H.R., J.D. Kirshman, J.E. Sealey, and J.H. Laragh. 1971. Hypertension of renal origin: evidence for two different mechanisms. Science 174:1344.

Bystrov, V.F., V.T. Ivanov, S.L. Portnova, T.A. Balashova, and Yu. A. Ovchinnikov. 1973. Refinement of the angular dependence of the peptide vicinal NH-CαH coupling constant. Tetrahedron 29: 873.

Chaiken, I.M., M.H. Freedman, J.R. Lyerla, Jr., and J.S. Cohen. 1973. Preparation and studies of ^{19}F-labeled and enriched ^{13}C-labeled semisynthetic ribonuclease-S′ analogues. J. Biol. Chem. 248: 884.

Craig, L.C. 1968. Conformation studies with polypeptides by rotatory dispersion and thin-film dialysis. Proc. Natl. Acad. Sci. 61: 152.

Craig, L.C., E.J. Harfenist, and A. C. Paladini. 1964. Dialysis studies. VII. The behavior of angiotensin, oxytocin, vasopressin, and some of their analogs. Biochemistry 3: 764.

Dadok, J., P. H. Von Dreele, and H. A. Scheraga. 1972. Decoupling proton magnetic resonance signals located under the H_2O peak. J. Chem. Soc., Chem. Comm. 1055.

d'Auriac, G. A., M. Baudouin, and P. Meyer. 1972. Mechanism of action of angiotensin in smooth muscle cell. Circulation Res. 31 (suppl. II): 151.

Deber, C.M., F.A. Bovey, J.P. Carver, and E.R. Blout. 1970. Nuclear magnetic resonance evidence for *cis*-peptide bonds in proline oligomers. J. Am. Chem. Soc. 92: 6191.

Deslauriers, R., C. Garrigou-Lagrange, A.-M. Bellocq, and I.C.P. Smith. 1973. Carbon-13 nuclear magnetic resonance studies on thyrotropin-releasing factor and related peptides. FEBS Lett. 31: 59.

Deslauriers, R., R. Walter, and I.C.P. Smith. 1972. A carbon-13 nuclear magnetic resonance study of oxytocin and its oligopeptides. Biochem. Biophys. Res. Comm. 48: 854.

Douglas, J.R., Jr., E.M. Johnson, Jr., G.R. Marshall, B.M. Jaffe, and P. Needleman. 1973. Stimulation of splenic prostaglandin release by angiotensin and specific inhibition by cysteine^{8}-AII. Prostaglandins 3: 67.

Eggena, P., I.L. Schwartz, and R. Walter. 1970. Threshold and receptor reserve in the action of neurohypophyseal peptides. J. Gen. Physiol. 56: 250.

Feeney, J., G.C.K. Roberts, J.H. Rockey, and A.S.V. Burgen. 1971. Conformation studies on oxytocin and lysine vasopressin in aqueous solution using high resolution NMR spectroscopy. Nature New Biol. 232:108.

Fermandjian, S., J.-L. Morgat, and P. Fromageot. 1971a. Studies of angiotensin-II conformations by circular dichroism. Eur. J. Biochem. 24: 252.

Fermandjian, S., J.-L. Morgat, P. Fromageot. 1971b. Crystallisation of angiotensinamide II. FEBS Lett. 16: 192.

Fermandjian, S., P. Fromageot, A.-M. Tistchenko, J.-P. Leicknam, and M. Lutz. 1972a. Angiotensin II conformations. Infrared and Raman Studies. Eur. J. Biochem. 28: 174.

Fermandjian, S., J.-L. Morgat, P. Fromageot, M. Lutz, and J.-P. Leicknam. 1972b. Structural aspects of angiotensin II. *In* M. Margoulies and F.C. Greenwood (eds), Protein and Polypeptide Hormones, Excerpta Medica, Amsterdam, pp. 460–468.

Ferreira, A.T., O.G. Hampe, and A.C.M. Paiva. 1969. The conformation of angiotensin II in aqueous solution. II. Dialysis and gel filtration behavior of [Asn^{1}-Val^{5}]-angiotensin II. Biochemistry 8: 3483.

Fessler, D.C., F. Sipos, G.S. Denning, Jr., D.T. Pals, and F.D. Masucci. 1972. Angiotensin II antagonism. Structure-activity relationships of 8-substituted angiotensin II analogs. J. Med. Chem. 15: 1015.

Finn, F.M., J. Dadok, and A.A. Bothner-By. 1972. Proton nuclear magnetic resonance studies of the association of ribonuclease S-peptide and analogs with ribonuclease S-protein. Biochemistry 11: 455.

Finn, F.M., and K. Hofmann. 1973. The S-peptide-S-protein system: a model for hormone-receptor interaction. Acc. Chem. Res. 6: 169.

Franze de Fernandez, M.T., A.E. Delius, and A.C. Paladini. 1968. Influence of pH on the conformation of angiotensin II and analog peptides. Biochim. Biophys. Acta 154: 223.

Gagnon, D., W.K. Park and D. Regoli. 1971. Specific antagonists for the myotropic action of angiotensin II and angiotensin I on the isolated rat colon. Brit. J. Pharmacol. 43: 409.

Glass, J.D., and A. Meister. 1970. 1-Amino-1,3-dicarboxycyclohexane (cycloglutamic acid), a new glutamic acid analog and a substrate of glutamine synthetase. Biochemistry 9: 842.

Glauser, S.C., H. Wagner, E.M. Glauser, and R.W. Sevy. 1970. A proposed structure and active site of angiotensin. Curr. Mod. Biol. 3: 221.

Glickson, J.D., W.D. Cunningham, and G.R. Marshall. 1972a. Proton magnetic resonance study of angiotensin II (Asn^{1}, Val^{5}) in aqueous solution, *In* J. Meienhofer (ed.), Chemistry and Biology of Peptides. Proceedings of 3rd American Peptide Symposium. Ann Arbor Science Publishing Co., Ann Arbor, Michigan, pp. 563–569.

Glickson, J.D., D.W. Urry, and R. Walter. 1972b. Method for correlation of proton magnetic resonance assignments in different solvents: conformational transition of oxytocin and lysine vasopressin from dimethylsulfoxide to water. Proc. Natl. Acad. Sci. 69: 2566.

Glickson, J.D., W.D. Cunningham, and G.R. Marshall. 1973. Proton magnetic resonance study of angiotensin II (Asn^{1}, Val^{5}) in aqueous solution. Biochemistry 12: 3684.

Glickson, J.D., J. Dadok, and G.R. Marshall. 1974. Proton magnetic double-resonance study of angiotensin II (Asn^1 Val^5) in aqueous solution employing correlation spectroscopy: Assignment of peptide NH resonances and transfer of saturation from water. Biochemistry 13: 11.
Hofmann, K., R. Andreatta, J.P. Buckley, W.E. Hageman, and A.P. Shapiro. 1968. Studies on polypeptides. XXXIX. Elimination of the imidazole portion of histidine as an essential site for biological function of angiotensin. J. Am. Chem. Soc. 90: 1654.
Jorgensen, E.C., and R.J. Weinkam. 1973. Conformation of angiotensin II in solution-physicochemical and synthetic studies. *In* H. Nesvadba (ed.), Proceedings of 11th European Peptide Symposium, Vienna, 1971, North-Holland, Amsterdam, pp. 311–323.
Karplus, S., and M. Karplus. 1972. Nuclear magnetic resonance determination of the angle ψ in peptides. Proc. Natl. Acad. Sci. 69: 3204.
Khairallah, P.A., A. Toth, and F.M. Bumpus. 1970. Analogs of angiotensin II. II. Mechanism of receptor interaction. J. Med. Chem. 13: 181.
Khosla, M.C., N.C. Chaturvedi, R.R. Smeby, and F.M. Bumpus. 1968. Synthesis of [1-isoleucine, 3-proline-, and 5- alanine-]- angiotensin II. Biochemistry 7: 3417.
Khosla, M.C., S. Kumar, R.R. Smeby, and F.M. Bumpus. 1972a. Solid-phase synthesis of [6-arginine]-, [4-histidine, 6-tyrosine]-, and [8-isoleucine]-angiotensins II. J. Med. Chem. 15: 627.
Khosla, M.C., R.A. Leese, W.L. Maloy, A.T. Ferreira, R.R. Smeby, and F.M. Bumpus. 1972b. Synthesis of some analogs of angiotensin II as specific antagonists of the parent hormone. J. Med. Chem. 15: 792.
Kopple, K.D., G.R. Wiley, and R. Tauke. 1973. A dihedral angle - vicinal proton coupling constant correlation for the α-β bond of amino acid residues. Biopolymers 12: 627.
Krejci, I., V. Pliska, and J. Rudinger. 1970. Change from agonism to antagonism in the action of some oxytocin analogues: interpretation by a receptor model. Brit. J. Pharmacol. 39: 217P.
Levy, G.C., and J.D. Cargioli. 1972. Carbon-13 chemical shifts on the TMS scale. J. Magnet. Reson. 6: 143.
Marshall, G.R. 1970. Conformation, computers, and biological activity. *In* B. Weinstein and S. Lande (eds.), Peptides: Chemistry and Biochemistry. Marcel Dekker, New York, pp. 151–162.
Marshall, G.R. 1971. Studies on the biologically-active conformations of angiotensin. Intra-Sci. Chem. Rep. 5: 305.
Marshall, G.R., and H.E. Bosshard. 1972. Angiotensin II. Studies on the biologically active conformation. Circulation Res. 30-31 (Suppl. II): 143.
Marshall, G.R., J. Beitch, R.A. Ellis, and J.M. Fritsch. 1972a. Macromolecular modeling system: the insulin dimer. Diabetes 21: 506.
Marshall, G.R., H.E. Bosshard, N.C. Eilers, P. Needleman. 1972b. Constraints on the receptor-bound conformation of angiotensin II. *In* J. Meienhofer (ed.), Chemistry and Biology of Peptides. Proceedings of 3rd American Peptide Symposium, Ann Arbor Science Publishing Co., Ann Arbor, Michigan, pp. 571-577.
Marshall, G.R., N. Eilers, and W. Vine. 1972c. Angiotensin II: A competitive inhibitor and analogs with restricted conformation. *In* S. Lande (ed.), Proceedings of 2nd American Peptide Symposium, Gordon and Breach, New York, Progress in Peptide Research, pp. 15–18.
Marshall, G.R., H.E. Bosshard, and J.D. Glickson. 1973a. Conformation of angiotensin II: differences between aqueous solution and the receptor. To be published.

Marshall, G.R., H.E. Bosshard, W.H. Vine, and J.D. Glickson. 1973b. NMR evidence against γ-turn and β-turn models of angiotensin II in aqueous solution. Nature New Biol. 245: 125.

Marshall, G.R., W. Vine, and P. Needleman. 1970. A specific competitive inhibitor of angiotensin II. Proc. Natl. Acad. Sci. 67: 1624.

Marshall, G.R., J. Fritsch, and H. Bosshard. 1973c. To be published.

Meister, A. 1968. Stereochemical mapping of the active site of glutamine synthetase. Fed. Proc. 27: 100.

Meyer, P., M. Baudouin, S. Fermandjian, M. Worcel, J.-L. Morgat, and P. Fromageot. 1972. Angiotensin receptors in smooth muscle cells. *In* J. Genest and E. Koiw (eds.), Hypertension '72, Springer-Verlag, New York, p. 495.

Needleman, P., R.J. Freer, and G.R. Marshall. 1972a. Angiotensin-receptor interaction: influence of pH on angiotensin inhibition by Phe^4-Tyr^8-angiotensin II in rat uterine smooth muscle. Arch. Internatn. Pharmacodyn. Ther. 200: 118.

Needleman, P., E.M. Johnson, Jr., W. Vine, E. Flanigan, and G.R. Marshall. 1972b. Pharmacology of antagonists of angiotensin I and II. Circulation Res. 31: 862.

Needleman, P., E.M. Johnson, Jr., W. Vine, E. Flanigan, and G.R. Marshall. 1972. Comparative pharmacology of angiotensin antagonists. *In* J. Meienhofer (ed.), Chemistry and Biology of Peptides. Proceedings of 3rd American Peptide Symposium, Ann Arbor Science Publishing Co., Ann Arbor, Michigan, pp. 501–507.

Needleman, P., A.H. Kauffman, J.R. Douglas, Jr., E.M. Johnson, Jr. and G.R. Marshall. 1973a. Specific stimulation and inhibition of renal prostaglandin release by angiotensin analogs. Am. J. Physiol. In press.

Needleman, P., G.R. Marshall, and J. Rivier. 1973b. Angiotensin II: synthesis and biological activity of 6–(1-methyl-histidine) and 6–(3-methyl-histidine) analogs. J. Med. Chem. 16: 968.

Nonomura, Y., Y. Hotta, and H. Ohashi. 1966. Tetrodotoxin and manganese ions: effects on electrical activity and tension in taenia coli of guinea pig. Science 152: 97.

Page, I.B., and McCubbin, J.W. 1969. Renal Hypertension, Year Book Medical Publishers, Chicago.

Paiva, A.C.M., V.L.A. Nouailhetas, M.E. Miyamoto, G.B. Mendes, and T.B. Paiva. 1973. New specific angiotensin antagonists. [8-Valine]-, [8-Isoleucine]-, and chlorambucil-des-1-aspartic, 8-valine-angiotensins I. J. Med. Chem. 16: 6.

Paiva, T.B., A.C.M. Paiva, R.J. Freer, and J.M. Stewart. 1972. Alkylating analogs of peptide hormones. 2. Synthesis and properties of *p*-[N,N-Bis (2-chloroethyl)amino]phenylbutyryl derivatives of angiotensin II. J. Med. Chem. 15: 6.

Paiva, T.B., A.C.M. Paiva, and H.A. Scheraga. 1963. The conformation of angiotensin II in aqueous solution. Biochemistry 2: 1327.

Paladini, A.C., A.E. Delius, M.T. Franze de Fernandez. 1963. Potentiation of the pressor effects of angiotensin in alkaline solution. Biochim. Biophys. Acta 74: 168.

Pals, D.T., F.D. Masucci, G.S. Denning, Jr., F. Sipos, and D.C. Fessler. 1971a. Role of the pressor action of angiotensin II in experimental hypertension. Circulation Res. 29: 673.

Pals, D.T., F.D. Masucci, F. Sipos, and G.S. Denning, Jr. 1971b. A specific competitive antagonist of the vascular action of angiotensin II. Circulation Res. 29: 664.

Park, W.K., J. Asselin, and L. Berlinguet. 1972. Solid phase peptide synthesis of 1-aminocyclopentanecarboxylic acid (ACPC) analogs of angiotensin II by the use of a new apparatus. *In* S. Lande (ed.), Progress in Peptide Research, Proceedings of 2nd American Peptide Symposium, Gordon and Breach, New York, pp. 49–58.

Park, W.K., and D. Regoli. 1971. Specific inhibitors for angiotensin II and angiotensin I. Brit. J. Pharmacol. 43: 418P.

Peach, M.J. 1971. Adrenal medullary stimulation induced by angiotensin I, angiotensin II, and analogues. Circulation Res. 28–29 (suppl. II): 107.

Peach, M.J. F.M. Bumpus, and P.A. Khairallah. 1969. Inhibition of norepinephrine uptake in hearts by angiotensin II and analogs. J. Pharmac. Exp. Ther. 167: 291.

Printz, M.P., G. Nemethy, and H. Bleich. 1972a. Proposed models for angiotensin II in aqueous solution and conclusions about receptor topography. Nature New Biol. 237: 135.

Printz, M.P., H.P. Williams, and L.C. Craig. 1972b. Evidence for the presence of hydrogen-bonded secondary structure in angiotensin II in aqueous solution. Proc. Natl. Acad. Sci. 69: 378.

Ramachandran, G.N., R. Chandrasekaran, and K.D. Kopple. 1971. Variation of the NH-CαH coupling constant with dihedral angle in the NMR spectra of peptides. Biopolymers 10: 2113.

Regoli, D. 1972. Studies on the intrarenal action of the renin-angiotensin system. *In* J. Genest and E. Koiw (eds.), Hypertension '72. Springer-Verlag, New York, p. 72.

Regoli, D., W.K. Park, and F. Rioux. 1973. II. Pharmacology of angiotensin antagonists. Can. J. Physiol. Pharmac. 51: 114.

Regoli, D., W.K. Park, F. Rioux, and C.S. Chan. 1971. Antagonists of angiotensin substitution of an aliphatic chain to phenyl ring in position 8. Rev. Can. Biol. 30: 319.

Rioux, F., W.K. Park and D. Regoli. 1973. I. Pharmacology of angiotensin Antagonists. Can. J. Physiol. Pharmac. 51: 108.

Rioux, F., D. Regoli, and W.K. Park, 1971. Competitive antagonists of angiotensin II on the isolated rat stomach strip. Rev. Can. Biol. 30: 333.

Rudinger, J., V. Pliska, and I. Krejci. 1972. Oxytocin analogs in the analysis of some phases of hormone action. Recent Progr. Hormone Res. 28: 131.

Saruta, T., R. Cook, and N.M. Kaplan. 1972. Adrenocortical steroidogenesis: Studies on the mechanism of action of angiotensin and electrolytes. *J.* Clin. Invest. 51: 2239.

Schattenkerk, C., and E. Havinga. 1965. Studies on polypeptides IV. Syntheses and activities of some angiotensin-like peptides. Rec. Trav. Chim. Pays-Bas 84: 653.

Schwyzer, R., and H. Turrian. 1960. The chemistry and pharmacology of angiotensin. Vit. Hormones 18: 237.

Seu, J.H., R.R. Smeby, and F.M. Bumpus. 1962. Synthesis of isoleucyl^5-alanyl^7-angiotensin II. J. Am. Chem. Soc. 84: 3883.

Shaw, E. 1970. Selective chemical modification of proteins. Physiol. Rev. 50: 244.

Smeby, R.R., K. Arakawa, F.M. Bumpus, and M.M. Marsh. 1962. A proposed conformation of isoleucyl^5-angiotensin II. Biochim. Biophys. Acta 58: 550.

Stewart, J.M., and R.J. Freer. 1972. Properties of angiotensin receptor in smooth muscle: a proposed model. *In* J. Meienhofer, Chemistry and Biology of Peptides, Proceedings 3rd American Peptide Symposium, Ann Arbor Science Publishing Co., Ann Arbor, Michigan, pp. 521–524.

Torchia, D.A., and F.A. Bovey. 1971. A nuclear magnetic resonance study of poly (L-proline) in aqueous and aqueous salt solutions. Macromolecules 4: 246.

Triner, L., Y. Vulliemoz, M. Verosky, and G.G. Nahas. 1970. Effect of catecholamine on adrenylcyclase activity in rat uterus. Life Sci. 9: 707.

Turker, R.K., M.M. Hall, M. Yamamoto, C.S. Sweet, and F.M. Bumpus. 1972. A new, long-lasting competitive inhibitor of angiotensin. Science 177: 1203.

Turker, R.K., M. Yamamoto, P.A. Khairallah, and F.M. Bumpus. 1971. Competitive antagonism of 8-Ala-angiotensin II to angiotensins I and II on isolated rabbit aorta and rat ascending colon. Eur. J. Pharmac. 15: 285.

van Breemen, C., B.R. Farinas, P. Gerba, and E.D. McNaughton. 1972. Excitation-contraction coupling in rabbit aorta. Studied by the Lanthanum method for measuring cellular calcium influx. Circulation Res. 30: 44.

Venkatachalam, C.M., and G.N. Ramachandran. 1967. Stereochemistry of polypeptide chains–comparison of different potential functions. *In* G.N. Ramachandran (ed.), Conformation of Biopolymers, Academic Press, New York, p. 83.

Vine, W.H., D.A. Brueckner, P. Needleman, and G.R. Marshall. 1973. Synthesis, biological activity, and ^{19}F nuclear magnetic resonance spectra of angiotensin II analogs containing fluorine. Biochemistry 12: 1630.

Vogler, K., R.O. Studer, W. Lergier, and P. Lanz. 1965. Synthese von All-D-Val^5-angiotensin II-Asp^1-β-amid. Helv. Chim. Acta 48: 1407.

Walaszek, E.J., and D.C. Dyer. 1966. Polypeptide receptor mechanisms: influence of pH. *In* E.G. Erdos, N. Back, and F. Sicuteri (eds.), Hypotensive Peptides, Springer-Verlag, New York, pp. 327–340.

Walter, R., I.L. Schwartz, J.H. Darnell, and D.W. Urry. 1971. Relation of the conformation of oxytocin to the biology of neurohypophyseal hormones. Proc. Natl. Acad. Sci. 68: 1355.

Walter, R., I.L. Schwartz, O. Hechter, T. Dousa, and P.L. Hoffman. 1972. Bromoacetyl-oxytocin, an irreversible inhibitor of neurohypophyseal hormone-stimulated adenylate cyclase, and a possible affinity label for hormone receptors. Endocrinology 91: 39.

Weinkam, R.J., and E.C. Jorgensen. 1971a. Angiotensin II analogs. VIII. The use of free radical containing peptides to indicate the conformation of the carboxyl terminal region of angiotensin II. J. Am. Chem. Soc. 93: 7033.

Weinkam, R.J., and E.C. Jorgensen. 1971b. Angiotensin II analogs. IX. Conformational studies of angiotensin II by proton magnetic resonance. J. Am. Chem. Soc. 93: 7038.

Yamamoto, M., R.K. Turker, P.A. Khairallah, and F.M. Bumpus. 1972. A potent competitive antagonist of angiotensin II. Eur. J. Pharmacol. 18: 316.

Zimmer, S., W. Haar, W. Maurer, H. Ruterjans, S. Fermandjian, and P. Fromageot. 1972. Investigation of the structure of angiotensin II using ^{13}C nuclear-magnetic-resonance spectra. Eur. J. Biochem. 29: 80.

Cardiovascular Evaluation of [1-Sarcosine-8-Isoleucine] Angiotensin II and Its Effects on Blood Pressure of Conscious Renal Hypertensive Dogs

Charles S. Sweet,[1] Carlos M. Ferrario, Anthony Kosoglov, and F. Merlin Bumpus

Research Division
Cleveland Clinic
Cleveland, Ohio

The pharmacology of angiotensin has been extensively investigated since its discovery and subsequent purification, but little was known about the receptors involved in its action until specific competitive antagonists became available. Khairallah, Toth, and Bumpus (1970) and Marshall, Vine, and Needleman (1970), working independently, reported that modification of the amino acid sequence of angiotensin II, particularly in position 8, resulted in peptides which would block the musculotropic effects of the parent peptide.

Since then several investigators (for review, see Bumpus *et al.* 1973) have reported different modifications of the peptide which have resulted in more potent and longer-acting inhibitors than the original peptides reported by Khairallah *et al.* (1970) and Marshall *et al.* (1970). [1-Sarcosine, 8-isoleucine] angiotensin II ([Sar^1, Ile^8]-ang II) is one of the more potent angiotensin II blockers based on its antagonistic activity on rabbit aortic strips. Such a potent specific inhibitor of angiotensin II has made it possible to use a different approach to elucidate the participation of the renin-angiotensin system in renal hypertension. Several experimental approaches were used to evaluate the *in vivo* pharmacology of [Sar^1, Ile^8]-ang II in dogs. The antagonistic effect of [Sar^1, Ile^8]-ang II against the pressor response to exogenous angiotensin II was evaluated in anesthetized normotensive dogs. Since angiotensin can potentiate the vasoconstrictor effect of normal sympathetic nerve activity and can increase blood pressure by a central mechanism,

[1]Present address: Merck Institute, West Point, Pa. 19486.

the antagonist was also evaluated for its ability to antagonize the effects of angiotensin in these systems. Finally, the antagonist was used to clarify the role of angiotensin II in three hypertensive models: acute hypertension in anesthetized dogs resulting from renal artery constriction, evolving hypertension in conscious dogs days after renal artery constriction, and chronic sustained hypertension produced by cellophane-induced perinephritis.

METHODS

Antagonism of the Vasoconstrictor Effect of Angiotensin II by [Sar^1, Ile^8]-ang II

Normotensive mongrel dogs of either sex weighing 15–20 kg were anesthetized with i.v. chloralose (100 mg/kg) and s.c. morphine (2 mg/kg). Following tracheal intubation, dogs were respired artificially by means of a Mark 8 respirator (Bird Co.). Arterial blood pressure was measured by a Statham P23db strain-gauge transducer connected to a recorder and attached to an arterial catheter inserted into the right femoral artery. Drugs were injected through a cannula in a femoral and saphenous vein. Prior to infusion of the analog, at least two complete dose-response curves to intravenous injections of [Val^5]-ang II amide (Hypertensin®, Ciba) were obtained. A range of doses of intravenous 1-norepinephrine (Levophed bitartrate®, Winthrop; dose in terms of base) were employed to determine vascular specificity. The pressor response to angiotensin II and norepinephrine were repeated at various intervals during infusion of the analog and up to 45 min post infusion. [Sar^1, Ile^8]-ang II (1 mg/ml) was dissolved in saline and stored in a freezer. On the day of the experiment an aliquot of the stock solution was diluted to a volume of 10 ml with saline and infused for 55 min into the left saphenous vein at a rate of 0.1 cm^3/min with a Harvard infusion pump.

Neurogenic Vasoconstrictor Effects of Angiotensin II in the Hind Paw

Since angiotensin II enhances the response to sympathetic nerve stimulation, the left hind paw of five dogs was perfused as previously described (Sweet, Kadowitz, and Brody, 1971). After administration of heparin sodium (400 U/kg, Lipo-hepin®, Riker Labs), the cranial tibial artery was cannulated and the hind paw perfused at constant flow by a Sigmamotor Pump (model T-8) with blood supplied from the left iliac artery. Flow was initially set to provide a perfusion pressure which approximated systemic pressure and was not changed thereafter. The lumbar sympathetic chain was approached through a flank incision and ligated at L-4. A Harvard electrode was placed on the chain distal to the ligature. The nerve was stimulated with pulses (2 msec duration, 8–10 volts, variable frequency) for 15-sec periods with a Grass Stimulator (model S-4). Intra-arterial injections of norepinephrine, angiotensin II, and tyramine were made in small volumes (0.025–0.1 cm^3) into the perfusion circuit. Angiotensin II (0.2 μg/min) was infused intra-arterially into the hind paw to augment the vasoconstrictor responses to tyramine and sympathetic nerve stimulation, and maintained during the simultaneous infusion of [Sar^1, Ile^8]-ang II (through separate cannulae) and the vasoconstrictor responses repeated.

Infusion of [Sar^1, Ile^8]-ang II into the Vertebral Artery

Angiotensin II can increase blood pressure by an effect on the central nervous system. Since this hypertensive response is produced by activation of the sympathetic nervous system, it was important to determine whether the blocker would antagonize this response. Five dogs were anesthetized with s.c. morphine (2 mg/kg) and i.v. chlorolose (100 mg/kg), and in each dog one vertebral artery was cannulated with a fine, nonobstructing, 22-gauge cannula near its origin. The other vertebral artery was left intact. Dogs were artificially respired with room air. Angiotensin II was infused into the vertebral artery (0.1 cm^3/min) at 0.002–0.006 μg/kg/min. These doses produced only insignificant increase in blood pressure when administered intravenously. After a central response was repeatedly demonstrated, [Sar^1, Ile^8]-ang II (0.025 μg/kg/min) was infused into the vertebral artery for 30 min. After stopping the infusion, the cardiovascular response to vertebral artery infusion of angiotensin II was retested.

Acute Renal Artery Constriction in Anesthetized Dogs

A low sodium diet (< 1 mEq/100 g) and removal of one kidney enhances the release of renin from the kidney during renal artery constriction (Bunag, Page, and McCubbin, 1966). Therefore, mongrel dogs were fed a low sodium diet (Prescription Diet, Hill Packing Co., Topeka, Kansas) for two weeks prior to the day of the experiment. A week before the experiment the right kidney was removed. On the day of the experiment the dogs were anesthetized with i.v. chlorolose (100 mg/kg) and s.c. morphine (2 mg/kg), and the left renal artery was approached retroperitoneally through a flank incision. An electromagnetic flow transducer (Micron No. RC-1000) was secured around the left renal artery and the flow signal recorded on a direct-writing polygraph. A clamp devised to constrict the renal artery (Ferrario *et al.*, 1971) was placed distal to the flow transducer. After an initial equilibration period, the clamp was adjusted such that systolic renal blood flow was reduced by 50%. Forty-five min after renal artery constriction, [Sar^1, Ile^8]-ang II was infused (0.4 μg/kg/min) until systemic blood pressure returned to preconstriction values. This time averaged 21 min in five experiments. The pressor responses to intravenous angiotensin and norepinephrine were also recorded before, during, and after infusion of the antagonist.

Acute Hypertensive Dogs

Surgery was performed on mongrel dogs of either sex weighing 15–20 kg. Under pentobarbital anesthesia (30 mg/kg i.v.) and sterile operative conditions, a Tygon cannula (0.040 inch i.d. × 0.085 inch o.d.) was inserted via the left iliac artery into the abdominal aorta. Another catheter was inserted through the right jugular vein into the right atrium. One week later, a clamp devised to constrict the renal artery (Ferrario *et al.*, 1971) was placed on the left renal artery and the contralateral kidney removed. After 3–5 days recovery, the dogs were placed unrestrained on a padded surface in a quiet room and blood pressure was recorded daily for several days until a stable pressure was obtained. Measurements were always made at the same time of day for 30–45 min. The indwelling catheter was attached to a Statham P23db strain-gauge transducer and blood pressure recorded on a direct-writing polygraph (Brush, Gould Instruments).

Tightening of the externally adjustable clamp after control blood pressure measurements were obtained has been described in detail (Ferrario *et al.*, 1971). Briefly, adjustment of the clamp was estimated roughly by using fluoroscopy with the dog lightly anesthetized with thiopental (25 mg/kg i.v.). This procedure allows visualization of the screw and measurement of the degree of the screw's displacement relative to the bottom plate in which the renal artery is encased. In the present experiments the clamp was adjusted so that the screw encroached on the area of the lumen by 50%. This procedure permitted convenient external adjustment without the use of traumatic surgery. Mean arterial blood pressure increased to hypertensive levels within days following adjustment of the clamp. All dogs recovered well from surgery, ate eagerly, and appeared alert and healthy in all respects.

Chronic Perinephretic Hypertensive Dogs

Other dogs were prepared as before except hypertension was produced by cellophane wrapping of one kidney and contralateral nephrectomy. Experiments were performed on these dogs when hypertension was established for at least 3 months.

Drug Infusion

Intravenous infusion of [Sar^1, Ile^8]-ang II (0.075–0.20 μg/kg/min) for 5 hr was made with a small electrolytically driven pump (Sage Instrument, Model 172) attached to the dog's leather vest. Synthetic angiotensin II, 1 μg (Hypertension,® Ciba), and norepinephrine, 10 μg, were dissolved in saline and injected into the jugular catheter.

Statistical analyses were performed using paired-comparison t tests. A probability level of $p<0.05$ was used as the criterion for significance.

RESULTS

Blockade of the Direct Vasoconstrictor Response to Angiotensin II by [Sar^1, Ile^8]-ang II

The blood pressure responses to three test doses of angiotensin II were significantly reduced during a 55-min infusion of [Sar^1, Ile^8]-ang II in five

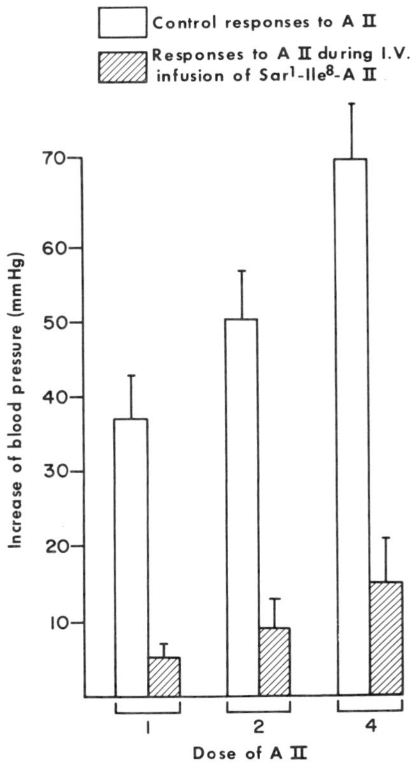

Fig. 1. Average pressor responses ± 1 s.e. to angiotensin II (1,2,4 μg) before and during the i.v. infusion of [Sar^1, Ile^8]-ang II (0.2 μg/kg/min) in five dogs.

anesthetized dogs (Fig. 1). Before infusion the pressor response to 1 μg, 2 μg and 4 μg of angiotensin II was 38 ± 6 (s.e.), 50 ± 7 (s.e.), and 69 ± 7 (s.e.) mmHg, respectively. During infusion of the blocker, 0.2 μg/kg/min for 55 min, the blood pressure responses to the three doses of angiotensin II were 5 ± 2, 9 ± 4, and 15 ± 6 (s.e.) mm Hg. The antagonist did not alter the vasoconstrictor response to norepinephrine (0.4 μg/kg) [89 ± 4 (s.e.) mmHg control, 87 ± 6 (s.e.) mmHg during infusion]. Sixty minutes after termination of the infusion, angiotensin II reactivity had returned to 75% of control. For example, the responses to two representative doses of angiotensin II, 0.1 μg/kg and 0.2 μg/kg, were 36 ± 7 (s.e.) mmHg and 49 ± 10 (s.e.) mmHg, respectively, 60 min after infusion of the analog. Intravenous infusion of [Sar^1, Ile^8] -ang II (0.2 μg/kg/min for 55 min) in these dogs did not significantly after baseline mean arterial pressure [95 ± 8 (s.e.) mmHg control; 98 ± 5 (s.e.) mmHg during infusion], although there was a transient pressor effect in all dogs.

Blockade of Angiotensin-Induced Facilitation of Adrenergic Transmission

The angiotensin-induced augmentation of the vasoconstrictor response to sympathetic nerve stimulation and its antagonism by [Sar^1, Ile^8]-ang II was demonstrated in the perfused dog hind paw. The vasoconstrictor response to stimulation of the lumbar sympathetic chain was enhanced during an intra-arterial infusion of angiotensin II (0.2 μg/min). The response to sympathetic stimulation at 5, 10, and 20 c/s increased 22 ± 6 (mean difference ± s.e., from control), 27 ± 6 and 29 ± 11 mmHg, respectively, from an average control value of 51 ± 4 (s.e.), 68 ± 6 (s.e.), and 100 ± 9 (s.e.) mmHg. During simultaneous infusion of [Sar^1, Ile^8]-ang II (0.8 μg/min) this angiotensin-induced increase in reactivity was abolished. The vasoconstrictor response decreased 23 ± 8 (mean difference ± s.e.), 27 ± 5, and 30 ± 8 mmHg at 5, 10, and 20 c/s from the stimulated levels during simultaneous infusion of both peptides.

Blockade of the Central Hypertensive Response to Angiotensin II

The interaction between angiotensin II and the central nervous system and its antagonism by the analog was investigated in a series of experiments. The effect of the analog on the neurogenic effects of angiotensin II was evaluated by comparing the pressor response to angiotensin infused into the vertebral artery of anesthetized dogs before and after infusion of the antagonist into the vertebral artery. The results of these experiments are summarized in Table 1. Mean arterial blood pressure increased 19 ± 3 (s.e.) mmHg during intra-vertebral infusion of angiotensin II. Following a 20-min infusion of [Sar^1, Ile^8]-ang II, the cardiovascular response to intravertebral angiotensin II was abolished. However, this response returned to control levels 30 min after the infusion was terminated.

Table 1. Effect of vertebral artery infusion of [Sar^1, Ile^3]-ang II (0.025 μg/kg/min) on the central hypertensive response to angiotensin II

	Control	2 min after [Sar^1,Ile^8]-ang II	30 min after [Sar^1,Ile^8]-ang II
Initial mean arterial blood pressure (mmHg)	117	122	121
Mean arterial blood pressure following intravertebral angiotensin II (mmHg)[a]	136	124	146
Mean difference ± s.e. (mmHg)	+19 ±3	+2 ±2	+25 ±4
P	< 0.05	N.S.	< 0.05

[a]Doses varied from 0.0015 to 0.004 μg/kg/min for 3 min.

Reversal of Acute Hypertension in Anesthetized Dogs with Renal Artery Constriction

The effect of the antagonist on the hypertensive response to endogenous angiotensin produced following acute renal artery constriction was studied in five anesthetized dogs. Systolic renal blood flow was reduced by 50% in the sole remaining kidney by means of a small adjustable renal artery clamp. Forty-five minutes after renal artery constriction, mean arterial pressure increased to 101 ± 9 (s.e.) mmHg from a control pressure of 82 ± 11 (s.e.) mmHg. Blood samples from peripheral arterial blood were collected before and after renal artery constriction and measured for plasma renin activity. Plasma renin activity increased an average of 0.76 ± 0.1 (s.e.) ng/ml/hr ($p < 0.02$) from a control value of 1.00 ± 0.15 (s.e.) ng/ml/hr after renal artery constriction.

Intravenous infusion of [Sar^1, Ile^8]-ang II (0.4 μg/kg/min for 20 min) produced a transient pressor response of 5–10 mmHg, but after 20 min of infusion, mean arterial blood pressure decreased 19 ± 2 mmHg (mean difference ± s.e.) ($p < 0.05$). Forty-five minutes after termination of the infusion, blood pressure returned toward hypertensive levels.

Effect of Renal Artery Constriction and Intravenous Infusion of [Sar^1, Ile^8]-ang II on Mean Arterial Blood Pressure in Conscious Dogs

Mean arterial blood pressure increased significantly within 3–7 days following tightening of the renal artery clamp (Table 2). The pressor response to intravenous angiotensin II (μg) was tested once the blood pressure was stable at the hypertensive level, and then after a 5-hr intravenous infusion of [Sar^1, Ile^8]-ang II. Infusion of [Sar^1, Ile^8]-ang II, lasting 5 hr, decreased mean arterial blood pressure on average of 18 ± 4 (s.e.) mmHg ($p < 0.05$) from a

Table 2. Effect of renal artery construction and intravenous infusion of [Sar^1,Ile^8]-ang II on mean arterial blood pressure in the conscious dog.

	Mean arterial pressure (mmHg)[a]	MD±S.E. (mmHg)[b]	*P*
Before	107 ± 3		
3–7 days after renal artery construction	141 ± 4	+34 ± 4	< 0.001
5 hr during infusion of analog	125 ± 5	−16 ± 3	< 0.01

[a]Values are means ±1s.e. of blood pressure changes as a result of renal artery constriction and infusion of [Sar^1,Ile^8]-ang II (range, 75–200 ng/kg/min for 5 hr) in eight conscious dogs.
[b]Mean difference ± s.e. (paired t comparison).

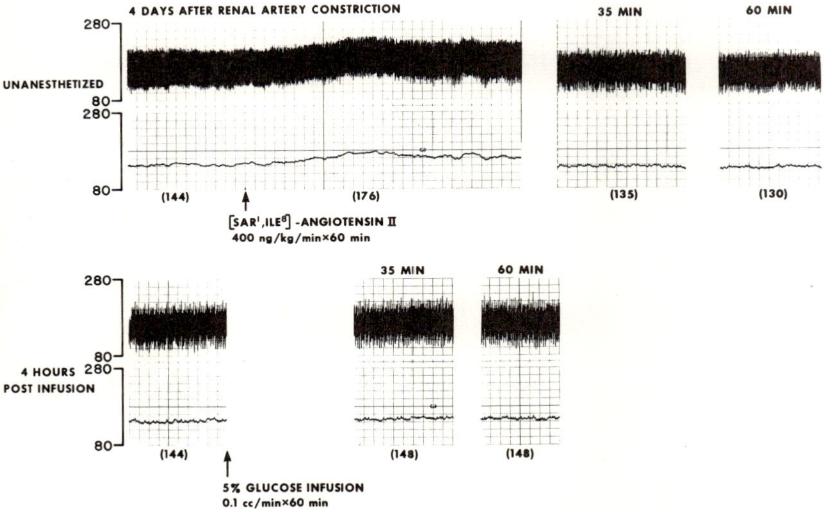

Fig. 2. Effect of [Sar¹, Ile⁸]-ang II on systemic arterial blood pressure of a conscious dog four days after renal artery constriction. Top panel, pulsatile and mean arterial pressure before infusion of antagonist and again at 35 min and 60 min during infusion of the antagonist (number in parentheses represents the mean arterial blood pressure); bottom panel, the same dog 4 hr later. An infusion of 5% glucose (vehicle) did not alter baseline blood pressure (144 mmHg control, 148 mmHg 60 min during infusion).

control value of 138 ± 4 (s.e.) mmHg (Table 2). The pressor response to angiotensin II before infusion of the antagonist was 38 ± 4 mmHg (s.e.) and 7 ± 2 (s.e.) mmHg ($p < 0.001$) after infusion. A 5-hr infusion was chosen, since with shorter infusion periods (1 hr), a transient hypertensive response preceded the antihypertensive effect. An example of a typical experiment is shown in Fig. 2. The antagonist initially increased and then decreased mean arterial pressure. In the same dog and under the same experimental conditions, a 1-hr intravenous infusion of vehicle did not alter baseline blood pressure.

Effect of [Sar¹, Ile⁸]-ang II on Blood Pressure of Chronic Renal Hypertensive Dogs

The effect of [Sar¹, Ile⁸]-ang II was tested in six dogs made hypertensive by the cellophane-wrapping technique and in seven other dogs made hypertensive by renal artery constriction (duration 28 days) (Table 3). [Sar¹, Ile⁸]-ang II was infused at rates (1–5 μg/kg/min i.v.) which completely blocked pressor response to angiotensin II. Two of the dogs were infused continuously for 24 hr (50 ng/kg/min). There was no fall in mean arterial pressure in these experiments. In seven dogs made hypertensive by renal artery constriction 28 days prior to the experiment, continuous intravenous infusion of the antagonist failed to lower arterial pressure.

Table 3. Effect of [Sar^1,Ile^8]-ang II on blood pressure of chronic renal hypertensive dogs.

	Mean arterial pressure, ±s.e. (mmHg)	MD±s.e. (mmHg)[a]	P
	Cellophane wrap (n=9)		
Before	154 ± 8		
During infusion[b]	173 ± 11	+18 ± 5	< 0.02
	Renal artery constriction (mean duration, 28 days; n=7)		
Before	131 ± 6		
During infusion[c]	143 ± 5	+12 ± 3	< 0.02

n, number of dogs
[a]Mean difference ± standard error (paired t comparison)
[b]Because of the large quantities of the analog required for dog evaluation, only two dogs were infused for 24 hr at 50 ng/kg/min. Two dogs were infused for 1 hr (1–5 μg/kg/min). Five dogs were infused for 5 hr at 200 ng/kg/min.
[c]200–400 ng/kg/min lasting 5–24 hr.

DISCUSSION

The various side groups of angiotensin II required for biological activity have been reviewed by Bumpus (1971). For a number of years the research effort in elucidating the structure-activity relationships of the polypeptide has been directed at the development of synthetic angiotensin II analogs which would inhibit the response to angiotensin II. Such compounds are presently available and have fulfilled a previous notable deficiency in the understanding of the actions of angiotensin II. From such studies it has been established that the aromatic groups in the 4, 6, and 8 positions are essential determinants for the biological effects of angiotensin II. Various analogs were synthethized with modifications of the 8 position and one analog, [Ile^5, Ala^8]-ang II, antagonized the effects of angiotensin on the guinea pig ileum (Kharallah, Toth, and Bumpus, 1970). Although this peptide was not active *in vivo,* Marshall, Vine, and Needleman, (1970) transposed the phenylalanyl and tyrosyl residues of angiotensin II and found that this peptide was an inhibitor of spasmogenic effects of angiotensin on isolated uterine muscle and inhibited the pressor action of angiotensin in rats. Several analogs have been synthetized recently (Turker *et al,* 1971a,b; Pals *et al.*, 1971; Regoli and Park, 1972; Needleman *et al.*, 1972; Saint-Louis and Regoli, 1972; Paiva *et al.*, 1973).

One of these analogs, (L-sarcosine, 8-isoleucine) angiotensin II was shown to be a potent antagonist against angiotensin II *in vitro* (Yamamoto *et al.*, 1972). In the present study this analog was shown to be an effective inhibitor against the direct and indirect effects of angiotensin. It is also evident that this analog produced a specific antagonism, since it did not antagonize the vasoconstrictor response to norepinephrine. Our observation that the hypertensive response to intravertebral infusions of angiotensin was blocked by the antagonist suggests that specific angiotensin receptor sites exist in those areas of the brain which are perfused by the vertebral artery. A similar conclusion can be inferred from the work of Solomon and Buckley (1972), who demonstrated blockade of the centrally mediated pressor response to angiotensin I and angiotensin II following intraventricular administration of two converting enzyme inhibitors.

The reversal of the vasoconstrictor responses to sympathetic nerve stimulation (previously enhanced by angiotensin II) following an infusion of [Sar^1, Ile^8]-ang II, was demonstrated in the dog hind paw. These experiments further demonstrate that the angiotensin antagonist can block not only the direct vasoconstrictor effects of angiotensin II but the indirect effects as well.

The antagonism of the cardiovascular effects of endogenous angiotensin has been demonstrated with various inhibitors of the renin-angiotensin system. Needleman *et al.* (1972) used Cys^8-angiotensin II and reported a significant lowering of blood pressure of anesthetized rats made acutely hypertensive by unclamping of a renal pedicle that had been temporarily occluded. Miller *et al.* (1972), prevented the rise in blood pressure of unanesthetized dogs following renal artery constriction when the nonapeptide Pyr-Trp-Pro-Arg-Pro-Gln-Ile-Pro-Pro was previously administered.

In the present experiments in anesthetized dogs, [Sar^1, Ile^8]-ang II completely reversed the hypertension caused by acute renal artery constriction and abolished the pressor response to angiotensin II. This strongly suggests that this hypertension is mediated entirely by endogenous angiotensin II. In conscious dogs made hypertensive by renal artery constriction and contralateral nephrectomy (duration < 7 days), mean arterial blood pressure decreased significantly during infusion of the blocker. However, blood pressure never completely returned to prehypertensive levels. Several explanations could account for this observation. It is possible that other humoral factors, in addition to angiotensin, may be operating to maintain blood pressure in these dogs. Although blockade of the vasculature receptor site was complete (as evidenced by the blockade of angiotensin II pressor response), it is conceivable that angiotensin may be exerting its effects at sites which are inaccessible to the antagonist. A third possibility is that some of the agonistic effects of the peptide antagonist may be masking what otherwise would be a complete return of blood pressure to preconstriction levels.

In contrast to the results obtained in the short-term hypertensive group, infusion of the blocker in other dogs with long-term renovascular hypertension (range, 12–44 days), was associated with increases rather than decreases in the blood pressure. The pressor response to 10 different infusions in seven hypertensive dogs (renal artery clamp) produced significant increases in blood pressure. The same results were obtained in other dogs with hypertension resulting from cellophane wrapping of one kidney and contralateral nephrectomy. Presently, it is not clear why blood pressure increased in these animals. Pals *et al.* (1971) and Saint-Louis and Regoli (1972) have reported that angiotensin II antagonist will transiently increase blood pressure due to the intrinsic activity of the compound. Page, Kaneko, and McCubbin (1966) reported that the vascular responsiveness to i.v. angiotensin II is not augmented in chronic hypertensive dogs. In the present experiments the antagonist was infused continuously for hours. Consequently, under these circumstances it is possible that the hypertensive response observed during infusion of the peptide antagonist may be a reflection of its intrinsic activity.

Our findings in conscious dogs with acute renal hypertension ($<$ 7 days) are in agreement with several workers (Pals *et al.*, 1971; Brunner *et al.*, 1971; Bumpus *et al.*, 1973; Saint-Louis and Regoli, 1972) who have reported that angiotensin antagonists can reduce blood pressure in hypertensive rats. These findings, which suggest an angiotensin involvement in the pathogenesis of the hypertension, could not be carried over to dogs with chronic hypertension. Although it is likely that the failure of the angiotensin antagonist to lower blood pressure in these latter experiments reflects the lack of participation of angiotensin II as the cause of the elevated blood pressure, the pressor effects observed during continuous infusion of the peptide limit the interpretation of results in chronic hypertensive dogs.

REFERENCES

Brunner, H.R., Kushman, J.D., Sealey, J.E., and Laragh, J.H. 1971. Hypertension of renal origin: evidence for two different mechanisms. Science 174:1344–1346.

Bumpus, F.M. 1971. Angiotensin structure activity relationships. *In* M. Margoulies and F.C. Greenwood (eds.), Structure-Activity Relationships of Protein and Polypeptide Hormones, Excerpta Medica, Amsterdam, p. 18.

Bumpus, F.M., Sen, S., Smeby, R.R., Sweet, C.S., Ferrario, C.M., and Khosla, M.C. 1973. Angiotensin II antagonists: their use in experimental hypertension. Circulation Res. Suppl. I to Circulation Res. Vols. 32 and 33, I: 150–158.

Bunag, R.D., Page, I.H., and McCubbin, J.W. 1966. Influence of dietary sodium on stimuli causing renin release. Am. J. Physiol. 211: 1383–1386.

Ferrario, C.M., Blumle, C., Nadzam, G.R., and McCubbin, J.W. 1971. An externally adjustable renal artery clamp. J. Appl. Physiol. 31:635, 637.

Khairallah, P.A., Toth, A., and Bumpus, F.M. 1970. Analogs of angiotensin II. II. Mechanism of receptor interaction. J. Med. Chem. 13:181–184.

Marshall, G.R., Vine, W., and Needleman, P. 1970. A specific competitive inhibitor of angiotensin II. Proc. Natl. Acad. Sci. 67:1624–1626.

Miller, E.D., Samuels, A.I., Haber, E., and Barger, A.C. 1972. Inhibition of angiotensin conversion in experimental renovascular hypertension. Science 177:1108–1109.

Needleman, P., Johnson, E.M., Jr., Vine, M., Flanigan, E., and Marshall, G.R. 1972. Pharmacology of antagonists of angiotensin I and II. Circulation Res. 31:862–867.

Page, I.H., Kaneko, Y., and McCubbin, J.W. 1966. Cardiovascular reactivity in acute and chronic renal hypertensive dogs. Circulation Res. 18:379–387.

Paiva, A.C.M., Nonailhetas, V.L.H., Miyamoto, M.E., Mendes, G.B., and Paiva, T.B. 1973. New specific angiotensin antagonists (8-valine)-(8-isoleucine) and chlorambucil-des-1-aspartic-8-valine-angiotensin I. J. Med. Chem. 16:6–8.

Pals, D.T., Masucci, F.D., Sipos, F., and Denning, G.S., Jr. 1971. A specific competitive antagonist of the vascular action of angiotensin II. Circulation Res. 29:664–672.

Regoli, D., and Park, W.K. 1972. Pressor and myotropic effect and antagonistic properties of several analogs of angiotensin II. Can. J. Physiol. Pharmac. 50:99–112.

Saint-Louis, J., and Regoli, D. 1972. Antagonists of angiotensin; effect on the blood pressure of normal and hypertensive rats. Rev. Can. Biol. 31:241–251.

Solomon, T.A., and Buckley, J.P. 1972. Inhibition of the central pressor effects of angiotensin I and II. Fifth International Congress on Pharmacology, p. 218.

Sweet, C.S., Kadowitz, P.J., and Brody, M.J. 1971. Another humoral substance that enhances adrenergic responsiveness during acute renal ischemia. Nature (Lond.) 231:263–264.

Turker, R.K., Hall, M.M., Sweet, C.S., and Bumpus, F.M., 1971a. A new long-acting competitive inhibitor of angiotensin. Science 15:285–291.

Turker, R.K., Yamamoto, M., Khairallah, P.A., and Bumpus, F.M. 1971b. Competitive antagonism of 8-ala-angiotensin II to angiotensin I and II on isolated rabbit aorta and rat ascending colon. Eur. J. Pharmac. 15:285–291.

Yamamoto, M., Turker, R.K., Khairallah, P.A., and Bumpus, F.M. 1972. A potent competitive antagonist of angiotensin II. Eur. J. Pharmac. 18: 316–322.

Feedback Failure of Renin Release in the Spontaneously Hypertensive Rat by DOCA and Sodium

Leo B. Czyzewski
Department of Pharmacology
Hoffmann-La Roche Inc.
Nutley, New Jersey

Pharmacologic properties of angiotensin include arteriolar vasoconstriction, resulting in increased peripheral resistance (Conn, 1955; Finnerty *et al.*, 1961; Segel *et al.*, 1963). Angiotensin can also affect the cardiovascular system via a central component(s) (Alexandre *et al.*, 1970; Andersson, Eriksson, and Fernandez, 1971; Fitzsimons, 1971; Hayden and Targett, 1971; Kawamura, 1972). A central mechanism and peripheral vascular smooth muscle effects potentially implicate the renin-angiotensin system in generating hypertensive diseases. The pharmacology of the renin-angiotensin system is outlined in Fig. 1.

In some forms of hypertension a failure of feedback suppression of renin release occurs. This failure has been demonstrated in patients with malignant hypertension (Catt *et al.*, 1971; McAllister *et al.*, 1971), renal artery stenosis and renal disease (Warren and Ferris, 1970), and suggested as a mechanism in hypertensive females using antiovulatory agents (Skinner, Lumbers, and Symonds, 1969; Saruta, Saade, and Kaplan, 1970).

Failure of suppression of renin release in various forms of hypertension may result in a continuous release of renin from the kidneys and could be analogous to a continuous angiotensin infusion. This could lead to the phenomenon of autopotentiation and has been reported in each of several species: rabbit (Gavras *et al.*, 1971; Dickinson and Lawrence, 1963; Yu and Dickinson, 1971); dog (McCubbin *et al.*, 1965; Belleau and Earley, 1967; Healy *et al.*, 1965); man (Laragh, Cannon, and Ames, 1964). The phenomenon of autopotentiation results from the continuous infusion of angiotensin at rates which initially have no effect on blood pressure, but after one or more days of continuous intravenous infusion results in progressively increas-

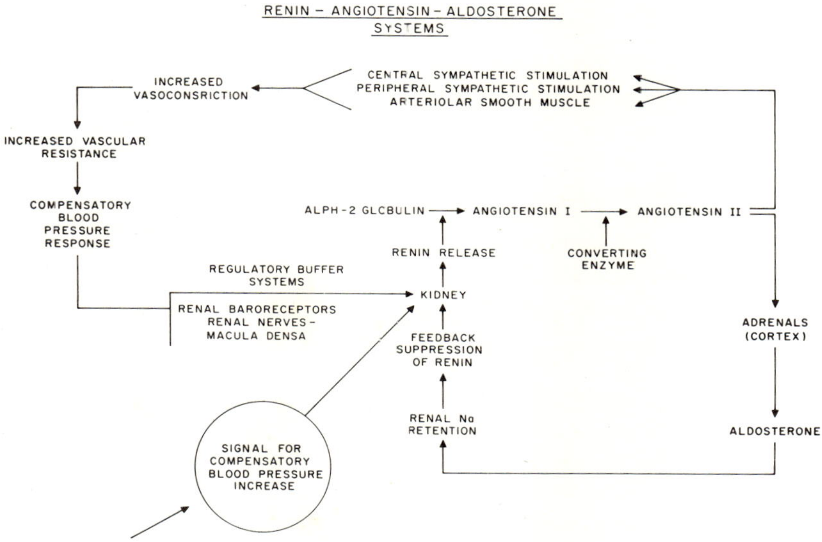

Fig. 1. A signal for compensatory blood pressure increase initiates a response in the kidney, inducing renin release from the juxtaglomerular apparatus. Renin cleaves a plasma protein to form angiotensin I in the circulating blood which is, in turn, converted to angiotensin II, primarily in the lungs. Angiotensin can qualitatively effect its response on blood pressure by central and peripheral influence, leading to increased vasoconstriction and the final compensatory blood pressure increase. Angiotensin also acts on the adrenal cortex to release aldosterone, which retains sodium and water in the kidney which, in turn, results in feedback suppression of renin release. Failure of suppression of renin release could result in continuous renin release and angiotensin formation which is analogous to continuous angiotensin infusion.

ing blood pressure. Angiotensin autopotentiation thus results in elevation of blood pressure, even though plasma levels of angiotensin II may be within the homeostatic range. For this reason normal or average levels of serum renin activity or angiotensin II may be meaningless in relating the pathogenic role(s) of this system to elevated blood pressure.

It has been suggested that the spontaneously hypertensive rat is an excellent model for the study of hypertensive disease, since the development of high blood pressure in this species resembles, in some ways, the progressive increase in blood pressure found in the patient with essential hypertension (Okamoto and Aoki, 1963; Okamoto *et al.,* 1966; Louis *et al.,* 1969; McAllister *et al.,* 1971). It was, therefore, decided to study the spontaneously hypertensive rat for possible abnormalities of the renin-angiotensin system and to relate the findings to the human condition.

The model system that was developed consisted of deoxycorticosterone acetate (DOCA)-induced sodium retention in the normal rat. This test system resulted in a feedback suppression of renin release and may be comparable to the system used in man (McCubbin *et al.,* 1965; Newsome and Bartter, 1968;

Warren and Ferris, 1970). The test system was applied to two strains of normotensive rats and to one strain of spontaneously hypertensive rats. This study will attempt to answer three questions: (1) is the serum renin activity in spontaneously hypertensive rats different from that of two normotensive rat strains, at various ages and stages of hypertension; (2) can a failure of the normal feedback suppression of renin release be a possible contributing mechanism of hypertension in spontaneously hypertensive rats; (3) can spironolactone change the rate of rise of blood pressure in the young maturing spontaneously hypertensive rat?

METHODS

The inbreeding of spontaneously hypertensive (SH) rats at appropriate intervals provided sufficient animals at 4, 8, 16, and 40 weeks of age. Normotensive Royal Hart Wistar rats were purchased from Royal Hart Laboratories, New Hampton, New York, and normotensive Charles River rats from Charles River Breeding Laboratories, Wilmington, Massachusetts.

Normotensive animals were permitted to acclimatize for one week prior to test day, while all rats were housed in individual cages (7 inch wide by 7 inch high by 9½ inch long) for at least three days prior to the experiment day. All animals were housed in a specially ventilated animal room maintained at 74°F and were exposed to a 12-hr light cycle from 6 a.m. to 6 p.m. by means of an automated control. Unless otherwise specified, all experimental rats were permitted free access to tap water and diet. The diet consisted of Purina laboratory rat chow.

Deoxycorticosterone acetate (DOCA) (Mann Research Laboratories) was administered as a single subcutaneous dose in 0.1 ml of olive oil at the times indicated in the results or, for the standard test procedure, 48 hr prior to decapitation. Placebo-treated animals received 0.1 ml of olive oil alone, unless otherwise specified. The DOCA-treated rats were only permitted free access to 0.9% NaCl solution, while the placebo group was limited to tap water *ad lib.* Optimal depression of serum renin activity was obtained two days following the administration of DOCA (40 mg/kg) and ingestion of 0.9% NaCl (DOCA-Na). This was used as the test model. Spironolactone (Calbiochem Laboratories, Calif.) was administered subcutaneously in 0.2 ml of olive oil and/or orally in approximately 0.2 ml of distilled water as outlined in the results.

A modification of the procedures of Williams, Harrison, and Grollman (1939) was used to record systolic blood pressure by cyclical occlusion of the tail artery pulse (occluding cuff and blood pressure system from Narco Bio-Systems Inc., Houston, Tex.). Blood pressure values were measured in unanesthetized rats previously warmed for approximately 5 min in an animal chamber (13 inch high by 12 inch diameter) which was maintained at 35°C by a PDU-50 power dial rheostat lamp (Lutron Electronics Co. Inc., Emmons,

Pa.). Both a sensing and occluding cuff were placed on the rat's tail after the animal was placed into a rat holder. The pneumatic sensing cuff, which was attached to a pneumatic pulse transducer (catalogue no. 92-600-70, Bio-Systems Inc., Houston, Tex.), sensed the pulse return. The pulse return was recorded on a two-channel polygraph (Hewlett Packard, model no. 7702B, Sanborn Division, Waltham, Mass.). The average of five systolic blood pressure readings, determined in succession on one day in each rat during the week prior to application of the test system, was used in calculating the mean and standard error for each group of rats. Correlations were determined for the mean systolic blood pressure and the serum renin activity.

On the test day the rats were sacrificed between 9 and 11 a.m. and a 4-sec free-flowing blood sample was obtained from the trunk immediately following decapitation. The blood sample was collected in siliconized plastic tubes (13 × 100 mm) immersed in ice, permitted to clot, and centrifuged at 10,000 × g for 20 min at 4°C. The serum was then frozen in 1-ml aliquots. In addition, a pooled serum sample representing each test group was prepared, frozen, and later used for establishing the standard angiotensin binding curves for the assay.

The techniques of incubations and radioimmunoassay of angiotensin I have been published previously (Pettinger, Marchelle, and Augusto, 1971) and were used with the following modifications. The pH of the serum sample was adjusted to 5.9 with 0.1 volume of 1.0 M sodium citrate. $2H_2O/HCl$ pH 5.0 buffer, and EDTA was added to give a final concentration of 3×10^{-3} M. The serum obtained from both placebo and DOCA-Na-treated rats was incubated for 24 hr at 37°C. The serum obtained from both the spironolactone and placebo experiments of this group were incubated for 2 hr at 37°C. The average of quadruplicate results from each serum sample was used to calculate the mean and standard error of each group of rats, and expressed as nanograms of angiotensin I accumulated per 100 ml per hour. Angiotensin I labeled with ^{125}I was purchased at monthly intervals from Schwarz-Mann, Orangeburg, N.Y.

RESULTS

Maximum suppression of serum renin activity occurred in normal rats within 2–4 days following the subcutaneous administration of DOCA (40 mg/kg) when combined with 0.9% NaCl ingestion (DOCA-Na) (Fig. 2). The serum renin activity returned to control levels within 1–2 weeks following the DOCA-Na challenge, indicating a sustained release of DOCA from the injection site.

The dose-response relations of DOCA administration *versus* suppression of serum renin activity are given in Fig. 3. Two days prior to decapitation DOCA was administered. The serum renin activity following DOCA administration at 4 mg/kg was significantly suppressed, while 40 mg/kg was followed

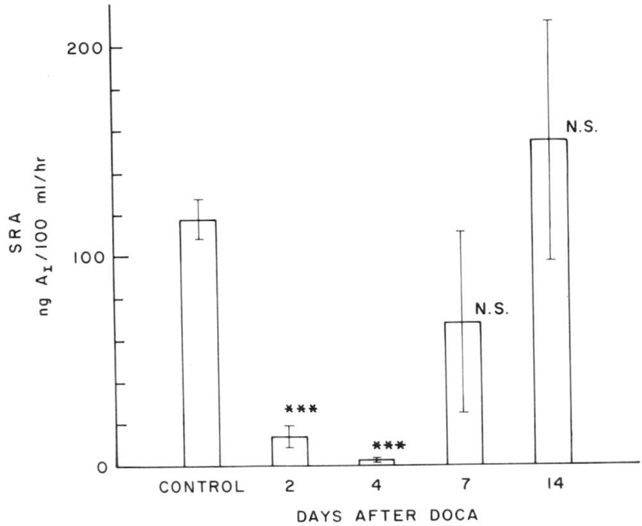

Fig. 2. Chronology of DOCA-induced suppression of serum renin activity (SRA) in normotensive male Royal Hart Wistar rats (250 ± 25 g). DOCA (40 mg/kg) was given s.c. as a single dose 14 days before decapitation in one group, seven days before in another, four days before in a third, and two days before in the fourth. The placebo was injected two days before decapitation in the control group. Each value is the mean ± s.e. for five rats. N.S., not significant; *** $P < 0.001$.

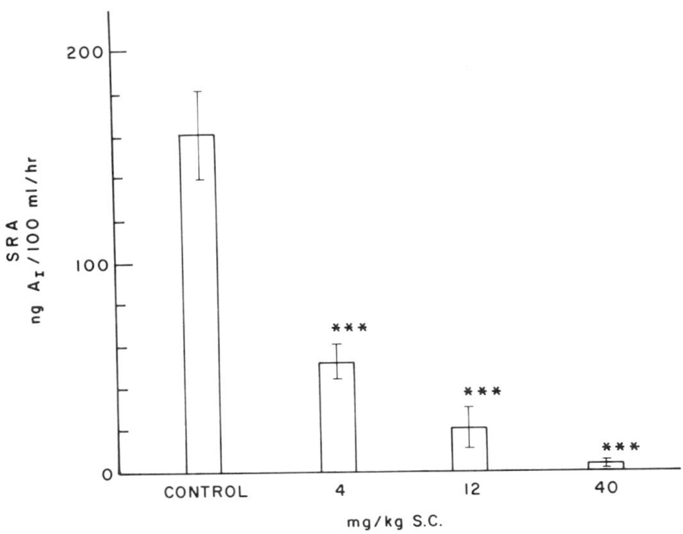

Fig. 3. Dose response of DOCA-Na induced suppression of serum renin activity (SRA) in normotensive male Royal Hart Wistar rats (250 ± 25 g), decapitated two days after DOCA administration. Each value is the mean ± s.e. of five animals. *** $P < 0.001$.

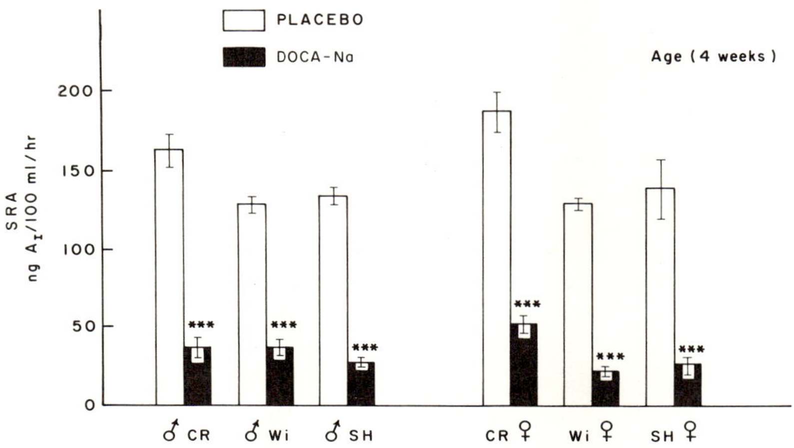

Fig. 4. Control serum renin activity (SRA) and DOCA-Na-suppressed SRA in Charles River (CR), Wistar (Wi), and SH male and female rats at four weeks of age. Each value is the mean ± s.e. in a minimum of five rats. All groups were done simultaneously. *** $P < 0.001$.

by a further suppression. This latter dose combined with 0.9% NaCl as drinking water was used as the model to test for failure of feedback suppression of renin release in both SH and normotensive rats.

The serum renin activity of placebo and DOCA-Na-treated male and female Charles River, Wistar, and SH rats at ages 1, 2, 4, and 10 months of age are given in Figs. 4–7.

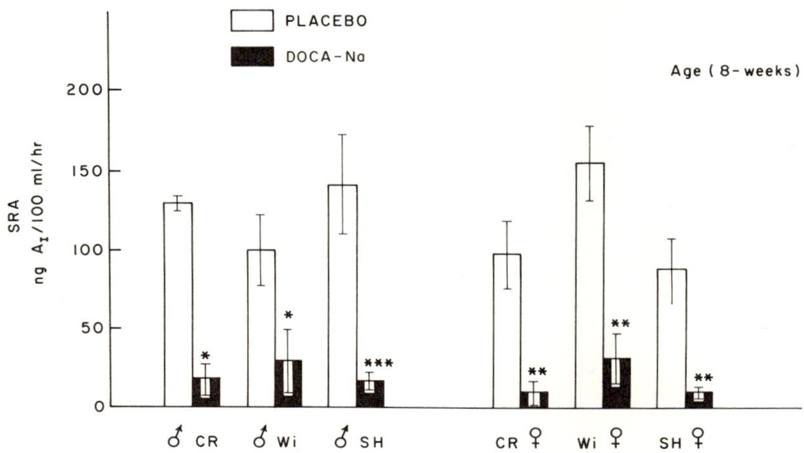

Fig. 5. Control serum renin activity (SRA) and DOCA-Na-suppressed SRA in Charles River (CR), Wistar (Wi), and SH male and female rats at eight weeks of age. Each value is the mean ± s.e. in a minimum of five rats. All groups were done simultaneously. * $P < 0.05$; ** $P < 0.01$; *** $P < 0.001$.

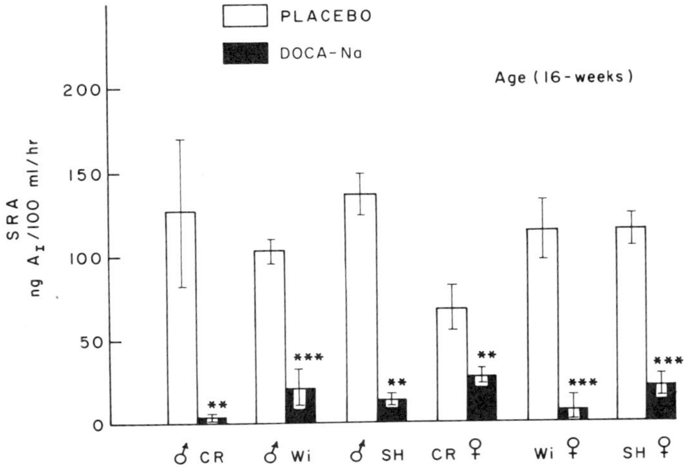

Fig. 6. Control serum renin activity (SRA) and DOCA-Na-suppressed SRA in Charles River (CR), Wistar (Wi), and SH male and female rats at 16 weeks of age. Each value is the mean ± s.e. in a minimum of five rats. All groups were done simultaneously. ** $P < 0.01$; *** $P < 0.001$.

The serum renin activity was compared in normotensive male Charles River and Wistar rats and showed that of the 4-week-old male Charles River (163.6 ± 9.7) to be greater ($P < 0.01$) than that of the 4-week-old male Wistar (129.0 ± 5.1) (Fig. 4), and the 40-week-old male Charles River (195.8 ± 21.1) to be greater ($P < 0.01$) than the 40-week-old male Wistar (112.8 ± 16.8) (Fig. 7). The serum renin activity (186.4 ± 12.2) from normotensive 4-week-old female Charles River rats was significantly higher ($P < 0.001$) than the value of 128.2 ± 2.7 obtained from female Wistar rats of the same age.

The serum renin activity, when compared within each sex of both normotensive strains, showed significant differences only in female Charles River rats. A comparison of 4-week-old Charles River female rats with 8, 16-, and 40-week-old Charles River females showed the following differences: 4-week 186.4 ± 12.2 *versus* 8-week 98.4 ± 20.9 ($P < 0.01$), *versus* 16 week 69.5 ± 14.3 ($P < 0.001$), *versus* 40 week 130.4 ± 17.7 ($P < 0.05$) (Figs. 4–7).

When compared either within each sex or between male and female, the serum renin activity within the spontaneously hypertensive rats was not significantly different at any of the ages studied (4, 8, 16, or 40 weeks) (Fig. 8).

A comparison of the serum renin activity between spontaneously hypertensive rats and the two normotensive strains showed the following significant differences: 4-week-old male SH 134.4 ± 4.2 *versus* Charles River male 163.6 ± 9.7 ($P < 0.05$) (Fig. 4); 40-week-old male SH 124.2 ± 13.9 *versus* Charles River male 195.8 ± 21.1 ($P < 0.05$) (Fig. 7); 4-week-old female SH 137.6 ± 17.7 *versus* Charles River females 186.4 ± 12.2 ($P < 0.05$) (Fig. 4); 16-week-old female SH 113.2 ± 12.0 *versus* Charles River female 69.5 ± 14.3 ($P <$

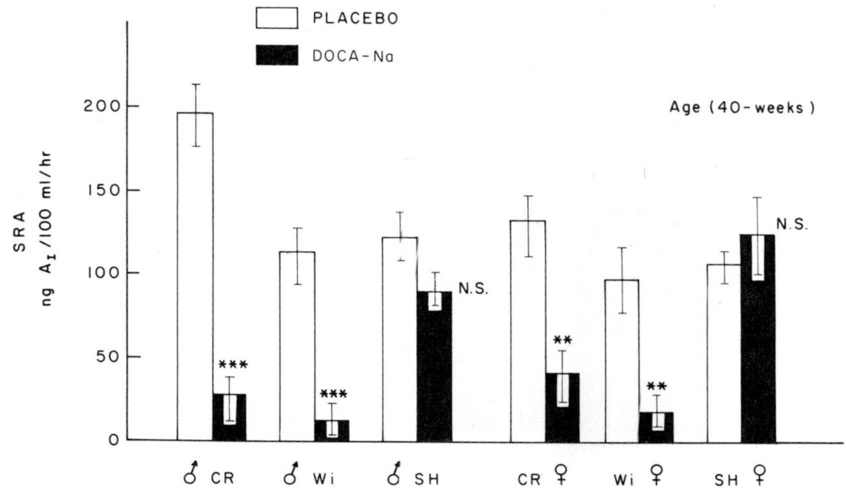

Fig. 7. Control serum renin activity (SRA) and DOCA-Na-suppressed SRA in Charles River (CR), Wistar (Wi), and SH male and female rats at 40 weeks of age. Each value is the mean ± s.e. in a minimum of five rats. All groups were done simultaneously. ** $P < 0.01$; *** $P < 0.001$; N.S., not significant.

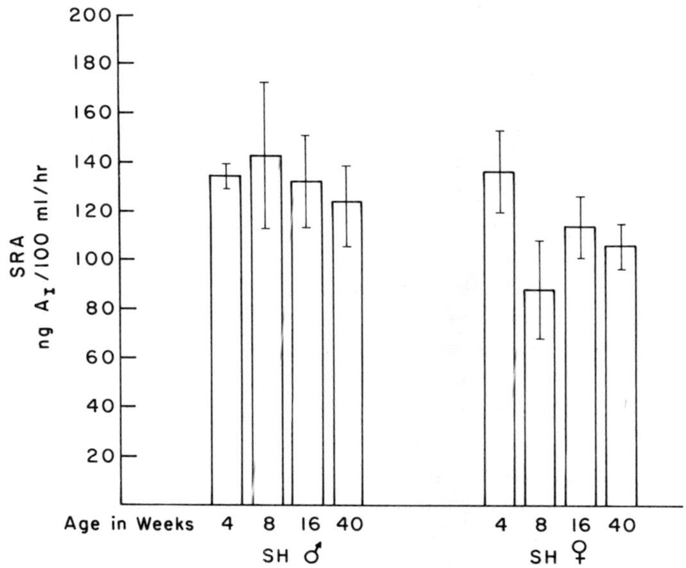

Fig. 8. The serum renin activity (SRA) in spontaneously hypertensive male and female rats.

0.05) (Fig. 6); 8-week-old female SH 87.6 ± 19.2 *versus* Wistar females 155.2 ± 20.5 ($P < 0.05$) (Fig. 5).

The serum renin activity was suppressed by DOCA-Na in both males and females of both normotensive strains at 1, 2, 4, and 10 months of age (Figs. 4–6); however, a failure of suppression of serum renin activity by DOCA-Na was observed in both male and female SH rats at 40 weeks of age (Fig. 7).

The systolic blood pressures were higher ($P < 0.01$) in female SH rats at one month of age than in Wistar or Charles River normotensive females of the same age (Fig. 9). There was a progressive increase in systolic blood pressure reaching 198 ± 5 mmHg at 40 weeks of age in the female SH rats. Similarly, the male SH rats reached 196 ± 11 mmHg at the same age. There were no significant differences in systolic blood pressure between SH and Charles River male rats at one month of age.

An analysis of correlation between serum renin activity and blood pressure in rats receiving either placebo (0.1 ml olive oil) or DOCA (40 mg/kg s.c. in 0.1 ml olive oil) was performed. The analyses were performed on each placebo and DOCA test group (serum renin activity) as presented in Figs. 4–10 which list the blood pressures and corresponding serum renin activities. Of the groups tested, four showed a negative correlation (blood pressure increasing and serum renin activity decreasing) between blood pressure and serum renin activity ($P < 0.05$). These were the Charles River female rats receiving the placebo at 40 weeks (Figs. 7,9) and DOCA at 16 weeks (Figs. 6,9), the Royal Hart (Wistar) female rats receiving the placebo at 16 weeks

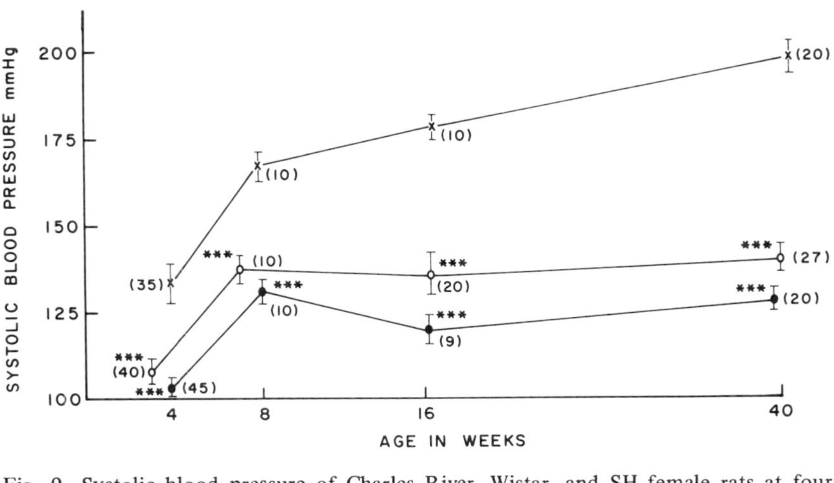

Fig. 9. Systolic blood pressure of Charles River, Wistar, and SH female rats at four, eight, 16, and 40 weeks of age. Each value is the mean ± s.e. The number of animals is given in parentheses. *** $P < 0.001$ indicates the significance of difference from the mean of comparably aged SH rats. Normotensive controls: Charles River (○), Royal Hart Wistar (•), and spontaneously hypertensive (X).

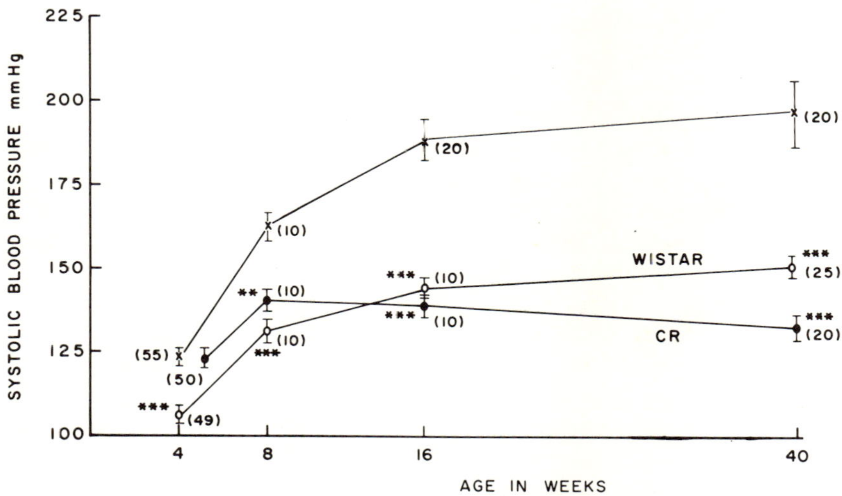

Fig. 10. Systolic blood pressure in male Charles River, Wistar, and SH rats at four, eight, 16, and 40 weeks of age. Each value is the mean ± s.e. The number of animals is given in parentheses. *** $P < 0.001$ indicates the significance of difference from the mean of comparably aged SH rats. Normotensive controls: Charles River (○), Royal Hart Wistar (●), and spontaneously hypertensive (X).

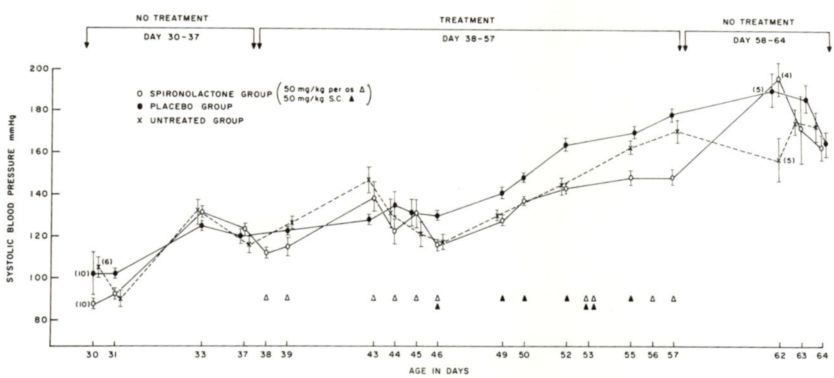

Fig. 11. The effects of spironolactone, placebo, and no treatment on systolic blood pressure in aging male SH rats. Spironolactone (25 or 50 mg/kg) given s.c. in 0.2 ml olive oil or given p.o. in 0.2 ml distilled water on consecutive days as indicated. Placebo group received equal volumes (s.c. or oral) of vehicle alone. Blood pressure determined immediately post-drug as indicated. Spironolactone caused a significantly lower ($P <$ 0.001) blood pressure than the untreated controls on days 55 and 57. The blood pressures of the placebo group were significantly higher than the untreated controls on days 46–57.

(Figs. 6,9), and the spontaneously hypertensive female rats receiving DOCA at 40 weeks (Figs. 7,9).

The oral and subcutaneous administration of spironolactone to male SH rats, at 25 mg/kg from day 38 to and including day 57, caused a decrease in blood pressure commencing on day 44 (Fig. 11). The systolic blood pressure of the spironolactone group was significantly lower ($P < 0.001$) than the placebo group from days 46–57. The spironolactone-treated SH rats were significantly lower ($P < 0.001$) than the untreated controls on days 55 and 57. Following day 57, both spironolactone and placebo treatments were stopped. On day 62 the blood pressure of the spironolactone group had significantly increased ($P < 0.001$) from 149 ± 1 to 196 ± 15 mmHg, while the placebo group showed a somewhat lesser increase. The systolic blood pressure of both the placebo (191 ± 8 mmHg) and spironolactone (196 ± 15 mmHg) groups on day 62 were significantly higher ($P < 0.001$) than the untreated controls (158 ± 10 mmHg) (Fig. 11).

The serum renin activity of 57-day-old spironolactone and placebo-treated animals was not significantly different. On day 64 (seven days following no treatment) the serum renin activity was not significantly differ-

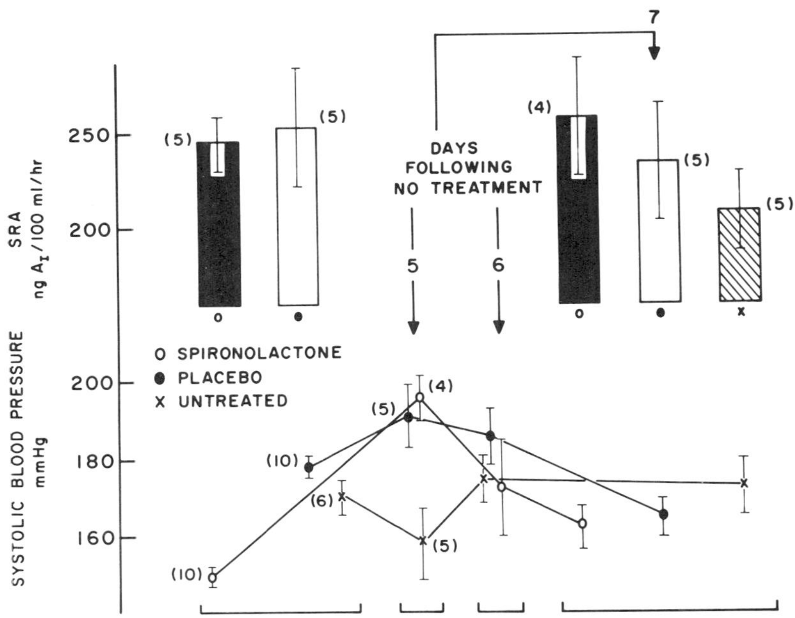

Fig. 12. The effects of spironolactone, placebo, and no treatment on serum renin activity (SRA) in aging male SH rats. On day 57, the last day of treatment, the SRA was not significantly different from values obtained on day 64, seven days following no treatment.

ent in either the spironolactone, placebo, or untreated groups, although the untreated controls appeared to have lower values (Fig. 12).

DISCUSSION

Warren and Ferris (1970) have shown that the induction of a positive sodium balance in man with several types of hypertension fails to suppress the serum renin activity to the extent that occurs in the normotensive population. The apparent failure of feedback suppression of renin release could result in continued angiotensin formation and elevation of blood pressure as a result of autopotentiation (Dickinson and Lawrence, 1963; McGregor and Smirk, 1968; Gavras *et al.,* 1971; McCubbin *et al.,* 1965; Laragh, Cannon, and Ames, 1964). The SH rat served as a model for these studies since it has biochemical and pharmacologic abnormalities similar to those in human subjects with essential hypertension (Aoki *et al.,* 1963; Folkow *et al.,* 1970; Haeusler and Haefely, 1970; Nagaoka *et al.,* 1970; Nagaoka, Kikuchi, and Aramaki, 1969a,b; Newsome and Bartter, 1968; Okamoto *et al.,* 1964; Nicholas, 1970; Villamil, Nachev, and Kleeman, 1970). In order to test for failure of feedback suppression of renin release in the SH rat, various combinations of DOCA and sodium chloride were used as the test system for the suppression of serum renin activity in both normal and SH rats.

The DOCA-Na challenge suppressed serum renin activity in both normotensive strains at 4, 8, 16, and 40 weeks of age and in the SH rats at 4, 8, and 16 weeks of age. However, at 40 weeks of age, a failure of feedback suppression of renin release was evidenced in both male and female SH rats. The failure of the negative feedback system in the 40-week-old SH rat could have become evident *at once,* or subtle changes could have been occurring at an earlier age but were not readily detectable by the test system used. The negative feedback failure could precede the onset of the hypertensive phase and result in a continuous renin release with consequent angiotensin formation. A continuous formation of small quantities of angiotensin II over prolonged periods of time could result in a progressive rise in blood pressure and may be the primary event initiating the onset of the hypertensive phase in the young SH rat. These findings (failure of feedback suppression of renin), together with no significant differences in serum renin activity in the spontaneously hypertensive rat (of either sex) at 4, 8, 16, or 40 weeks of age, could be explicable in terms of the autopotentiation phenomenon. The continuous infusion of angiotensin at a rate which initially has no effect on blood pressure will result in progressively increasing blood pressure after one or more days of continuous infusion (Gavras *et al.,* 1971; Dickinson and Lawrence, 1963; McCubbin *et al.,* 1965). The increase in blood pressure which results from such an infusion is said to be a result of the autopotentiation phenomenon. At the termination of the angiotensin infusion, the elevated blood pressure will return to control levels, the rate of return being dependent upon the length of time angiotensin II was infused (Brown, Duke, and Joels, 1963; Dickinson and Lawrence, 1963; Laragh, Cannon, and Ames, 1964; McCubbin *et al.*, 1965).

The initial failure of the feedback suppression system in the SH rat could result in a rate of angiotensin formation which causes no initial increase in blood pressure; however, after a period of time, a progressive blood pressure increase could occur as a result of autopotentiation. Therefore, a continued low rate of angiotensin formation would not be readily detectable in the SH rat and, hence, would be in agreement with the normal values of serum renin activity in the SH rat reported in this study. An initial low rate of angiotensin formation could, however, result in increased blood pressure, depending upon the initial onset of the lesion and the length of time an inappropriate renin release was in progress. The failure to detect differences in the serum renin activity of the SH rat at all ages studied does not necessarily negate the renin-angiotensin system from a role in the development of the hypertensive phase in this species, but must be considered with regard to the autopotentiation phenomenon described for angiotensin II. It has been reported that in certain individuals with mild essential hypertension, the angiotensin II levels have been reported to be both below and above the normal value as well as showing no variation (McCubbin *et al.*, 1965; Catt *et al.*, 1971). Whether failure of feedback suppression of renin release is responsible for the varied levels of angiotensin found in certain individuals is unknown. However, angiotensin's known pharmacologic activities, coupled with inappropriate renin release, suggest a potential mechanism for rapid acceleration of pathologic lesions in malignant hypertension.

In the SH rat the onset of this abnormality (failure of feedback suppression of renin release) correlates with both the biochemical and pharmacologic abnormalities (Aoki *et al.*, 1963; Sivertsson and Olander, 1968; Nagaoka *et al.*, 1969a; Folkow *et al.*, 1970; Haeusler and Haefely, 1970; Nagaoka *et al.*, 1970) which are similar to human subjects with essential hypertension (Sivertsson and Olander, 1968). These findings appear to be in accord with the failure of feedback suppression of renin release which occurs in several forms of hypertensive disease. This failure has been demonstrated in hypertensive patients with renal artery stenosis, renal disease, and malignant hypertension (McAllister *et al.*, 1971), and in patients with essential hypertension who develop high angiotensin levels with no apparent deficiency of extracellular fluid volume (Catt *et al.*, 1971).

The normal levels of serum renin activity found in the SH rat at the ages studied may, in fact, represent two- or three-fold relative elevations of serum renin activity for this model. For example, a well-known reciprocal relationship between effects of angiotensin and renin release does exist. The effects of angiotensin are aldosterone release from the adrenals with consequent sodium retention and renin suppression (Gross, 1960; Biron *et al.*, 1961; Davis *et al.*, 1961; Conn, Rovner, and Cohen, 1965), increased sodium content of vascular smooth muscle (Villamil *et al.* 1970), supersensitivity to vasoconstrictor substances (Nicholas, 1970), and elevation of blood pressure, the latter three effects having been reported to occur in the SH rat (McGregor and Smirk, 1968; Nagaoka *et al.*, 1969a; Folkow *et al.*, 1970; Haeusler and Haefely, 1970).

It would appear, according to observed and reported effects and the reciprocal relationships of renin release to these effects, that the serum renin activity should be significantly lower in the SH rat and patients with essential hypertension if the feedback suppression loop were functional. Therefore, normal levels of serum renin activity in the SH rat and in human patients with essential hypertension may actually be a result of inappropriate renin release.

Long-term spironolactone treatment has been successfully used in hypertensive patients to effect a lowering of blood pressure (Spark and Melby, 1968; Brown *et al.*, 1972). The present experiments showed that spironolactone did lower the rate of rise in blood pressure when compared with both placebo controls (days 46–56) and to untreated controls (days 55 and 56), suggesting a true hypotensive effect in the young maturing SH rat. The blood pressure of the spironolactone group significantly increased following cessation of drug treatment, suggesting a rebound effect. The blood pressure of the spironolactone group then returned to values not significantly different from either the placebo or untreated controls. Whether the effect of spironolactone is exerted through its aldosterone antagonistic response still remains to be resolved, since (1) patients with hypertension and accompanying high aldosterone secretion rates failed to show improvement following adrenalectomy (no aldosterone adenoma present) (Laragh, Ledingham, and Sommers, 1967; Katz, 1967), (2) aldosterone secretion rate and plasma renin activity may be normal in primary aldosteronism (Conn *et al.*, 1965; Del Greco *et al.*, 1967) (Figs. 11 and 12).

These results demonstrate that the SH rat can be used as a model for the study of the changes that occur as essential hypertension progresses to the malignant phase. Spironolactone treatment in the young maturing SH rat can lower the rate of rise of blood pressure. In addition, one of the changes taking place in the SH rat is a significant loss of responsiveness of the negative feedback system concerned with renin release, an effect becoming evident at 40 weeks of age. The failure of feedback suppression of renin release in the 40-week-old SH rat may be analogous to an inappropriate renin release, and may be comparable with that in the malignant hypertensive individual where it has been shown that a feedback failure of renin release does occur (McAllister *et al.*, 1971).

ACKNOWLEDGEMENTS

Figures 2–10 are reproduced by permission of the authors and the publishers of *American Journal of Physiology.*

REFERENCES

Alexandre, J.M., J. Menard, C. Chevillard, and H. Schmitt. 1970. Increased plasma renin activity induced in rats by physostigmine and effects of alpha- and beta-receptors blocking drugs thereon. Eur. J. Pharmac. 12:127–131.

Andersson, B., L. Eriksson, and O. Fernandez. 1971. Reinforcement by Na^+ of centrally mediated hypertensive response to angiotensin II. Life Sci. 10:633–638.

Aoki, K., H. Tankawa, T. Fujinami, A. Miyazaki, and Y. Hashimoto. 1963. Pathological studies on the endocrine organs of the spontaneously hypertensive rats. Jap. Heart J. 4:426–442.

Belleau, L.J., and L.E. Earley. 1967. Autoregulation of renal blood flow in the presence of angiotensin infusion. Am. J. Physiol. 213:1590–1595.

Biron, P., E. Koiw, W. Nowaczynski, J. Brouillet, and J. Genest. 1961. The effects of intravenous infusions of valine-5 angiotensin II and other pressor agents on urinary electrolytes and corticosteroids, including aldosterone. J. Clin. Invest. 40:338–347.

Brown, A.M., H.N. Duke, and N. Joels. 1963. The part played by cerebral anaemia in the response to occlusion of the common carotid arteries in the cat. J. Physiol. 165:266–273.

Brown, J.J., D.L. Davies, J.B. Ferriss, R. Fraser, E. Haywood, A.F. Lever, and J.I.S. Robertson. 1972. Comparison of surgery and prolonged spironolactone therapy in patients with hypertension, aldosterone excess, and low plasma renin. Brit. Med. J. 2:729–734.

Catt, K.J., E. Cran, P.Z. Zimmet, J.B. Best, M.D. Cain, and J.P. Coghlan. 1971. Angiotensin II blood levels in human hypertension. Lancet 1:459–463.

Conn, J.W. 1955. Primary aldosteronism. J. Lab. Clin. Med. 45:661–664.

Conn, J.W., E.L. Cohen, D.R. Rovner, and R.M. Nesbit. 1965. Normokalemic primary aldosteronism. A detectable cause of curable 'essential' hypertension. J. Am. Med. Ass. 193:200–206.

Conn, J.W., D.R. Rovner, and E.L. Cohen. 1965. Normal and altered function of the renin-angiotensin-aldosterone system in man. Ann. Int. Med. 63:266–284.

Davis, J.O., C.C.J. Carpenter, C.R. Ayers, J.E. Holman, and R.C. Bahn. 1961. Evidence for secretion of an aldosterone-stimulating hormone by the kidney. J. Clin. Invest. 40:684–696.

Del Greco, F., N.H. Simon, S. Goodman, and J. Roguska. 1967. Plasma renin activity in primary and secondary hypertension. Medicine (Balt.) 46:475–490.

Dickinson, C.J., and J.R. Lawrence. 1963. A slowly developing pressor response to small concentrations of angiotensin. Its bearing on the pathogenesis of chronic renal hypertension. Lancet 1:1354–1356.

Finnerty, F.A., G.D. Massaro, V. Chupkovich, and J. Tuckman. 1961. Evaluation of the pressor, cardiac and renal hemodynamic properties of angiotensin II in man. Circulation Res. 9:256–263.

Fitzsimons, J.T. 1971. The effect on drinking of peptide precursors and of shorter chain peptide fragments of angiotensin II injected into the rat's diencephalon. J. Physiol. 214:295–303.

Folkow, B., M. Hallback, Y. Lundgren, and L. Weiss. 1970. Background of increased flow resistance and vascular reactivity in spontaneously hypertensive rats. Acta Physiol. Scand. 80:93–106.

Gavras, H., A.F. Lever, J.J. Brown, R.F. Macadam, and J.I.S. Robertson. 1971. Acute renal failure, tubular necrosis, and myocardial infarction induced in the rabbit by intravenous angiotensin II. Lancet 2:19–22.

Gross, F. 1960. Adrenocortical function and renal pressor mechanisms in experimental hypertension. *In* K.D. Bock and P. Cottier (eds.), Essential Hypertension: An International Symposium. Springer-Verlag, Berlin, p. 92.

Haeusler, G., and W. Haefely. 1970. Pre- and postjunctional supersensitivity of the mesenteric artery preparation from normotensive and hypertensive rats. Naunyn-Schmiedebergs Arch. Pharmak. Exp. Path. 266:18–33.

Hayden, J., and M.A. Targett. 1971. Central components of the renin-angiotensin system. Brit. J. Pharmac. 41:177–186.

Healy, J.K., C. Barcena, B.J.M. O'Connell, and G.E. Schreiner. 1965. Renal and pressor action of angiotensin in the normal dog. Am. J. Physiol. 208:1093–1099.

Katz, F.H. 1967. Primary aldosteronism with suppressed plasma renin activity due to bilateral nodular adrenocortical hyperplasia. Ann. Int. Med. 67:1035–1042.

Kawamura, H. 1972. A study of hypertension. The effects of angiotensin II on the MAO activity and roles of calcium ion on the catecholamine contents in the rat hypothalamus and striatum. Jap. Circulation J. 36:349–362.

Laragh, J.H., P.J. Cannon, and R.P. Ames. 1964. Interaction between aldosterone secretion, sodium and potassium balance, and angiotensin activity in man: studies in hypertension and cirrhosis. Can. Med. Ass. J. 90:248–256.

Laragh, J.H., J.G.G. Ledingham, and S.C. Sommers. 1967. Secondary aldosteronism and reduced plasma renin in hypertensive disease. Trans. Ass. Am. Physicians 80:168.

Louis, W.J., R. Tabei, S. Spector, and A. Sjoerdsma. 1969. Studies on the spontaneously hypertensive rat. Genealogy, effects of varying salt intake, and kinetics of catecholamine metabolism. Circulation Res. 24–25 (suppl. I):93–102.

McAllister, R.G., Jr., C.W. Van Way, K. Dayani, W.J. Anderson, E. Temple, A.M. Michelakis, W.S. Coppage, and J.A. Oates. 1971. Malignant hypertension: effect of therapy on renin and aldosterone. Circulation Res. 28 (suppl. II):160–174.

McCubbin, J.W., R.S. DeMoura, I.H. Page, and F. Olmsted. 1965. Arterial hypertension elicited by subpressor amounts of angiotensin. Science 149:1394–1395.

McGregor, D.D., and F.H. Smirk. 1968. Vascular responses in mesenteric arteries from genetic and renal hypertensive rats. Am. J. Physiol. 214:1429–1433.

Nagaoka, A., H. Kawaji, Y. Imai, and H. Fukui. 1970. Systemic edema, thrombosis, and other hypertensive lesions observed in the spontaneously hypertensive rat at advanced age. Jap. J. Pharmac. 20:509–516.

Nagaoka, A., K. Kikuchi, and Y. Aramaki. 1969a. Depressor responses of the spontaneously hypertensive rats to the antihypertensive agents. Jap. J. Pharmac. 19:401–408.

Nagaoka, A., K. Kikuchi, and Y. Aramaki. 1969b. Electrolyte pattern of the aorta in the spontaneously hypertensive rats. Jap. J. Pharmac. 19:462–464.

Newsome, H.H., and F.C. Bartter. 1968. Plasma renin activity in relation to serum sodium concentration and body fluid balance. J. Clin. Endocr. 28:1704–1711.

Nicholas, T.E. 1970. Potentiation of the effects of noradrenaline and of sympathetic stimulation of the perfused rat caudal artery by angiotensin. J. Pharm. Pharmac. 22:37–41.

Okamoto, K., and K. Aoki. 1963. Development of a strain of spontaneously hypertensive rats. Jap. Circulation J. 27:282–293.

Okamoto, K., K. Aoki, S. Nosaka, and M. Fukushima. 1964. Cardiovascular diseases in the spontaneously hypertensive rat. Jap. Circulation J. 28:943–952.

Okamoto, K., R. Tabei, M. Fukushima, S. Nosaka, Y. Yamori, K. Ichijima, H. Haebara, M. Matsumoto, T. Maruyama, Y. Suzuki, and M. Tamegai. 1966. Further observations of the development of a strain of spontaneously hypertensive rats. Jap. Circulation J. 30:703–716.

Pettinger, W.A., M. Marchelle, and L. Augusto. 1971. Renin suppression by DOC and NaCl in the rat. Am. J. Physiol. 221:1071–1074.

Saruta, T., G.A. Saade, and N.M. Kaplan. 1970. A possible mechanism for hypertension induced by oral contraceptives. Archs Int. Med. 126:621–626.

Segel, N., T.J. Baylet, A. Paton, P.W. Dykes, and J.M. Bishop. 1963. The effects of synthetic vasopressin and angiotensin on the circulation in cirrhosis of the liver. Clin. Sci. 25:43–55.

Sivertsson, R., and R. Olander. 1968. Aspects of the nature of the increased vascular resistance and increased 'reactivity' to noradrenaline in hypertensive subjects. Life Sci. 7:1291–1297.

Skinner, S.L., E.R. Lumbers, and E.M. Symonds. 1969. Alteration by oral contraceptives of normal menstrual changes in plasma renin activity, concentration and substrate. Clin. Sci. 36:67–76.

Spark, R.F., and J.C. Melby. 1968. Aldosteronism in hypertension, the spironolactone response test. Ann. Int. Med. 69:685–691.

Villamil, M.F., P. Nachev, and C.R. Kleeman. 1970. Effect of prolonged infusion of angiotensin II on ionic composition of the arterial wall. Am. J. Physiol. 218:1281–1286.

Warren, D.J., and T.F. Ferris. 1970. Renin secretion in renal hypertension. Lancet 1:159–162.

Williams, J.R., T.R. Harrison, and A. Grollman. 1939. Simple method for determining the systolic blood pressure of the unanesthetized rat. J. Clin. Invest. 18:373–376.

Yü, R., and C.J. Dickinson. 1971. The progressive pressor response to angiotensin in the rabbit–the role of the sympathetic nervous system. Arch. Internatn. Pharmacodyn. 191:24–36.

Influence of the Adrenergic Nervous System on Renal Water Excretion and Renal Renin Secretion

Robert W. Schrier, Judith Harbottle, and Tomas Berl
Department of Medicine
University of Colorado Medical Center
Denver, Colorado

There is now considerable experimental evidence which suggests that the adrenergic nervous system is involved in both the control of water excretion and renin secretion. The purpose of the present investigation is to examine the mechanisms involved in these effects. Alpha-adrenergic stimulation with the endogenous catecholamine, norepinephrine, is known to be associated with an increase in renal water excretion (Smythe, Nickel, and Bradley, 1952; Baldwin, Gombos, and Chasis, 1963; Fisher, 1968; Lieberman, Klein, and Kleeman, 1970; Klein *et al.,* 1971) and, in contrast, beta-adrenergic stimulation with isoproterenol has been demonstrated to be associated with an antidiuretic effect (Lehr, Mallow, and Krukowski, 1967; Lees, 1968; Lees and Lockett, 1965). Studies therefore were designed to differentiate between (1) a direct effect of adrenergic stimulation on the water permeability of the renal tubule, (2) an effect mediated by alterations in renal hemodynamics, and (3) an effect mediated by changes in the release of antidiuretic hormone (ADH). In Table 1 are shown the effects of intravenous isoproterenol on systemic and renal hemodynamics and sodium excretion in both intact dogs and acutely hypophysectomized dogs undergoing a water diuresis. In both groups of animals the intravenous infusion of isoproterenol was associated with a marked increase in cardiac output and a fall in total peripheral resistance. A decrease in systemic arterial pressure also occurred in both groups of animals, but the renal perfusion pressure was maintained constant throughout the experiments by the adjustment of a suprarenal aortic clamp. In neither group of animals was the intravenous infusion of isoproterenol associated with significant changes in glomerular filtration rate, renal vascular resistance, or urinary sodium excretion. Although the systemic and renal hemodynamics and electrolyte excretions were similar (Table 1), the effects

Table 1. Effect of intravenous isoproterenol on systemic and renal hemodynamics and sodium excretion

	Control	P	Iso[a]	P	Control
In intact dogs (N=10)					
Cardiac output (liter/min)	3.7 ± 0.4	< 0.001	5.8 ± 0.05	< 0.001	3.7 ± 0.4
Systemic arterial pressure (mmHg)	152 ± 1.7	< 0.005	143 ± 5.4	< 0.01	151 ± 2.0
Renal perfusion pressure (mmHg)	131 ± 3.6	NS	131 ± 3.3	NS	131 ± 3.5
Glomerular filtration rate (ml/min)	54 ± 2.5	< 0.05	58 ± 2.2	NS	58 ± 2.6
Renal vascular resistance [mmHg/ (ml/min)]	0.449 ± 0.04	NS	0.428 ± 0.03	NS	0.430 ± 0.03
Urinary sodium excretion (μEq/min)	14 ± 3	NS	14 ± 3	NS	19 ± 3
In hypophysectomized dogs (N=8)					
Cardiac output (liter/min)	3.6 ± 0.4	< 0.001	4.9 ± 0.4	< 0.001	3.5 ± 0.3

Systemic arterial pressure (mmHg)	135 ± 6.7	< 0.05	114 ± 3.0	< 0.02	139 ± 6.5
Renal perfusion pressure (mmHg)	112 ± 2.6	NS	110 ± 4.2	NS	111 ± 4.6
Glomerular filtration rate (ml/min)	35 ± 2.6	NS	34 ± 2.6	NS	34 ± 2.7
Renal vascular resistance [mmHg/ (ml/min)]	0.546 ± 0.04	NS	0.567 ± 0.03	NS	0.578 ± 0.04
Urinary sodium excretion (μEq/min)	13 ± 4	NS	12 ± 4	< 0.01	16 ± 4

[a]Iso, isoproterenol.

on urinary osmolality and free-water clearance in the two groups of animals were strikingly different (Fig. 1). In intact animals the intravenous infusion of isoproterenol was associated with a significant increase in urinary osmolality and a decrease in free-water clearance which was reversible after cessation of the infusion. In contrast, as shown on the right-hand side of Fig. 1, in the acutely hypophysectomized animals no alteration in urinary osmolality or

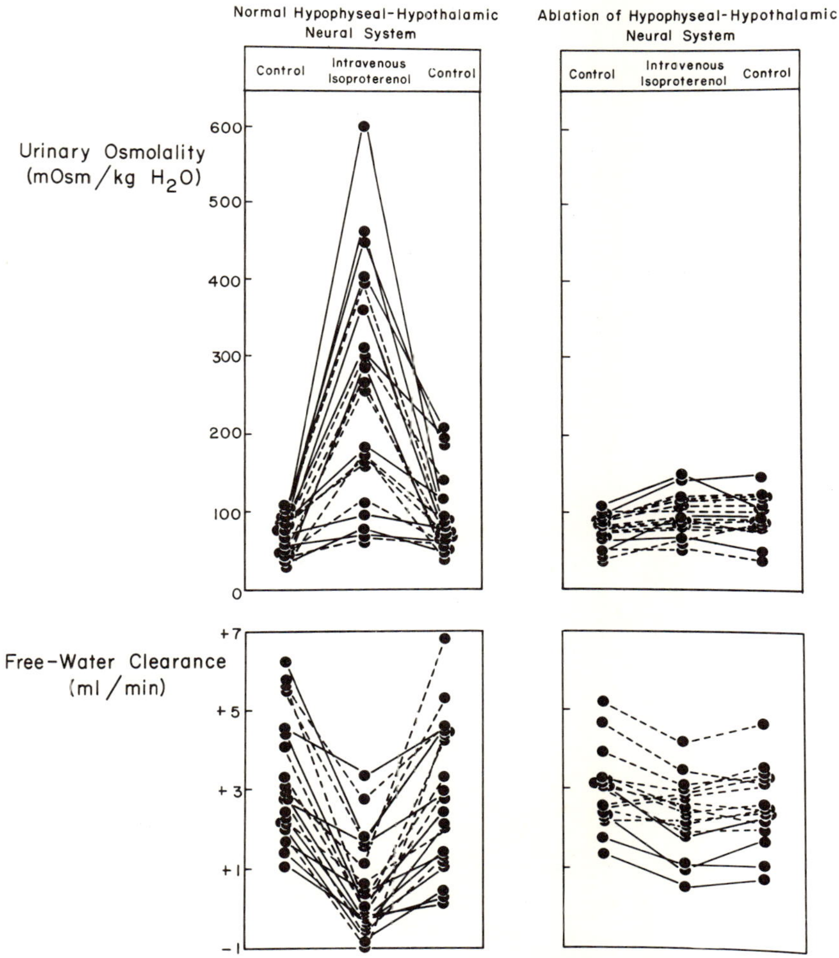

Fig. 1. Effect of beta-adrenergic stimulation with intravenous isoproterenol to increase urinary osmolality and decrease free-water clearance in the intact dog (left-hand side), but not in dogs in which the source of vasopressin has been abolished (right-hand side). In this and subsequent figures the solid and broken lines indicate results from innervated and denervated kidneys respectively. [From Schrier *et al.* (1972) by permission of publisher.]

Table 2. Effect of intrarenal isoproterenol on renal hemodynamics, electrolyte excre and renal diluting capacity

	Control		Iso[a]		Control
Glomerular filtration rate (ml/min)	44.3 ± 2.8	NS	47.0 ± 3.4	NS	45.8 ± 3.5
Renal vascular resistance [mmHg/ (ml/min)]	0.503 ± 0.05	NS	0.474 ± 0.05	NS	0.512 ± 0.05
Urinary sodium excretion (μEq/min)	23 ± 5.4	< 0.005	36 ± 7.8	NS	29 ± 5.7
Free-water clearance (ml/min)	3.48 ± 0.26	< 0.05	3.82 ± 0.33	NS	3.52 ± 0.30
Urinary osmolality (mOsm/kg H_2O)	57 ± 3	NS	59 ± 4	NS	60 ± 5

[a]Iso, isoproterenol.

free-water clearance was observed during the intravenous infusion of isoproterenol. The results in innervated and denervated kidneys were not significantly different and are indicated by the solid and broken lines, respectively. These results therefore suggested that the primary effect of systemic beta-adrenergic stimulation on renal water excretion is mediated by increased release of endogenous vasopressin (Schrier, Lieberman, and Ufferman, 1972). The possibility existed, however, that, in addition to this extrarenal effect, intrarenal beta-adrenergic stimulation might exert a direct effect on renal tubular water permeability. This is an attractive hypothesis, since the effect of vasopressin on water permeability of the renal tubule appears to be mediated by stimulating adenyl cyclase to catalyze the formation of cyclic AMP, an enzyme which in several tissues has been shown to be stimulated by beta-adrenergic stimulation (Turtle and Kipnis, 1967). In an effort to examine this possibility further, studies were performed in which isoproterenol was infused directly into the renal artery. The results of these studies are shown in Table 2. In these studies systemic effects, including changes in arterial pressure, cardiac output, and total peripheral resistance, were not observed during the infusion of isoproterenol into the renal artery, and recent studies have demonstrated that the kidney is an important site of inactivation of isoproterenol (Lifschitz *et al.*, 1973). This set of experimental circumstances therefore allowed a large amount of the beta-adrenergic agonist, isoproterenol, to be delivered to the renal circulation while avoiding any extrarenal hemodynamic changes which might alter the release of endogenous vasopressin. This dose of intrarenal isoproterenol (0.018–0.036 μg/kg/min) was comparable to the doses used in the intravenous studies and was not associated with consistent changes in glomerular filtration rate or renal vascular resistance. The slight increase in urinary sodium excretion was not reversible after cessation of the infusion. Since the concentration of isoproterenol in the renal circulation in these experiments was greater than the level achieved during intravenous infusion of the drug, a similar or even more pronounced antidiuretic effect might have been expected in these intrarenal experiments, providing that such an effect was due at least partially to a direct action of beta-adrenergic stimulation to increase water permeability of the renal tubular epithelial cells. No antidiuresis, however, was observed when isoproterenol was infused directly into the renal artery and, in fact, when the results from the infused kidney were compared with results from the contralateral control kidney, intrarenal isoproterenol was found to increase rather than decrease free-water clearance. The mean urinary osmolality remained at minimal levels of 57 ± 3, 59 ± 4, and 60 ± 5 mOsm/kg H_2O before, during, and after the intrarenal infusion of isoproterenol (Schrier *et al.*, 1972).

While these results do not provide evidence for a direct effect of isoproterenol on renal tubular water permeability, it cannot be excluded that larger intrarenal doses of this beta agonist might exert such an effect. If so, then the intrarenal beta-adrenergic receptors mediating such an effect must be less sensitive than the beta-adrenergic receptors in the heart and peripheral vasculature which were significantly stimulated during the intravenous infusion of isoproterenol. Moreover, the *in vivo* demonstration of such an intrarenal beta-adrenergic receptor affecting water permeability of the renal tubule will be difficult, since larger intrarenal doses of isoproterenol produce systemic effects and thus do not allow for the differentiation between an antidiuretic effect initiated by extrarenal *versus* intrarenal pathways. On the basis of these studies we therefore conclude that the primary effect of beta-adrenergic stimulation involves the integrity of the hypothalamo-neurohypophyseal system and the release of vasopressin. The present results have also failed to provide evidence of a major role of alterations in renal hemodynamics, renal sympathetic tone, and solute excretion, or a direct effect of isoproterenol on the water permeability of the renal tubular epithelium.

Studies were also performed to examine the mechanism of the effect of alpha-adrenergic stimulation with intravenous norepinephrine to increase renal water excretion. While previous investigations in man (Smythe *et al.*, 1952; Baldwin *et al.*, 1963; Fisher, 1968) and experimental animals (Liberman *et al.*, 1970; Klein *et al.*, 1971) have clearly demonstrated such an effect, the mechanism of this diuretic effect of alpha-adrenergic stimulation has not been well delineated. Since norepinephrine has been found to antagonize the *in vitro* effect of vasopressin on water transport in the toad bladder (Strauch and Langdon, 1969; Handler, Bensinger, and Orloff, 1968) a direct antagonistic effect of alpha-adrenergic stimulation on the vasopressin-mediated osmotic movement of water has been proposed. As with beta-adrenergic stimulation, this hypothesis is attractive since the effect of vasopressin appears to be mediated by stimulating adenyl cyclase to catalyze the formation of cyclic AMP, a process which has been reported to be inhibited by alpha-adrenergic stimulation in several tissues of the body (Turtle and Kipnis, 1967; Porte, 1967) including the kidney (Beck *et al.*, 1972). The results from previous *in vivo* studies (Smythe *et al.*, 1952; Baldwin *et al.*, 1963; Fisher, 1968; Liberman *et al.*, 1970; Klein *et al.*, 1971), however, have not allowed definitive conclusions, since the increase in renal arterial pressure, which occurs during the intravenous infusion of norepinephrine, could itself account for the water diuresis (Selkurt, Womack, and Dailey, 1965; Thurau and Deetjen, 1962). In addition, the alterations in systemic hemodynamics during intravenous norepinephrine administration could directly or indirectly lead to a suppression of endogenous vasopressin release. Somewhat against a suppression of vasopression release accounting for the diuretic effect of intravenous norepinephrine is the finding that this effect has been observed both in man (Fisher, 1968) and dog (Klein *et al.*, 1971) during the infusion of exogenous vasopressin. Submaximal doses of vasopressin were, however, used in these previous studies and no evidence was provided that maximal suppression of endogenous vasopressin was present at the time the norepinephrine was infused (Fisher, 1968; Klein *et al.*, 1971). Against the background of these previous *in vivo* investigations the present studies were undertaken in anesthetized hydropenic dogs in which the renal arterial pressure was controlled during the intravenous infusion of norepinephrine (0.5 μg/kg/min) by the adjustment of a suprarenal aortic clamp. The results of these studies are shown in Fig. 2 (Schrier and Berl, 1973). In spite of the constancy of renal perfusion pressure intravenous norepinephrine was consistently associated with an increase in free-water clearance and a decrease in urinary osmolality. The results were similar in innervated and denervated kidneys. As in previous studies (Smythe *et al.*, 1952; Baldwin *et al.*, 1963; Fisher, 1968) this effect of

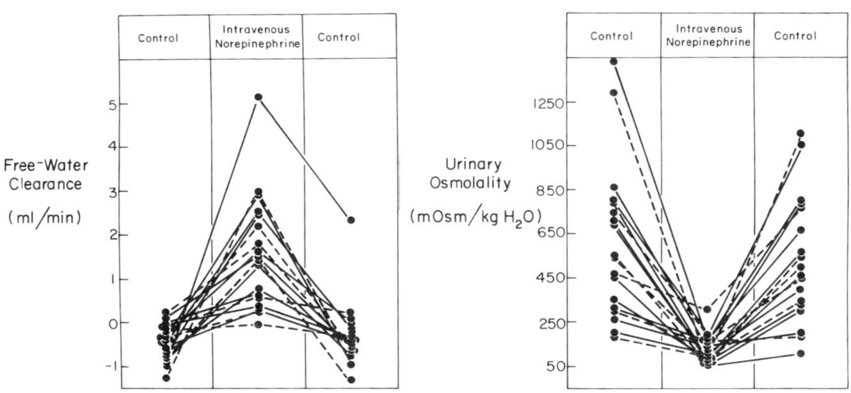

Fig. 2. Effect of intravenous norepinephrine to increase free-water excretion and decrease urinary osmolality in intact animals. [From Schrier *et al.* (1972) by permission of publisher.]

norepinephrine to increase solute-free-water excretion was not accounted for by either an increase in glomerular filtration rate or solute excretion rate. These results therefore suggested that this effect of norepinephrine was due to a direct effect on the renal tubule or an effect mediated by suppression of endogenous vasopressin. Studies were therefore performed in acutely hypophysectomized animals receiving replacement glucocorticoid hormone and a constant exogenous infusion of vasopressin in an effort to examine the possibility of an *in vivo* competitive inhibition between norepinephrine and vasopressin. Initial studies failed to demonstrate an effect of norepinephrine on urinary dilution in acutely hypophysectomized animals receiving larger doses of vasopressin (80 μU/kg/min). The results of studies in which smaller doses of vasopressin (20–40 μU/kg/min) were used are shown in Fig. 3 (Schrier and Berl, 1973). As in the previous studies the renal perfusion pressure was maintained constant during the norepinephrine infusion by the adjustment of a suprarenal aortic clamp. In contrast to the results in intact animals norepinephrine failed to alter free-water clearance or urinary osmolality in acutely hypophysectomized animals receiving exogenous vasopressin. The different effect of intravenous infusion of norepinephrine on water excretion in intact and hypophysectomized animals was not associated with differences in systemic and renal hemodynamics (Table 3). Taken together, these results therefore suggest that the primary effect of norepinephrine to increase renal-water excretion is related to suppression of endogenous vasopressin release. Additional studies were, however, undertaken to examine the effect on renal-water excretion of infusing norepinephrine directly into the

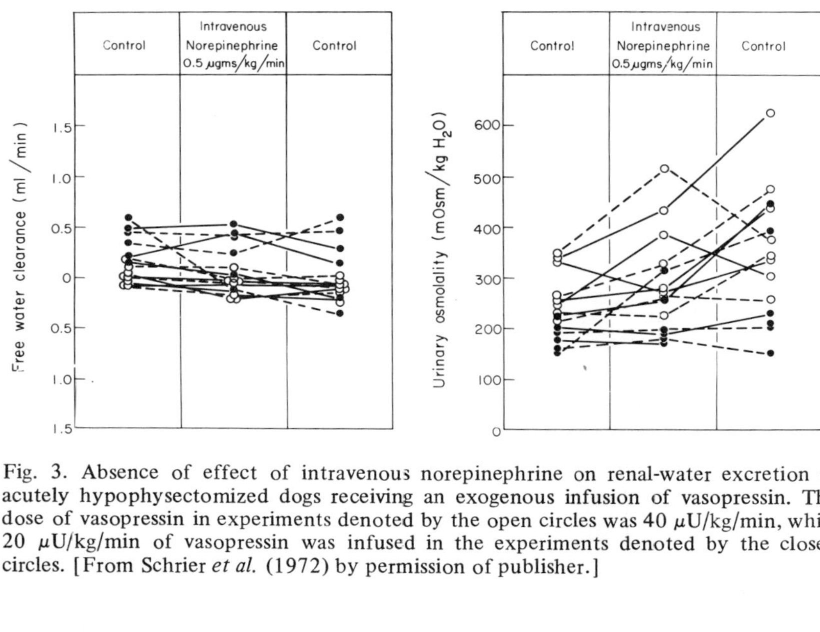

Fig. 3. Absence of effect of intravenous norepinephrine on renal-water excretion in acutely hypophysectomized dogs receiving an exogenous infusion of vasopressin. The dose of vasopressin in experiments denoted by the open circles was 40 μU/kg/min, while 20 μU/kg/min of vasopressin was infused in the experiments denoted by the closed circles. [From Schrier *et al.* (1972) by permission of publisher.]

renal artery. The dose used delivered an amount of the catecholamine to the renal circulation equivalent to that reaching the renal circulation during the intravenous infusion of norepinephrine. The effect of norepinephrine on renal hemodynamics and solute excretion was not significantly different from that observed in the intravenous studies and, as in the hypophysectomized animals, a consistent alteration in renal-water excretion was not observed (Schrier and Berl, 1973).

Additional studies were then designed to determine the afferent mechanism(s) whereby alpha- and beta-adrenergic stimulation alter the release of endogenous vasopressin. The possibility existed that catecholamines, such as norepinephrine and isoproterenol, directly alter the release of vasopressin. Alternatively, the changes in cerebral perfusion pressure which occur during alpha- and beta-adrenergic stimulation could directly influence the release of vasopressin. In order to study the first possibility norepinephrine and isoproterenol were infused directly into the carotid artery in a dose estimated to deliver a high concentration of the catecholamine to the cerebral circulation while avoiding the systemic hemodynamic consequences of the agents. In these studies the carotid infusion of norepinephrine (Berl *et al.*, 1974) or isoproterenol (Berl *et al.*, 1974) was not associated with alterations in renal-water excretion. The effect of changes in cerebral perfusion pressure on renal-water excretion was also examined. In Fig. 4 is illustrated a pump-perfusion method which was used to change arterial pressure in the cerebral circulation. In these animals the arterial baroreceptors were denervated to avoid any baroreceptor-mediated influence on renal-water excretion. In these perfusion studies 20–40 mmHg alterations in cerebral pressure were not associated with changes in renal-water excretion (Berl *et al.*, 1973).

Since in recent experiments we have demonstrated that the interruption of parasympathetic afferent, but not efferent, pathways is associated with alterations in vasopressin release (Schrier and Berl, 1972), the possibility was examined that the influence of beta- and alpha-adrenergic stimulation on vasopressin release is mediated by changes in baroreceptor neural tone. In these studies neither the diuretic effect of alpha-adrenergic stimulation (Fig. 5) nor the antidiuretic effect of beta-adrenergic stimulation (Fig. 6) was observed in animals with denervated carotid sinuses and bilateral cervical vagotomy. The effect of norepinephrine and isoproterenol on renal-water excretion was, however, observed in sham-operated animals, as shown on the left-hand side of both figures. These studies therefore provide substantial evidence that the effect of catecholamines on vasopressin release is primarily mediated by alterations in baroreceptor neural tone. These alterations in baroreceptor tone may be initiated by changes in systemic hemodynamics. Support for this possibility is derived from the recent demonstration that intravenous prostaglandin E_1, which produces similar systemic hemodynamic effects as isoproterenol but does not possess beta-adrenergic properties, is

Table 3. Effect of intravenous norepinephrine on systemic and renal hemodynamics and sodium excretion

	Control		Norepi[a]		Control
			In intact dogs (N=9)		
Cardiac output (liter/min)	3.8 ± 0.4	NS	4.2 ± 0.7	NS	3.5 ± 0.5
Systemic arterial pressure (mmHg)	121 ± 8	< 0.005	142 ± 7	< 0.005	117 ± 8
Renal perfusion pressure (mmHg)	117 ± 7	NS	117 ± 6	NS	112 ± 7
Glomerular filtration rate (ml/min)	50 ± 6	NS	50 ± 3	NS	54 ± 3
Renal vascular resistance [mmHg/(ml/min)]	0.495 ± 0.05	NS	0.495 ± 0.06	NS	0.439 ± 0.05
Urinary sodium excretion (μEq/min)	22 ± 8	NS	11 ± 2	< 0.01	33 ± 8

	In hypophysectomized dogs receiving vasopressin (N=7)				
Cardiac output (liter/min)	3.1 ± 0.4	NS	2.9 ± 0.1	NS	3.2 ± 0.4
Systemic arterial pressure (mmHg)	115 ± 9	< 0.001	152 ± 6	< 0.001	111 ± 7
Renal perfusion pressure (mmHg)	109 ± 5	NS	109 ± 6	NS	104 ± 4
Glomerular filtration rate (ml/min)	42 ± 3	< 0.02	45 ± 3	< 0.02	40 ± 3
Renal vascular resistance [mmHg/(ml/min)]	0.586 ± 0.04	NS	0.600 ± 0.03	NS	0.563 ± 0.03
Urinary sodium excretion (μEq/min)	8 ± 3	NS	12 ± 6	NS	23 ± 8

[a]Norepi, norepinephrine.

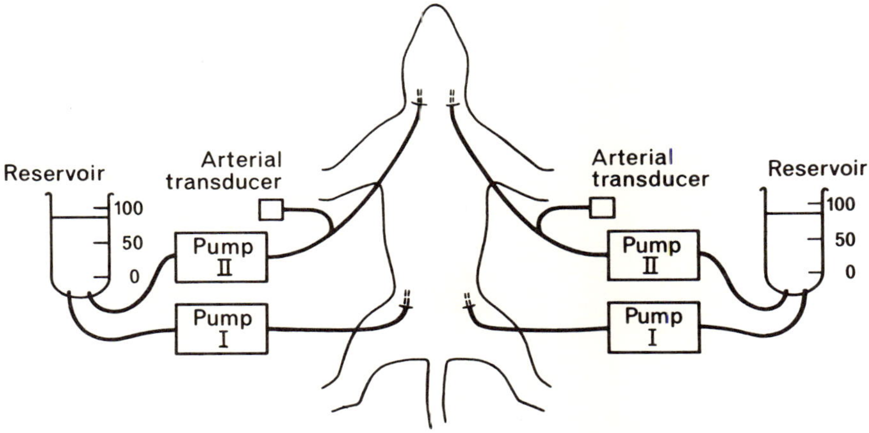

Fig. 4. Pump-perfusion method of increasing cerebral arterial pressure in animals with denervated arterial baroreceptors.

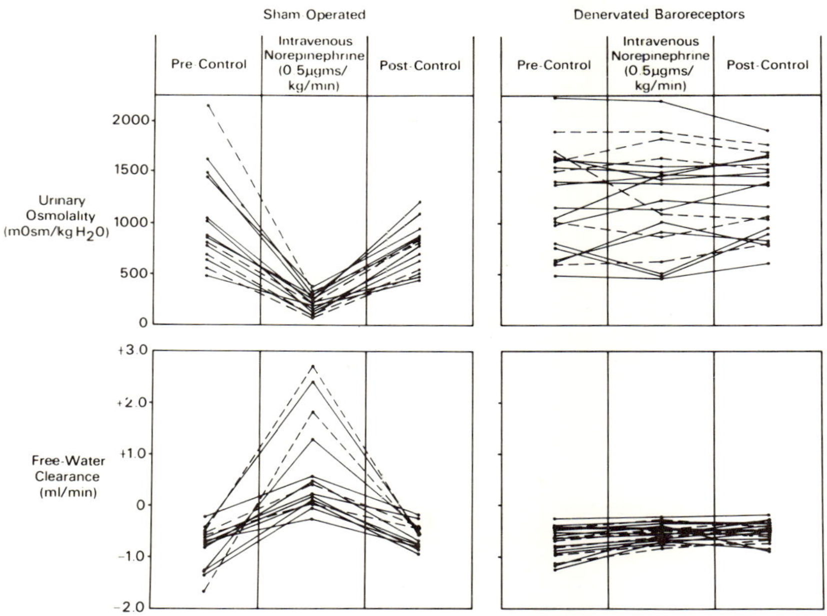

Fig. 5. Absence of effect of intravenous norepinephrine on urinary osmolality and free-water clearance in animals with denervated baroreceptors (right-hand side). The decrease in urinary osmolality and increase in free-water clearance in sham-operated dogs receiving intravenous norepinephrine are shown on the left-hand side of the figure. [From Berl *et al.* (1974) by permission of publisher.]

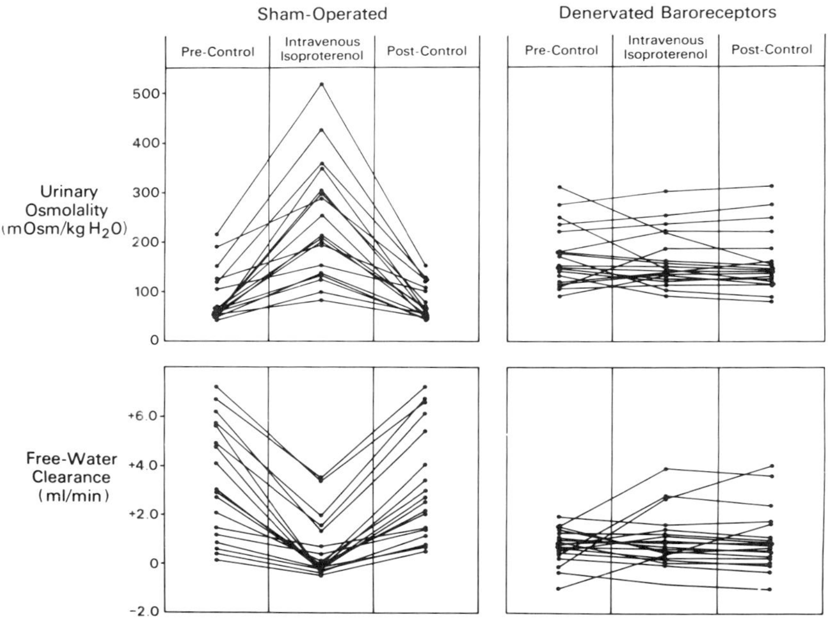

Fig. 6. Effect of intravenous isoproterenol to increase urinary osmolality (upper left) and decrease free water clearance (lower left) in sham-operated but not baroreceptor-denervated animals (upper and lower left). [From Berl *et al.* (1974) by permission of publisher.]

associated with a similar antidiuresis as intravenous isoproterenol (Berl and Schrier, 1973).

Since isoproterenol also stimulates renin secretion (Reid, Schrier, and Earley, 1972) and angiotensin has been purported to stimulate the release of vasopressin (Bonjour and Malvin, 1970), the possibility also had to be considered that such a pathway was involved in the antidiuretic effect of beta-adrenergic stimulation. This possibility seems unlikely, however, since we have been unable to demonstrate that angiotensin either infused intravenously or into the carotid artery is associated with an effect on renal-water excretion (Cadnapaphornchai *et al.*, 1973).

Additional studies were designed to delineate the mechanism whereby beta-adrenergic stimulation with isoproterenol increases the renal secretion of renin. While the stimulation of the adrenergic nervous system during carotid occlusion (Bunag, Page, and McCubbin, 1966), renal nerve stimulation (Vander, 1965; Ganong 1972a,b), and hemorrhage (Blaine, Davis, and Witty, 1970; Blaine and Davis, 1971) are known to stimulate renin secretion, the mechanism(s) of these effects is not known. These events, however, are frequently associated with significant diminutions in glomerular filtration rate, and thus an associated diminution in the rate of sodium transport to the macula densa could account for the increase in renin secretion (Vander, 1967). Alternatively, the renal vasoconstriction during adrenergic stimulation could diminish pressure at the level of some intrarenal pressure receptors which influence release of renin from the juxtaglomerular cells (Vander, 1967). However, the demonstration that beta-adrenergic stimulation with isoproterenol increases renin secretion in the absence of renal vasoconstriction suggests that pathways other than the baroreceptor and macula densa mechanisms may be involved. A direct effect of beta-adrenergic stimulation on the juxtaglomerular cells has been hypothesized, since these cells are richly innervated by adrenergic nerve endings (Wagermark, Ungerstedt, and Ljungquist, 1968). In the majority of previous studies a direct intrarenal effect of isoproterenol has not been possible to document, since the large doses of the drug which have been infused into the renal artery may alter systemic hemodynamics. The use of beta-adrenergic blocking agents, such as propranolol, also exert generalized systemic, rather than selective, intrarenal blockade. Our experiments were therefore designed to compare the effect of intravenous *versus* renal arterial infusions of the beta-adrenergic agonist, isoproterenol, on renin secretion. The doses of isoproterenol infused into the renal artery were such that no systemic hemodynamic alterations occurred. As shown in Fig. 7, a significant increase in renin secretion was observed only during the intravenous infusion of isoproterenol. Since the kidney was exposed to a much higher concentration of the beta-adrenergic agonist during the renal arterial infusions but no increase in renin secretion occurred, these

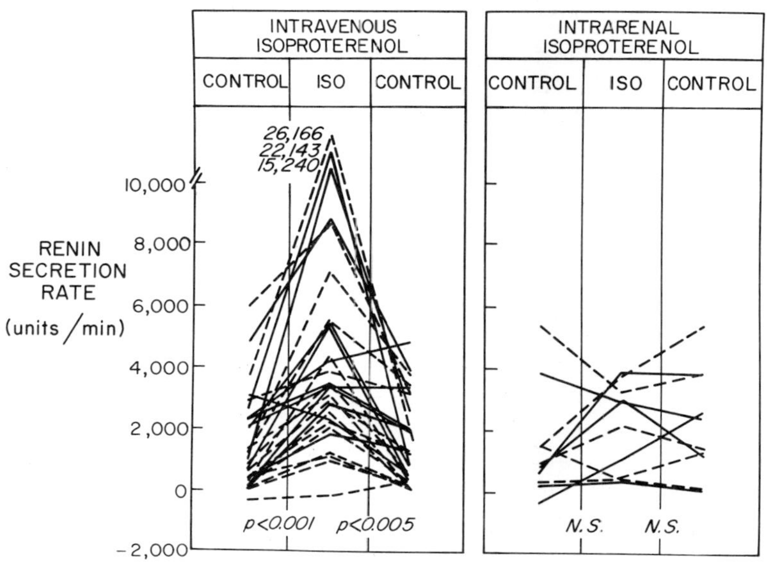

Fig. 7. Effect of intravenous but not intrarenal isoproterenol to increase renin secretion.

results suggest that the primary effect of beta-adrenergic stimulation to increase renin secretion is mediated by an extrarenal mechanism. Constancy of glomerular filtration rate and urine flow in animals undergoing a water diuresis suggested that alterations in sodium delivery to the macula densa probably were not responsible for the increase in renin secretion. Renal perfusion pressure was kept constant in all of these experiments and the effect was observed in denervated as well as innervated kidneys. These results therefore suggest that the primary effect of beta-adrenergic stimulation to increase renin secretion is mediated by an extrarenal mechanism involving an as yet undefined circulating substance. Although intravenous isoproterenol stimulates the release of vasopressin, the presence of vasopressin was not necessary for the effect on renin secretion to be observed since acute hypophysectomy did not abolish this effect (Reid *et al.*, 1972).

In summary, it has been demonstrated that both intravenous isoproterenol and norepinephrine exert profound effects on renal-water excretion in the absence of alterations in renal perfusion pressure. These effects of alpha- and beta-adrenergic stimulation were found not to be mediated by direct effects on the water permeability of the renal tubular epithelium or alterations in solute excretion rate or renal hemodynamics. Rather, the diuretic effect of alpha-adrenergic stimulation with intravenous norepinephrine was demonstrated to be mediated by suppression of vasopressin, while the antidiuretic effect of beta-adrenergic stimulation with intravenous isoproterenol was found to be mediated by stimulation of vasopressin release. The alterations in systemic hemodynamics during the intravenous infusion of norepinephrine and isoproterenol may initiate these nonosmotic influences on vasopressin release by altering afferent baroreceptor tone. This same pathway may be involved in the mediation of other nonosmotic influences on vasopressin release such as emotional and physical stress and changes in volume status. The present studies also indicate that the primary effect of beta-adrenergic stimulation to increase renin release is mediated by an extrarenal rather than an intrarenal mechanism. This effect on renin secretion was demonstrated to occur in the absence of alterations in renal arterial pressure, renal nerves, and renal hemodynamics, and thus may involve a change in concentration of some circulating renin-stimulating hormone.

ACKNOWLEDGMENTS

The authors are indebted to Lisbeth Streiff, Vicki Neel, and Dorothy Byrd for technical assistance and to Mrs. Linda Benson for secretarial assistance. This work was supported by grants HE 13319-01 and AM 12753 from the National Institutes of Health, and by NGR 05-025-007 from the National Aeronautics and Space Administration, and grants from the Bay Area Heart Association and the Hoechst Pharmaceutical Company.

REFERENCES

Baldwin, D.S., E.A. Gombos, and H. Chasis. 1963. Changes in sodium and water excretion induced by epinephrine and 1-norepinephrine in normotensive and hypertensive subjects. J. Lab. Clin. Med. 47:540.

Beck, N.P., S.W. Reed, H.V. Murdaugh, and B.B. Davis. 1972. Effects of catecholamines and their interaction with other hormones on cyclic 3′,5′-adenosine monophosphate of the kidney. J. Clin. Invest. 51:939.

Berl, T., J.A. Harbottle, P. Cadnapaphornchai, and R.W. Schrier. 1974. Mechanism of stimulation of vasopressin release during beta adrenergic stimulation with isoproterenol. J. Clin. Invest. 53: 857.

Berl, T., J.A. Harbottle, P. Cadnapaphornchai, and R.W. Schrier. 1974. Mechanism of suppression of vasopressin (ADH) by norepinephrine (NE). J. Clin. Invest. 53: 219.

Berl, T., and R.W. Schrier. 1973. Mechanism of effect of prostaglandin E_1 on renal water excretion. J. Clin. Invest. 52:463.

Blaine, E.H., and J.O. Davis. 1971. Evidence for a renal vascular mechanism in renin release: new observations with graded stimulation by aortic constriction. Circulation Res. 28–29 (suppl. II):118.

Blaine, E.H., J.O. Davis, and R.T. Witty. 1970. Renin release after hemorrhage and after suprarenal aortic constriction in dogs without sodium delivery to the macula densa. Circulation Res. 27:1081.

Bonjour, J.P., and R.L. Malvin. 1970. Stimulation of ADH release by the renin-angiotensin system. Am. J. Physiol. 218: 1555.

Bunag, R.D., I.H. Page, and J.W. McCubbin. 1966. Neural stimulation of release of renin. Circulation Res. 19:851.

Cadnapaphornchai, P., T. Berl, J.A. Harbottle, and R.W. Schrier. 1973. Evaluation of effect of angiotensin II (Angio) on renal water excretion. Clin. Res. 21:679 (abstr.).

Fisher, D.A. 1968. Norepinephrine inhibition of vasopressin antidiuresis. J. Clin. Invest. 47:540.

Ganong, W.F. 1972a. Sympathetic effects on renin secretion: mechanism and physiological role. *In* T. Assaykeen (ed.), Control of Renin Secretion, Plenum Press, New York, p. 17.

Ganong, W.F. 1972b. Effects of sympathetic activity and ACTH on renin and aldosterone secretion. *In* J. Genest (ed.) Hypertension 1972. Springer-Verlag, Berlin, p. 4.

Handler, J.S., R. Bensinger, and J. Orloff. 1968. Effect of adrenergic agents on toad bladder response to ADH, 3′,5′-AMP, and theophylline. Am. J. Physiol. 215:1024.

Klein, L.A., A.B. Liberman, M. Laks, and C.R. Kleeman. 1971. Interrelated effects of antidiuretic hormone and adrenergic drugs on water metabolism. Am. J. Physiol. 221:1657.

Lees, P. 1968. The influence of beta-adrenoceptive receptor blocking agents on urinary function in the rat. Brit. J. Pharmac. 34: 429.

Lees, P., and M.F. Lockett. 1965. Some actions of isoprenaline and orciprenaline on perfused cat kidneys. Brit. J. Pharmac. 25:152.

Lehr, D., J. Mallow, and M. Krukowski. 1967. Copious drinking and simultaneous inhibition of urine flow elicited by beta-adrenergic stimulation and contrary effect of alpha-adrenergic stimulation. J. Pharmac. Exp. Ther. 158:150.

Liberman, B., L.A. Klein, and C.R. Kleeman. 1970. Effect of adrenergic blocking agents on the vasopressin inhibiting action of norepinephrine. Proc. Soc. Exp. Biol. Med. 133:131.

Lifschitz, M.D., D. Keller, A. Goldfien, and R.W. Schrier. 1973. Mechanism of renal clearance of isoproterenol. Am. J. Physiol. 224: 733.

Porte, D., Jr. 1967. A receptor mechanism for the inhibition of insulin release by epinephrine in man. J. Clin. Invest. 46:86.

Reid, I.A., R.W. Schrier, and L.E. Earley. 1972. An effect of extrarenal beta adrenergic stimulation on the release of renin. J. Clin. Invest. 51:1861.

Schrier, R.W., and T. Berl. 1972. Mechanism of the antidiuretic effect associated with interruption of parasympathetic pathways. J. Clin. Invest. 51:2613.

Schrier, R.W., and T. Berl. 1973. Mechanism of effect of alpha adrenergic stimulation with norepinephrine on renal water excretion. J. Clin. Invest. 52:502.

Schrier, R.W., R. Lieberman, and R.C. Ufferman. 1972. Mechanism of antidiuretic effect of beta-adrenergic stimulation. J. Clin. Invest. 51:97.

Selkurt, E.E., I. Womack, and W.N. Dailey. 1965. Mechanism of natriuresis and diuresis during elevated renal arterial pressure. Am. J. Physiol. 209:95.

Smythe, C.McC., J.F. Nickel and S.E. Bradley. 1952. The effect of epinephrine (USP), l-epinephrine, and l-norepinephrine on glomerular filtration rate, renal plasma flow, and the urinary excretion of sodium, potassium and water in normal man. J. Clin. Invest. 31: 499.

Strauch, B.S., and R.G. Langdon. 1969. Tyramine, catechol amines, and the action of vasopressin stimulation of water efflux in toad bladders. Archs Biochem. Biophys. 129:227.

Thurau, K., and P. Deetjen. 1962. Die Diurese bei arteriellen Drucksteigerungen: Bedeutung der Hämodynamik des Nierenmarkes für die Harnkonzentrierung. Pflügers Arch. Ges. Physiol. 274:567.

Turtle, J.R., and D.M. Kipnis. 1967. An adrenergic receptor mechanism for the control of cyclic 3′,5′ adenosine monophosphate synthesis in tissues. Biochem. Biophys. Res. Comm. 28:797.

Vander, A.J. 1965. Effect of catecholamines and the renal nerves on renin secretion in anesthetized dogs. Am. J. Physiol. 209:659.

Vander, A.J. 1967. Control of renin release. Physiol. Rev. 47:359.

Wagermark, J., U. Ungerstedt, and A. Ljungquist. 1968. Sympathetic innervation of the juxtaglomerular cells of the kidney. Circulation Res. 22:149.

Aldosterone Antagonists in Laboratory Animals

Lorenz M. Hofmann
Department of Biological Research
Searle Laboratories
Chicago, Illinois

In the search for steroidal spirolactones, a variety of tests using spironolactone (S) as the standard in adrenalectomized rats and intact dogs were examined and indications of utility stressed for uncovering mineralocorticoid blocking activity (MBA), assessing potency and specificity relative to S. Following s.c. administration of 12 μg deoxycorticosterone acetate (DCA) or 0.2 μg aldosterone in rats (4-hr test) and 0.25 mg DCA or 10 μg aldosterone i.m. in dogs (5-hr test), a marked reduction in the urinary log (Na × 10)/K ratio occurs which is reversed in a dose-related manner with S at oral dosages of 0.3, 0.9, and 2.7 mg/rat and 1 or 2 and 8 mg/kg in the dog. Using these test procedures, the α-SH and α-SCH_3 metabolites of S were found to possess significant MBA. In other studies with intact dogs, the onset of anti-DCA activity of S occurred within 1 and 1–2 hr following intraduodenal and oral administration, respectively, with durations of activity exceeding 6 hr. Within 20–40 min after i.v. S, an elevation of the urinary Na/K ratio was observed which lasted for the remaining 280 min of the experiment. Methods, dosages (2.5–20 mg/kg), and data are reported on the use of the renal-hypertensive dog for demonstrating the antihypertensive effects of hydrochlorothiazide and S, alone or in combination.

Spironolactone [3-(3-oxo-7α-acetylthio-17β-hydroxy-4-androsten-17α-yl) propionic acid γ-lactone] is a clinically available steroidal 17-spirolactone specifically indicated in the treatment of hypertensive and edematous states related to elevated circulating levels of mineralocorticoids. A number of tests using adrenalectomized rats and intact dogs are elaborated upon in this report in order to indicate, in part, the methodology employed in the uncovering of other possibly clinically useful spirolactones. For illustrative purposes, the mineralocorticoid-blocking properties of recently identified sulfur-containing metabolites of S are reported.

MATERIALS AND METHODS

Adrenalectomized Rat

This animal model as developed by Kagawa (1960) is routinely used to evaluate mineralocorticoid antagonism activity (1) relative to a single standard 50% blocking dose of S, (2) for multiple dosage bioassays *versus* S, and (3) for demonstrating lack of effects of spirolactones on electrolyte excretion in the absence of adrenalcorticoids. Deoxycorticosterone acetate, a potent synthetic mineralocorticoid, is usually employed to elicit a marked retention of sodium in these tests with adrenalectomized rats. In all tests in which blocking properties of spirolactones are assessed the index employed is the reversal (increase) of the log(Na×10)/K ratio[1] response induced by DCA or aldosterone.

Screening tests. In these tests, male rats (150–200 gm) are bilaterally adrenalectomized and maintained for 24 hr on sugar cubes and tap water. Food and water are withdrawn during the test period. Groups of four animals are then treated successively with the following standardized injections: 12 μg of DCA in 0.1 ml of corn oil, 2.4 mg of the spirolactone to be tested or 0.33 mg of S in 0.5 ml of corn oil, and, lastly, 2.5 ml of 0.85% saline. A pooled urine sample from each group of rats is collected over a 4-hr period and diluted to 50 ml with distilled water. Electrolyte concentrations (mEq/1) are transformed into logs and the urinary Na/K ratios are reported as log(Na×10)/K. A 0.30 log unit change represents a two-fold change in the basic urinary measurement. At the 2.4-mg dose a spirolactone's qualitative anti-DCA activity is evidenced by a log(Na×10)/K ratio equal to that elicited by the 0.33 mg dose of spironolactone. This standard dose of S exhibits a 50% blockade of the depressed Na/K ratio induced by DCA.

Bioassay. To illustrate the utility of this assay, the anti-DCA potency and confidence limits of the C_7, α-SCH_3 metabolite was established relative to S. Both spirolactones were administered orally at dosages of 0.3, 0.9, and 2.7 mg/rat in 0.5 ml of corn oil. The relative potency of this metabolite was calculated from a six-point (two drugs × three doses) bioassay with dose-dependent increases in the urinary log(Na×10)/K ratio employed as the index of the DCA-blocking response. The 95% confidence limits of the mean potency ($\bar{x}$) was calculated as $\bar{x} \pm t$ (s.e.). In all of the bioassays reported, chi-square analyses indicated parallelism of the dose-response curves and validated each assay.

Aldosterone-treated Dog:

The dog was selected as the second species for comparative studies of the mineralocorticoid blocking activity of spirolactones. Five female dogs (16–24 kg) accustomed to repeated bladder catherterization and standardized diu-

[1] Multiplication of Na concentrations by 10 eliminates negative log Na/K values.

retic testing procedures and maintained on a normal diet were treated randomly at weekly intervals as (a) control with or without 10 μg aldosterone in 0.2 ml sesame oil intramuscularly and (b) 2 and 8 mg/kg dosages of S or its C_7, α-SH metabolite. All drug studies included pretreatment with aldosterone.

The experimental procedure was as follows. At − 30 min, aldosterone was injected in the hind limb, and 30 min later (at zero time) each animal was catheterized for complete emptying of the bladder and the spirolactone administered orally in a gelatin capsule followed by an oral load of tap water (10 ml/kg) via a stomach tube. The animals were placed in metabolism cages and urine collected (including catheterization sample) at 2½ hr. A second oral load of tap water (5 ml/kg) was given and a second 2½-hr period of urine collection obtained with bladder catheterization at the end of the 5-hr test. The compiled excretion data for Na and K are reported as μEq/kg for the entire 5-hr test. The relative antialdosterone potency and 95% confidence limits of the metabolite relative to S was calculated from a four-point (two drugs × two doses) bioassay.

Onset and Duration of Action:

Onset and duration of renal effects of S were studied in dogs given an oral or intraduodenal dose of 100 mg (8 mg/kg) and an intravenous dose as a bolus injection of approximately 65 mg followed by a constant infusion of 35 mg over an 80-min period. Three female dogs with chronic indwelling catheters (i.d.) in the duodenum were treated randomly as (a) control with or without 0.25 mg DCA (a dose equivalent in response to 10 μg aldosterone) in 0.5 ml corn oil i.m. and (b) 10 and 100 mg of S. Spironolactone was dissolved in 1.5 ml of propylene glycol, administered through the i.d. catheter, and then flushed in with an additional 1 ml of solvent. When given orally, the same solution of S was placed in a gelatin capsule. Both DCA and drug treatments were given simultaneously at the initiation of a 6-hr test and immediately followed by a 10-ml/kg oral load of tap water. Routine bladder catheterizations were carried out as previously described along with total urine collections at 1, 2, 3, 4 and 6 hr. Drug effects were compared with DCA controls for the same time periods.

Standard renal clearance studies with i.v. S were carried out in four female dogs which were trained to lie on a padded board for periods of up to 8 hr. After an initial oral load of 10 ml/kg tap water, 5% dextrose was infused i.v. at a rate of 4.5 ml/min. After a 1-hr period of equilibration, two 20-min control periods (−40–0 min) were obtained prior to the start of i.v. S (5 mg/kg plus an infusion of 2.67 mg/kg/80 min), and then followed by 16 consecutive 20-min clearance periods or for a total of 320 min post-treatment. Each dog was run in a complete control study of 420 min for period to period comparisons. Inulin clearances were used as an index of glomerular filtration rate (GFR). Free-water clearance (C_{H_2O}) was calculated as urine flow minus osmolar clearance.

Antihypertensive Response

Male or female renal-hypertensive dogs may be used as a test model for demonstrating the antihypertensive activity of spirolactones and/or hydrochlorothiazide. Following right nephrectomy, the left kidney's capsular tissue was removed and the organ securely wrapped in cellophane. The two operations were carried out over a three-week period with intermittent antibiotic therapy. The animals were maintained on a normal laboratory diet. Twice-daily recordings of blood pressure at 9 a.m. and 2 p.m. were obtained from an indwelling cannula in the abdominal aorta from Monday through Friday of each week. Hypertensive levels were established during a period in which no drugs were given. No consistent differences in blood pressures were observed for any given Friday *versus* any of the Monday through Thursday measurements. The maximum antihypertensive response to treatment occurred on the fifth day (Friday) and therefore, Friday (prior to treatment) to Friday comparisons were made in order to assess the antihypertensive effects of hydrochlorothiazide (HC) and S. In general, the protocol consisted of alternating one week of control and one week of treatment. In random selection, the treatment consisted of a single daily oral administration of HC or S in a gelatin capsule after the 9 a.m. reading from Monday through Friday. On the following Monday (72 hr post-treatment) blood pressure levels were usually approaching pretreatment levels. The dosages of HC or S employed were 2.5, 5, 10, and 20 mg/kg *alone* and in combinations of 2.5, 5, and 10 mg/kg. The antihypertensive responses were evaluated on the basis of reductions in systolic and diastolic pressures as well as mean arterial pressure (diastolic + 1/3 pulse pressure). The results from a female (6.8 kg) renal-hypertensive dog are presented with the view of illustrating the pharmacodynamics of these drugs in this test model.

RESULTS AND DISCUSSION

Five sulfur metabolites of S isolated in man by Karim and Brown (1972) and aldadiene, the dethioacetylated Δ^6 derivative, were screened for anti-DCA activity. In Table 1 the relative activities of each metabolite are presented as median effective doses (MED) in mg/rat at which there occurs a 50% blockade of the renal effects of 12 μg DCA. In decreasing orders of magnitude, three of these metabolites (α-SH, α-SCH_3, aldadiene) exhibited significant anti-DCA activities. The three other metabolites possess minor, if any, anti-DCA activity as evidenced by MED values greater than 2.4 mg/rat, i.e., their log(Na×10)/K ratio responses produced were less than that elicited by a standard 0.33 mg/rat dose of S.

In the bioassay of the α-SCH_3 metabolite *versus* S, the administration of DCA resulted, as expected, in the retention of sodium and enhanced potassium excretion together with a marked reduction in the urinary Na/K ratio (Table 2). Both spirolactones exhibited dose-dependent increases in the Na/K

Table 1. Spironolactone and metabolites: ratios of activities for 50% blockade of DCA-response in adrenalectomized rats

Spirolactones	6β-	7α-	MED (mg/rat)[a]	Relative activity
(S):		–SCOCH$_3$	0.33	1
	Δ^6		0.86	0.38
		–SH	0.22	1.50
		–SCH$_3$	0.34	0.97
	–OH	–SCH$_3$	> 2.4[b]	< 0.14
		–SCH$_3$ ↓ 0	> 2.4[b]	< 0.14
	–OH	–SCH$_3$ ↓ 0	> 2.4[b]	< 0.14

[a]MED, median effective dose for blockade of 12 μg DCA during a 4-hr test. MED × 5 ≃ mg/kg.
[b]Minor, if any, anti-DCA activity.

ratio as a result of enhanced excretion of sodium and/or potassium retention. This metabolite is equivalent (1.06 times) in potency to S as a mineralocorticoid antagonist. The 95% confidence limits (0.77 and 1.47) bracketed unity, indicating no significant differences in potency between these spirolactones. In this assay a 0.2-μg/rat dose of aldosterone can be substituted for

Table 2. Spironolactone and its α-SCH$_3$ metabolite: anti-DCA response in adrenalectomized rats

			Mean log urinary response/4 hr		
Treatment	mg/rat	*N*	Na × 10	K	(Na × 10)/K
Control		8	1.97[b]	0.78[b]	1.19[b]
DCA[a]		6	1.49 ± 0.24	0.93 ± 0.15	0.56 ± 0.15
S	0.3	6	1.46	0.84	0.62
S	0.9	6	1.52	0.83	0.70
S	2.7	6	1.81[b]	0.71[b]	1.11[b]
α-SCH$_3$	0.3	6	1.42	0.81	0.60
α-SCH$_3$	0.9	6	1.60	0.73[b]	0.87[b]
α-SCH$_3$	2.7	6	1.71	0.72[b]	0.98[b]

N number of groups (four rats/group).
[a]Mean ± 95% confidence limits for DCA controls.
[b]$P < 0.05$, relative to DCA controls.

the 12 μg DCA, resulting in quantitatively comparable effects upon the patterns of sodium and potassium excretion.

Further studies in the adrenalectomized rat were conducted with S over a wide range of dosages from 0.1 to 3.2 mg/animal or approximately 0.5–16 mg/kg (Table 3). In the absence of exogenous mineralocorticoids the compound failed to alter the urinary excretion patterns of Na or K. All urinary parameters were indistinguishable from untreated controls. These observations illustrate the specific requirement of at least normal circulating levels of mineralocorticoids for manifestation of the renal effects of spirolactones.

Spironolactone and its α-SH metabolite were assayed in the intact dog. The effects of these spirolactones together with the expected retention of sodium with a corresponding reduction in the urinary Na/K ratio following injection of aldosterone alone are summarized in Table 4. Potassium output was unaltered following aldosterone. The significant natriuresis elicited at the 8-mg/kg dosage by both S (150% increase) and this metabolite (85% increase) resulted in elevations of the Na/K ratio to approximately nonaldosterone control levels. Dose-dependent increases in this latter parameter indicated that the α-SH metabolite possessed 0.70 of the potency of S. The 95% confidence limits were between 0.09 and 2.33, indicating that the antialdosterone potency of this metabolite was not statistically different from that of S. Urine volumes were not reported. In all controls and treatments the urine flow rates remained relatively constant within 10 ± 1 (s.e.) ml/kg/5 hr. In this assay model the effects of 1-, 2-, or 8-mg/kg dosages of S are routinely compared with that of other spirolactones. In most assays the 2-mg/kg dosage of S significantly reverses the sodium-retaining effect of aldosterone. The time of onset of the natriuretic response is within the initial 2½ hr of the assay.

Times of onset and duration of mineralocorticoid blocking and diuretic responses of S are reported for use as reference values when undertaking

Table 3. Spironolactone: renal effects in the absence of mineralocorticoids

		Mean log urinary response/4 hr		
Treatment	mg/rat	(Na × 10)/K	K	(Na × 10)/K
Control[a]		2.06 ± 0.22	0.64 ± 0.23	1.42 ± 0.14
S	0.1	2.24	0.78	1.46
S	0.4	2.24	0.80	1.44
S	1.6	2.12	0.72	1.40
S	3.2	1.93	0.64	1.29

12 groups of animals for controls and 3 groups per dosage of S. mg/rat × 5 ≃ mg/kg dosage of S.

[a]Mean ± 95% confidence limits for non-DCA-treated controls.

Table 4. Spironolactone and its α-SH metabolite: antialdosterone response in the dog

Treatment	mg/kg	Aldosterone (μg)	Mean urinary response/5 hr[a]			
			N	Na	K	log(Na × 10)/K
Control			10	604 ± 117[b]	228 ± 85	1.472 ± 0.125[b]
Control		10	10	271 ± 112	264 ± 74	0.958 ± 0.207
S	2	10	5	284 ± 183	212 ± 88	1.074 ± 0.122
S	8	10	5	685 ± 187[b]	274 ± 109	1.420 ± 0.139[b]
α-SH	2	10	5	220 ± 191	146 ± 44[b]	1.041 ± 0.336
α-SH	8	10	5	503 ± 238[b]	252 ± 112	1.297 ± 0.285[b]

[a]Na and K excretion in μEq/kg. Mean ± 95% confidence limits for controls (two experiments per dog) with and without 10 μg aldosterone. Same five dogs with single oral drug treatment.
[b]$P < 0.05$ relative to aldosterone control.

Table 5. Spironolactone onset of anti-DCA response following oral and intraduodenal administration in the dog

			Hours after treatment[a]								
			0–1			1–2			0–6		
Treatment	mg	Route	Na	K	Na/K	Na	K	Na/K	Na	K	Na/K
Control			60	61	0.89	52	39	1.06	343[b]	204	1.20[b]
DCA			43	58	0.75	33	56	0.72	149	277	0.71
S	10	i.g.	24	76	0.45	19	62	0.57	158	330	0.62
S	100	i.g.	37	37	0.96	52	28[b]	1.15[b]	329[b]	196	1.28[b]
S	10	i.d.	42	64	0.73	66[b]	39[b]	1.07[b]	236	269	0.85
S	100	i.d.	77	57	1.24[b]	56[b]	14[b]	1.61[b]	354[b]	142[b]	1.40[b]

[a]Mean from three dogs. N=6 for each control. N=3 for each S experiment. Na and K in μEq/kg and Na/K as log(Na×10)/K.

[b]$P < 0.05$ relative to DCA control. 95% confidence limits for (Na, K, Na/K) = (43, 27, 0.28), (22, 18, 0.24) and (88, 123, 0.21) for hours 0–1, 1–2 and 0–6 respectively.

profile testing of other spirolactones. Of the three parameters, the urinary Na/K ratio was selected over individual cation changes (↑Na, ↓K) as the response index for assessing times of onset and duration of action. Following the intraduodenal and oral administration of 100 mg of S, initial anti-DCA activity occurred within 1 and 1–2 hr, respectively, with each duration time exceeding 6 hr. The compiled data are presented in Table 5. This dosage of S reversed completely the sodium retention induced by DCA to untreated control levels. The 10 mg (ca. 0.8 mg/kg) dosage of S was without effect, by either route, on total 6-hr cation levels. However within 1–2 hr after intraduodenal administration of this lower dose, significant anti-DCA activity was evident which lasted for the remainder of the test. Apparently, the differences in activity observed are a consequence of enhanced and/or more rapid absorption following direct installation into the duodenum as compared with oral delivery of the drug.

In the i.v. studies with S exogenous mineralocorticoids were not administered in order to assess the diuretic pattern of the drug in the presence of normal circulating levels of adrenalcorticoids. For brevity, the mean values from the four dogs are presented in Table 6 as averages of two consecutive 20-min clearance periods starting 40 min before and continuing for 80 min after the initial bolus injection. Thereafter, hourly clearance averages are reported up to 200 min post-treatment and, finally, the last 40 min of the 7-hr experiment. Within 20–40 min after i.v. S, a consistent elevation in the urinary Na/K ratio was observed which lasted throughout the remaining 280 min of the test. This response was initially as a consequence of potassium retention, later combined with a natriuretic response, and thereafter only the enhanced sodium output sustained the elevation in the Na/K ratio (Table 7).

Table 6. Intravenous spironolactone: onset and duration of diuretic action in the conscious dog

	−40–0	0–40	40–80	80–140	140–200	280–320
	C S	Drug infusion		C S	C S	C S
C_{inulin} (ml/min)	74,68	77,66	78,65	76,66	82,65	78,68
Urine (ml/min)	3.3,3.5	3.6,3.2	4.0,3.4	4.4,4.1	4.5,4.8	4.6,4.7
C_{H_2O} (ml/min)	2.6,2.4	2.7,2.4	3.0,2.7	3.3,2.9	3.4,3.0	3.5,3.5
Na (μEq/min)	20,21	27,35	32,46	43,70	46,90	50,146
K (μEq/min)	12,8.4	13,7.6	14,5.9	16,7.0	16,8.6	13,13
Na/K (μEq/min)	1.8,2.4	2.3,4.2	3.0,7.8	3.4,9.9	3.3,10.2	4.4,11.1

20-min clearance periods during 420 min of 5% dextrose infusion.
S, 5 mg/kg at 100 min with infusion of 2.67 mg/kg/80 min.
S, total dose 95–110 mg; effects monitored for 320 min.
C, controls for same four dogs.
No significant change in urine flow and inulin or free-water clearance.

Table 7. Intravenous spironolactone: onset and duration of diuretic action in the conscious dog

	0–20 min	Onset		Maximum		Duration
Urine	% Δ	min	% Δ	min	% Δ	min–onset
Na	40 ↑	80-100	63 ↑	300-320	192 ↑	> 220
K	32 ↓	20-40	51 ↓	60-80	60 ↓	180
Na/K	59 ↑	20-40	108 ↑	180-200	209 ↑	> 280

20-min clearance periods (C.P.) during 420 min of 5% dextrose infusion.
Four female dogs: corresponding C.P. comparisons; controls versus S.
All onset values $P < 0.05$.
S, 5 mg/kg at 100 min with infusion of 2.67 mg/kg/80 min.
D, total dose 95–110 mg; effects monitored for 320 min.

This diuretic pattern following S occurred in the absence of changes in urine flow and inulin or free-water clearance.

The maximum antihypertensive effects of S and HC at daily dosages within the range of diuretic levels are presented in Table 8. These maximum reductions in blood pressure occurred on the fifth day of treatment and, with the exception of the highest dosage (20 mg/kg), returned to or near control hypertensive levels within 72 hr after the last dosage. An additional 48 hr (five days post-treatment) were required for the blood pressure to return to untreated hypertensive levels following the 20-mg/kg dosage of either drug. Spironolactone was without effect at the lowest dosage (2.5 mg/kg) and yet, when combined with an equal amount of HC, a marked decrease (25%) occurred in systolic, diastolic, and mean blood pressures. Synergism cannot be ascribed to this combined dosage level because of the paucity of data. Available data from this animal and from other responsive dogs with moderate hypertension (about 150 mmHg, mean arterial pressure) indicate that a daily dosage of 5 mg/kg, alone or in combination, is an optimum regimen for demonstrating the antihypertensive effects of these drugs over a five-day period. Combining 5-mg/kg dosages of these drugs produces an antihypertensive response which is usually greater in magnitude than a 10-mg/kg dose of either agent alone. Unimportant reductions in body weight were observed during treatment. Hyporesponsiveness to intra-arterial injections of norepinephrine (0.5, 1, 2 μg/kg) have been observed in some experiments on the fifth day of treatment as compared with responses obtained on Friday p.m. of the control week. These findings (unreported) are tentative and would have to be explored further before ascribing to this observation a possible mode of antihypertensive action of HC and S.

SUMMARY

A variety of tests have been examined and methods reported in adrenalectomized rats for (a) initial screening of spirolactones for mineralocorticoid-

Table 8. Antihypertensive effects of hydrochlorothiazide and spironolactone in a renal hypertensive dog

Dosage[a] (mg/kg)		Control			Treatment			Recovery			% ΔC versus T		
		Blood pressure (mmHg)[b]											
S	HC	*s*	*d*	$\bar{X}$	*s*	*d*	$\bar{X}$	*s*	*d*	$\bar{X}$	s	*d*	$\bar{X}$
20		330	210	250	310	165	213	290	130	183	− 6	−21	−15
10		340	210	253	292	190	224	310	205	240	−14	−10	−11
5		330	210	250	282	180	214	320	215	250	−14	−14	−14
2.5		332	212	252	312	208	243	335	215	255	− 6	− 2	− 4
	20	348	238	275	242	152	182	275	185	215	−30	−36	−34
	10	318[c]	200[c]	239[c]	280	175	210	310	205	240	−12	−12	−12
	5	340	228	265	245	140	175	275	170	205	−28	−38	−34
	2.5	325[d]	215[d]	252[d]	292	180	217	310[e]	210[e]	243[e]	−10	−16	−14
10	10	340[f]	210[f]	253[f]	238	148	178	315	195	235	−30	−30	−30
5	5	338	212	254	210	128	155	275	170	205	−38	−40	−39
2.5	2.5	345	225	265	258	165	196	295	225	248	-25	−27	−26

Female beagle, 6.8 kg.

[a]Compound given in a capsule for five days after each 9 a.m. recording.

[b]Systolic (*s*), diastolic (*d*), and mean (X) blood pressures recorded for control on Friday preceding treatment on following Monday. Treatment blood pressures recorded on a Friday immediately before and 5 hr after fifth dosage. Recovery on following Monday at 9 a.m., i.e., 72 hr after fifth dosage. Control and treatment blood pressures calculated from recordings at 9 a.m. and 2 p.m. for each day.

[c]Pressures on Monday at 9 a.m. just prior to 10 mg/kg HC regimen were s=360, d=230 and $\bar{X}$=273 mmHg. Based upon these levels this dose of HC decreased s by 22%, d by 24%, and $\bar{X}$ by 23%.

[d]Control values from 2 p.m. recording on Friday.

[e]Recovery at 96 hr after fifth dosage on following Tuesday at 9 a.m.

[f]Control values from 9 a.m. recording on Friday.

blocking activity, (b) multiple dosage bioassays for potency evaluations relative to spironolactone, and (c) for assessing the specificity, i.e., lack of an effect of spirolactones on electrolyte excretion in the absence of adrenalcorticoids. Test methods were also reported using the intact dog for assessing antialdosterone potencies of spirolactones and times of onset and duration of mineralocorticoid blocking, and diuretic responses following oral, intraduodenal, and intravenous administration of spironolactone. In addition, methods are discussed and data reported on the use of the renal-hypertensive dog for demonstrating the antihypertensive effects of hydrochlorothiazide and spironolactone, alone or in combination.

ACKNOWLEDGMENTS

The skilled research assistance of Mrs. H. Pedrera and Mr. O. Suleymanov is gratefully acknowledged.

REFERENCES

Kagawa, C.M. 1960. Blocking the renal electrolyte effects of mineralocorticoids with an orally active steroidal spirolactone. Endocrinology 67: 125.

Karim, A., and E.A. Brown. 1972. Isolation and identification of novel sulfur-containing metabolites of spironolactone (Aldactone®). Steroids 20: 41.

Laboratory Comparison of Three Loop Diuretics

R. Z. Gussin[1]
American Cyanamid Company
Lederle Laboratories
Pearl River, New York

The precise renal tubular sites of action of various diuretics have been the subject of considerable controversy. General agreement exists for impairment of sodium reabsorption in the Henle loop by ethacrynic acid, furosemide, and triflocin, but there is little accord concerning additional sites. The use of clearance data to establish the site of activity is complicated when multiple sites are involved, stop-flow requires modification to prevent the influence of distal tubular impairment on proximally derived samples, and micropuncture studies are plagued by many problems including variable filtration rates, retrograde contamination of samples during collection, and inaccessibility of deeper nephrons. Therefore it appears that the proximal and distal portions of the nephron will remain the battlefields of nephrologists for some time to come.

Elucidation of the renal tubular sites of action and the mechanism of action of diuretic agents has evolved through the use of numerous methods of study. Table 1 lists some of the models and methods which have been utilized. From this massive scientific assault on kidneys, toad bladders, red blood cells, barnacle muscle fibers, frog skin, rats, cats, dogs, chickens, and a variety of other systems has emerged an extensive and confusing picture concerning the sites and mechanisms of the action of diuretics. Three diuretics of relatively recent vintage weathered this storm with a reasonable degree of agreement on at least one site of action. They are ethacrynic acid, furosemide, and triflocin. The structures of these diuretics are shown in Fig. 1.

Considerable evidence is available to implicate the Henle loop as a major site of action of these agents. The most convincing is their ability to decrease both free-water clearance (C_{H_2O}) in hydrated subjects, both animals and man, and solute-free water reabsorption (Tc_{H_2O}) in hydropenic subjects.

[1] Present address: McNeil Laboratories, Inc., Fort Washington, Pa. 19034

Table 1. Some models and methods for the laboratory evaluation of diuretics

Electrolyte and water clearance in various animal species
Stop-flow
Micropuncture and microperfusion
Kidney tissue gradient
Toad bladder and frog skin
Red blood cell
Isolated renal tubules
Chronic caval dogs
Intrarenal blood flow distribution
Barnacle muscle fiber
ATPase
Renal renin secretion
Oxygen consumption by renal tissue
Carbonic anhydrase
Kidney slices

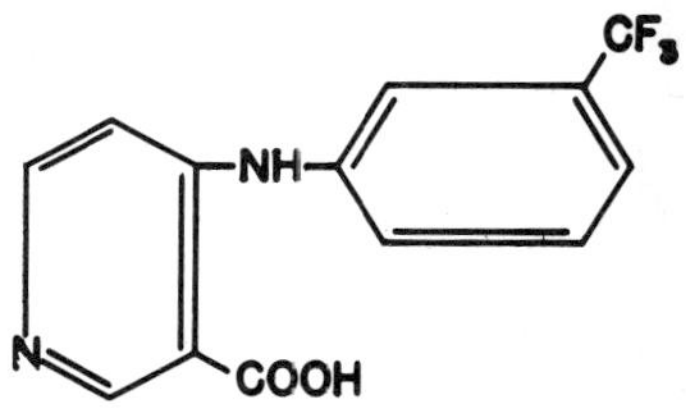

TRIFLOCIN

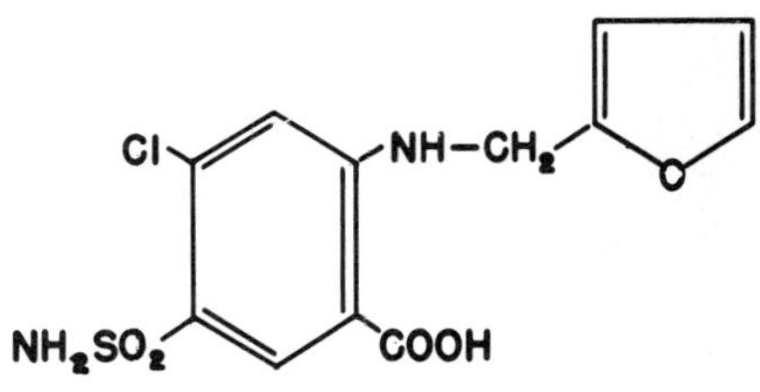

FUROSEMIDE

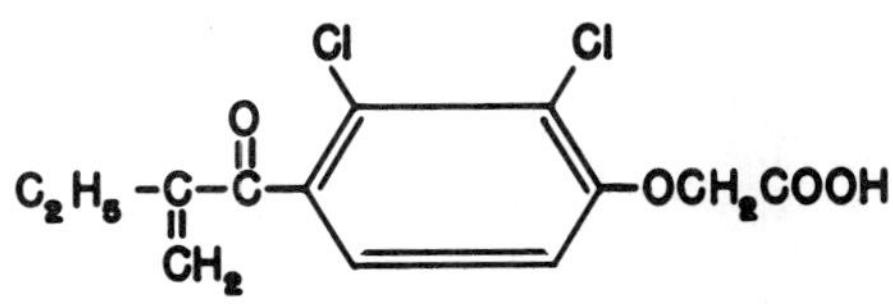

ETHACRYNIC ACID

Fig. 1. Structures of ethacrynic acid, furosemide, and triflocin.

The ability of ethacrynic acid to lower C_{H_2O} and Tc_{H_2O} was first reported by Beyer *et al.* (1965) in dogs, and by Goldberg *et al.* (1964), Earley and Friedler (1964), and Cannon *et al.* (1965) in man. A site of action for furosemide in the Henle loop was reported almost simultaneously with that for ethacrynic acid (Suki, Rector, and Seldin, 1965; Seldin *et al.*, 1966). Triflocin, a newer agent than the other two, was first reported to act in the Henle loop by Gussin *et al.* (1969).

Unfortunately the agreement on sites of action for ethacrynic acid, furosemide, and triflocin ends when one considers any renal tubular site other than the Henle loop. Table 2 illustrates the diversity of opinion concerning sites of action of the three diuretics.

Probably the greatest controversy exists over the presence or absence of a proximal tubular site. A decade ago the excretion of greater than 15% of the filtered sodium was accepted as evidence that a diuretic affected proximal tubular reabsorption. However, micropuncture studies revealed that much less than 85% of the filtered sodium may be reabsorbed in the proximal tubule (Cortney *et al.*, 1965; Bennet, Brenner, and Berliner, 1968). In fact, as much as 40–50% of the filtered sodium may pass beyond this tubular area. Therefore, a diuretic must cause the loss of more than 50% of the filtered sodium if this parameter is to be used to estimate proximal activity. Although the three diuretics under discussion are highly efficacious, they rarely produce a fractional sodium excretion of such magnitude.

Free-water clearance (C_{H_2O}) and solute-free water reabsorption (Tc_{H_2O}) have often been used to describe the tubular sites of action of diuretics. These parameters are very useful to describe a single pure site of action, but become confusing when a drug acts at multiple sites. A diuretic which interferes solely with proximal tubular reabsorption will deliver increased amounts of sodium to diluting segments in the ascending limb of Henle's loop and the distal convoluted tubule. Providing that these sites are unimpaired, additional amounts of free water will be formed by removal of sodium. If one or both of these sites is impaired, less than the usual amounts of sodium will be removed, and the effect will serve to mask the influence on free-water clearance of the depressed sodium reabsorption in the proximal tubule. Diuretics acting at distal diluting sites only will decrease C_{H_2O}, and conclusive evidence for an effect on the medullary diluting segment can be provided by demonstration of depressed Tc_{H_2O} in hydropenic subjects. Once again, however, multiple sites of activity complicate the picture. A diuretic agent acting at only the medullary diluting site will lower both C_{H_2O} in hydrated subjects and Tc_{H_2O} in hydropenic subjects. This is also true for a diuretic acting at both diluting sites. Ethacrynic acid, furosemide, and triflocin all can decrease C_{H_2O} and Tc_{H_2O}. They must, therefore, act at the medullary diluting site, but whether or not they have an effect at the distal cortical diluting site is not as clear. As demonstrated in Table 3, hydrochlorothiazide (HCTZ) produced an additional fall in C_{H_2O} after it had been reduced by triflocin. Since HCTZ does not depress Tc_{H_2O}, and so is assumed to act at

Table 2. Some proposed sites of diuretic activity

Ethacrynic acid		Furosemide		Triflocin	
Proposed site	Reference	Proposed site	Reference	Proposed site	Reference
PT	Gussin & Cafruny, 1966	HL	Morrin, 1966	HL	Gussin *et al.*, 1969
HL	Gussin & Cafruny, 1966	DT	Fraser *et al.*, 1967	PT	Gussin *et al.*, 1969
DT	Gussin & Cafruny, 1966	PT	Eknoyan *et al.*, 1970	DT	Gussin *et al.*, 1969
PT	Eknoyan *et al.*, 1970	PT	Morgan *et al.*, 1970	HL	Lockhart *et al.*, 1972
PT	Clapp *et al.*, 1971	HL	Morgan *et al.*, 1970	HL	Kaulker, 1973
PT	DiBona, 1971	PT	Duarte, 1972	DT	Kaulker, 1973
HL	DiBona, 1971			CD	Kaulker, 1973
PT	Duarte, 1972				

Abbreviations: PT, proximal tubule; HL, Henle loop; DT, distal tubule; CD, collecting ducts.

Table 3. Effect of triflocin and hydrochlorothiazide on electrolyte and water excretion in a hydrated dog receiving an infusion of 2.5% glucose + 2.5% mannitol i.v.

	Urine		mOsm/liter			
Time (min)	Flow (ml/min)	pH	Plasma	Urine	C_{osm}[a] (ml/min)	C_{H_2O}[a] (ml/min)
0-10	6.95	5.90	291	160	3.82	3.13
10-20	7.30	5.83	290	157	3.94	3.36
20-30	8.60	5.83	296	151	4.39	4.21
30-40	8.60	5.91	302	151	4.30	4.30
Triflocin 10 mg/kg prime i.v., plus 20 mg/kg/hr in the infusion						
40-50	11.40	5.61	297	203	7.79	3.61
50-60	12.90	5.78	292	230	10.17	2.73
60-70	12.90	5.85	294	229	10.05	2.45
70-80	12.50	6.00	296	233	9.84	2.66
HCTZ 2.5 mg/kg prime i.v., plus 3.0 mg/kg/hr in the infusion						
80-90	12.90	6.41	293	254	11.18	1.72
90-100	12.20	6.45	290	271	11.39	0.81
100-110	11.70	6.42	288	268	10.89	0.81
110-120	9.70	6.39	286	270	9.15	0.55

Hydration was accomplished by the oral administration of 30 ml H_2O per kg body weight 2 hr prior to urine collection and again 1.5 hr prior to urine collection. In addition 2.5% glucose + 2.5% mannitol was infused at 10 ml/min.
[a]C_{osm}, osmolar clearance; C_{H_2O}, free-water clearance.

the cortical diluting segment, the results with the combination of drugs could be interpreted as demonstrating an effect of the thiazide on a site which was unaffected by triflocin, presumably the cortical diluting site. However, it could also be interpreted as displaying the combined effect of two diuretics acting at different sites within a biochemical chain of events but still at the same anatomical tubular area.

Additional attempts to establish sites of activity other than the Henle loop for ethacrynic acid, furosemide, and triflocin have involved the use of stop-flow and micropuncture techniques. The stop-flow procedure was utilized by Beyer *et al.* (1965) to examine renal tubular sites of action of ethacrynic acid. These investigators concluded that the diuretic interfered with reabsorption of sodium in both distal and proximal portions of the nephron. The post-drug stop-flow occlusions in this study were performed significantly after drug administration, thus allowing the entire nephron to be exposed to drug. As pointed out by Gussin and Cafruny (1966) and by Orloff (1966), a major problem exists with the use of this type of classical stop-flow experiment to predict sites of action of diuretics. Since all urine from the proximal portion of the nephron must pass the distal tubule during collection, the capacity of the distal tubule to reabsorb sodium following administration of the drug could alter concentrations of electrolytes in samples derived from the proximal tubule. In order to solve this problem, Gussin and Cafruny modified the stop-flow method to exclude the contribution of the distal tubule to the composition of proximal samples. The stop-flow technique of Malvin, Wilde, and Sullivan (1958) was modified as follows: one ureter was occluded and ethacrynic acid was injected at the same time; the contralateral ureter was occluded 2 min after administration of the drug. The rationale was to limit the drug primarily to the proximal portion of the nephron on one side and to allow it to pass into the entire nephron on the other side. Stop-flow patterns of urine samples from the two kidneys could then be obtained and compared. Two requirements for a drug to be amenable to study by this procedure are entrance of the drug into the tubular lumen by proximal tubular secretion and a rapid onset of action. These two criteria are met by the three drugs under consideration. The results of a typical experi-

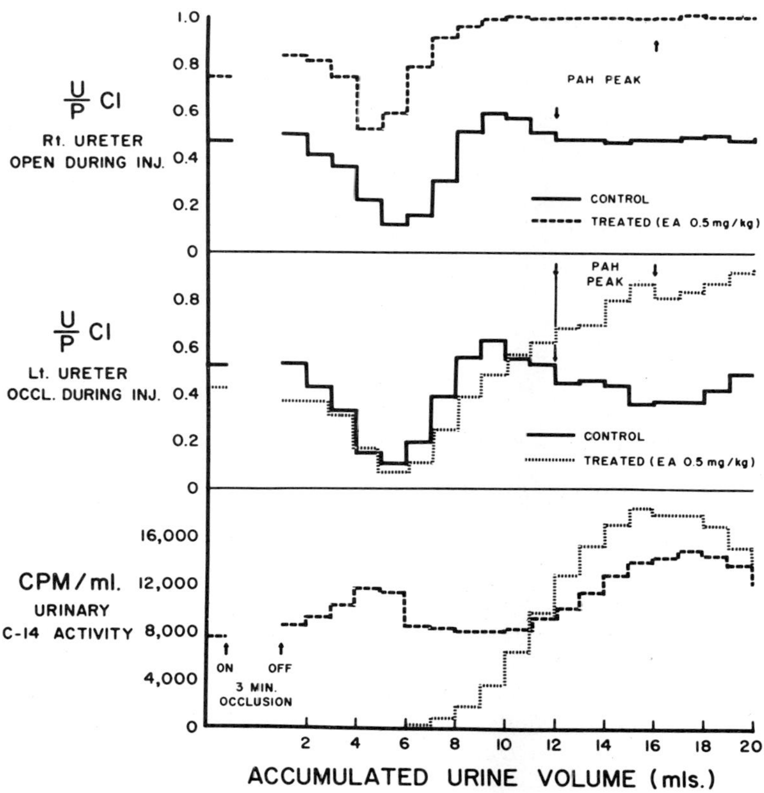

Fig. 2. Effect of ethacrynic acid (EA) on stop-flow patterns with ureter open or closed at the time of drug injection (Gussin and Cafruny, 1966).

ment with ethacrynic acid are shown in Fig. 2. Effects of ethacrynic acid on sodium and chloride levels of urine collected by the conventional stop-flow procedure (open side) were similar to those reported by Beyer *et al.* (1965). Urinary concentration (and *U*/*P* ratios) of these electrolytes was greater in all samples after drug. When the modified stop-flow procedure was used and the drug was limited to the proximal portion of the nephron, an increase in urinary concentration and urine/plasma (U/P) ratios of sodium and chloride was noted only in urine samples derived largely from proximal segments of the nephron. Similar results were obtained for triflocin (Fig. 3) and furosemide (Small and Cafruny, unpublished).

Based on the preceding findings it would appear that ethacrynic acid, furosemide, and triflocin are all capable of impairing sodium and chloride reabsorption in both proximal and distal portions of the nephron. However, conflicting reports have appeared, particularly when data were obtained by micropuncture techniques. Dirks, Cirksena, and Berliner (1966) were not able to demonstrate a net decrease in proximal tubular sodium reabsorption after ethacrynic acid. On the contrary, when urinary fluid and electrolyte losses were not replaced, proximal sodium reabsorption was actually enhanced. Clapp and Robinson (1968) obtained similar results in their initial experiments, but in later experiments, when urinary sodium and water losses were replaced and glomerular filtration rate (GFR) maintained, the ability of ethacrynic acid to depress proximal tubular sodium reabsorption became apparent. Controversy also exists amongst the micropuncturists in regard to a proximal tubular site of action of furosemide. Dirks *et al.* (1966), using dogs, and Deetjen (1966), using rats, failed to demonstrate proximal activity. Deetjen did, however, observe an abnormally large increase in proximal tubular diameter after furosemide and claimed that, although GFR remained constant, flow rate through the proximal tubule decreased and contact time of the fluid with the proximal tubular epithelium increased. This prolonged contact time could have masked a partially inhibited transport mechanism. Brenner *et al.* (1969) reported a proximal site of action of furosemide using the recollection micropuncture technique in rats. Their data were analyzed by comparison of pre- and post-furosemide samples at equivalent GFR's.

Lockhart, Dirks, and Carriere (1972) studied triflocin by recollection micropuncture in dogs and Kauker (1973) examined this diuretic by micropuncture in rats. Both of these studies failed to reveal proximal tubular activity while confirming activity at more distal areas of the nephron. However, whereas the study by Lockhart and co-workers in dogs implicated primarily the Henle loop, Kauker's study in rats indicated some activity in the loop but the greatest alterations in fluid and electrolyte reabsorption were reported to occur in the distal convoluted tubules and collecting ducts. Lockhart *et al.* also proposed the possibility of altered reabsorption in the collecting ducts, but assumed that this would be subordinate to a loop effect.

In contrast to the decreased fractional phosphate excretion in man after triflocin reported by Agus and Goldberg (1970), (Fig. 4) a study in our

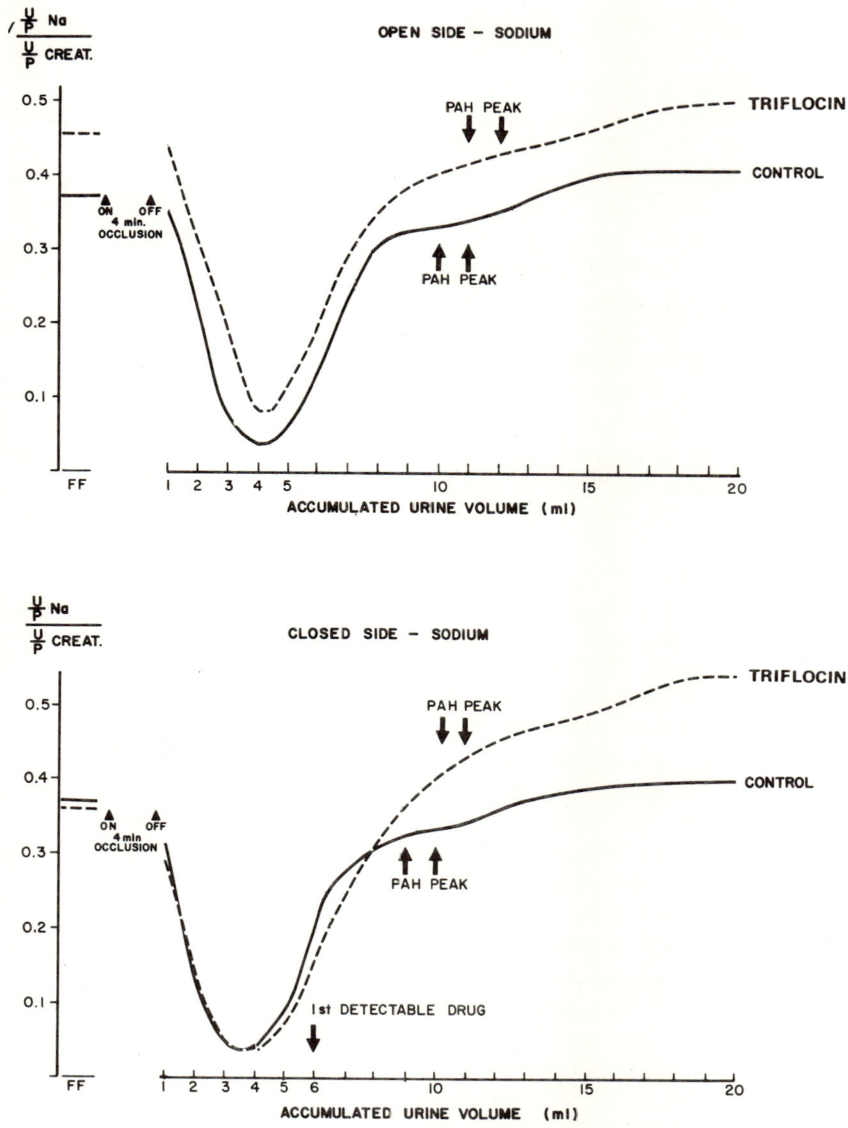

Fig. 3. Effect of triflocin on stop-flow patterns with ureter open or closed at the time of drug injection (Gussin *et al.*, 1969).

laboratory demonstrated that triflocin produced a dose-related increase in phosphate excretion in rats (Fig. 5). The magnitude of this effect was essentially the same as that with furosemide. An unexpected and interesting finding was the dose-related increase in phosphate excretion with ethacrynic acid. Ethacrynic acid was originally reported to lack diuretic activity in rats (Beyer *et al.*,

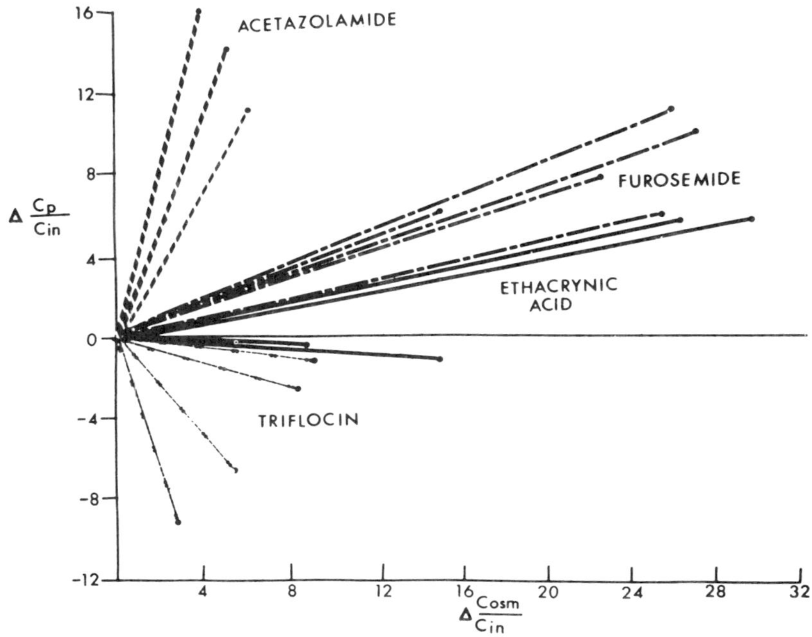

Fig. 4. Comparative effects of various diuretic agents on fractional excretion of phosphate as an index of proximal action of these drugs (Agus and Goldberg, 1970).

1965), although a later study (Zins *et al.*, 1968) did demonstrate activity with high doses given by intravenous infusion. In the study displayed in Fig. 5 orally administered ethacrynic acid failed to produce a natriuresis at a time when phosphate excretion was significantly elevated. This finding presents the interesting possibility that, in the rat, ethacrynic acid impairs proximal reabsorption of phosphate, and probably sodium, but that the excess sodium is reabsorbed at unimpaired reabsorptive areas further down the tubule. The findings concerning the effect of triflocin and ethacrynic acid on phosphate excretion may point out an additional complicating factor in evaluating renal tubular sites of action of diuretics; that is, a diuretic may not only lack activity at a specific tubular site, but it may stimulate reabsorptive mechanisms at that site and partially or totally antagonize the result of impairment of reabsorption at another site. In addition, the responses may be quite different depending on the experimental species.

Finally, a striking difference exists between triflocin and the other two loop-acting diuretics under discussion in regard to effects on intrarenal distribution of blood flow. Table 4 illustrates a composite of the results from two studies; Birtch *et al.* (1967) examined the influence of furosemide and ethacrynic acid on intrarenal blood flow, and Lockhart *et al.* (1972) exam-

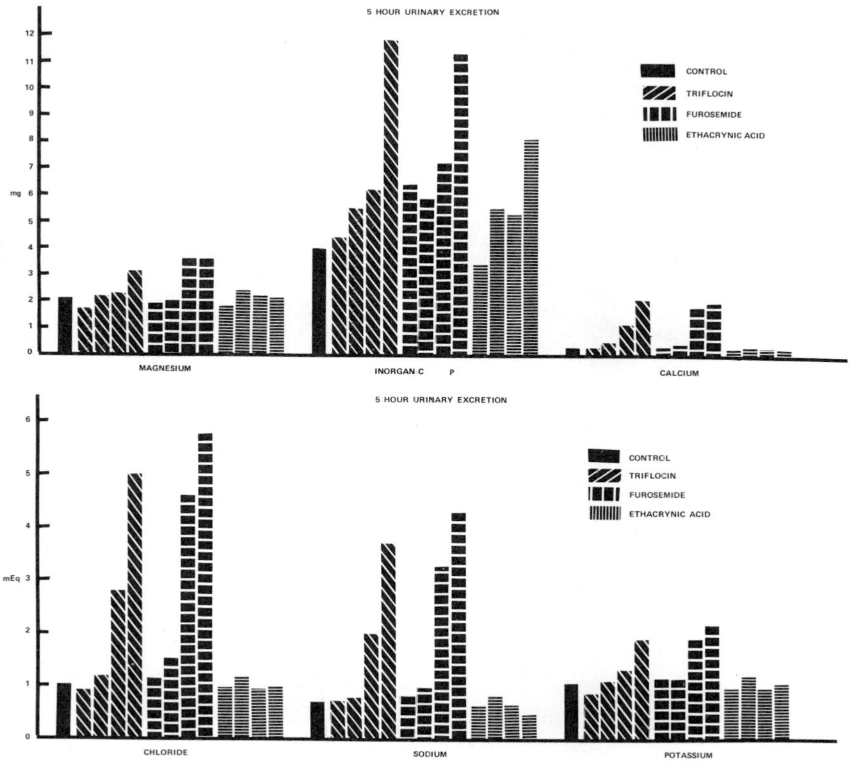

Fig. 5. Urinary electrolyte excretion after administration of 0.5, 5, 25, or 100 mg/kg of triflocin, furosemide, or ethacrynic acid to rats.

ined triflocin. Both groups of investigators used ^{85}Kr washout to estimate blood flow in various compartments of kidneys of anesthetized dogs. Birtch *et al.* (1967) demonstrated an increase in cortical flow and a concomitant decrease in outer medullary and juxtamedullary cortical flow after furosemide or ethacrynic acid. Lockhart *et al.* (1972) showed a striking reduction in outer cortical flow in most instances after administration of triflocin. This change in intrarenal flow distribution after triflocin resulted in the replacement of the two-component washout curve with a single-component curve. The effects of all three agents on intrarenal blood flow were supported in the two studies by autoradiograms and by the injection of silicone rubber. The contrary influence of triflocin on intrarenal blood flow as compared with ethacrynic acid and furosemide make the relationships of blood flow redistribution to diuretic effect extremely difficult to establish.

Table 4. Effects of ethacrynic acid, furosemide, and triflocin on the distribution of renal blood flow in the dog

	Flow rate (ml/min/g compartment)		
	Cortex		Outer medulla
Control	5.4		1.3
Ethacrynic acid	7.0		0.2
Control	5.9		2.4
Ethacrynic acid	7.9		0.2
Control	4.9		1.2
Furosemide	10.0		0.2
Control	6.2		1.3
Furosemide	9.3		0.2
Control	6.9		1.7
Triflocin		2.3[a]	
Control	6.4		1.1
Triflocin	6.9		1.4
Control	4.2		1.1
Triflocin		3.0[a]	
Control	5.9		1.5
Triflocin		1.7[a]	
Control	6.9		1.0
Triflocin	3.8		1.1

Values shown in this table are a composite of data published by Birtch *et al.* (1967) and Lockhart *et al.* (1972).
[a]A single component replaced the first two normal components.

ACKNOWLEDGMENTS

The author wishes to thank Mrs. M. A. Ronsberg and Mrs. I. Selander for their assistance in preparation of the manuscript.

REFERENCES

Agus, Z. S., and M. Goldberg. 1970. Renal mechanisms of the natriuretic and antiphosphaturic effects of triflocin–a new diuretic. J. Lab. Clin. Med. 76: 280.

Beyer, K. H., J. E. Baer, J. K. Michaelson, and H. F. Russo. 1965. Renotropic characteristics of ethacrynic acid: a phenoxyacetic saluretic-diuretic agent. J. Pharmac. Exp. Ther. 147: 1.

Bennett, C. M., B. M. Brenner, and R. W. Berliner. 1968. Micropuncture studies of nephron fuction in the rhesus monkey. J. Clin. Invest. 47: 203.

Birtch, A. G., R. M. Zakheim, L. G. Jones, and A. C. Barger. 1967. Redistribution of renal blood flow produced by furosemide and ethacrynic acid. Circulation Res. 21: 869.

Brenner, B. M., R. I. Keimowitz, F. S. Wright, and R. W. Berliner. 1969. An inhibitory effect of furosemide on sodium reabsorption by the proximal tubule of the rat nephron. J. Clin. Invest. 48: 290.

Cannon, P. J., H. O. Heinemann, W. B. Stason, and J. H. Laragh. 1965. Ethacrynic acid. Effectiveness and mode of diuretic action in man. Circulation 31: 5.

Clapp, J. R., and R. R. Robinson. 1968. Distal sites of action of diuretic drugs in the nephron. Am. J. Physiol. 215: 2218.

Clapp, J. R., G. A. Nottebohm, and R. R. Robinson. 1971. Proximal site of action of ethacrynic acid: importance of filtration rate. Am. J. Physiol. 220(5) 1355.

Cortney, M. A., M. Mylle, W. E. Lassiter, and C. W. Gottschalk. 1965. Renal tubular transport of water, solute, and PAH in rats loaded with isotonic saline. Am. J. Physiol. 209: 1199.

Deetjen, P. 1966. Micropuncture studies on site and mode of diuretic action of furosemide. Ann. N. Y. Acad Sci. 139: 408.

Dirks, J. H., W. J. Cirksena, and R. W. Berliner. 1966. Micropuncture study of the effect of various diuretics on sodium reabsorption by the proximal tubules of the dog. J. Clin. Invest. 45: 1875.

DiBona, G. F. 1971. Micropuncture studies on the site of action of ethacrynic acid in the rat. J.Pet.176: 255.

Duarte, C. G. 1972. Renal dissociation in urinary phosphate during ethacrynic acid and furosemide administration: dependence on filtered load. Federation proceedings, 31: 716.

Early, L. E., and R. M. Friedler. 1964. Renal tubular effects of ethacrynic acid. J. Clin. Invest. 43: 1495.

Eknoyan, G., *et al.* 1970. Combined ascitic-fluids and furosemide infusion in the management of ascites. New Eng. J. Med. 282: 713.

Fraser, A. G., J. F. Gowie, A. T. Lambie, and J. S. Robson. 1967. The effects of furosemide on the osmolality of the urine and the composition of renal tissue. J Pet 158: 475.

Goldberg, M., D. K. McCurdy, E. L. Foltz, and L. W. Bluemle, Jr. 1964. Effects of ethacrynic acid (a new saluretic agent) on renal diluting and concentrating mechanisms: evidence for site of action in the loop of Henle. J. Clin. Invest. 43: 201.

Gussin, R. Z., and E. J. Cafruny. 1966. Renal sites of action of ethacrynic acid. J. Pharmac. Exp. Ther. 153: 148.

Gussin, R. Z., J. R. Cummings, E. H. Stokey, and M. A. Ronsberg. 1969. CL 65,562 (4-(α,α,α-trifluoro-m-toluidino)-nicotinic acid), A novel 'high ceiling' diuretic. J. Pharmac. Exp. Ther. 167: 194.

Kauker, M. L. 1973. Micropuncture study of the effect of triflocin on tubular reabsorption in rats. *J. Pharmac. Exp. Ther.* 184: 472.

Lockhart, E. A., J. H. Dirks, and S. Carriere. 1972. Effects of triflocin on renal tubular reabsorption and blood flow distribution. Am. J. Physiol. 223: 89.

Malvin, R. L., W. S. Wilde, and L. P. Sullivan. 1958. Localization of nephron transport by stop-flow analysis. Am. J. Physiol. 194: 135.

Morgan, T., M. Tadokuro, and P. Martin, *et al.* 1970. Effect of furosemide on Na^+ and K^+ transport studies by microperfusion of the rat nephron. Am. J. Physiol. 218, 292.
Orloff, J. 1966. Pitfalls in the use of stop-flow for the localization of diuretic action, with special reference to Na reabsorption. Ann. N.Y. Acad. Sci. 139: 344.
Seldin, D. W., G. Eknoyan, W. M. Suki, and F. C. Rector, Jr. 1966. Localization of diuretic action from the pattern of water and electrolyte excretion. Ann. N. Y. Acad. Sci. 139: 328.
Small, A., and E. J. Cafruny. 1965. The renal sites of action of furosemide. Pharmacologist. 7: 165.
Suki, W., F. C. Rector, Jr., and D. W. Seldin. 1965. The site of action of furosemide and other sulfonamide diuretics in the dog. J. Clin. Invest. 44: 1458.
Zins, G. R., R. A. Walk, R. Z. Gussin, and C. R. Ross. 1968. The diuretic activity of ethacrynic acid in rats. J. Pharmac. Exp. Ther. 163: 210.

A Water Diuretic: How and Why

Virgil D. Wiebelhaus, Genevieve Sosnowski, Alfred R. Maass, and Francis T. Brennan
Smith Kline and French Laboratories
Division of Smith Kline Corporation
Philadelphia, Pennsylvania

We have felt for some time that the spectrum of diuretics which are now available offer the clinician virtually all the desired choices both as to the electrolyte to be influenced and the site of action desired. On the other hand, the only water diuretics available are glucocorticoids and alcohol. Alcohol acts primarily by suppression of the secretion of antidiuretic hormone (ADH). Under special circumstances, i.e., adrenal insufficiency in man or adrenalectomy in laboratory animals, water-diuretic responses to the administration of glucocorticoids can be demonstrated. The diverse pharmacology of the steroids renders them unsuitable for sustained use for diuretic purposes, and the serious use of alcohol for medicinal purposes has never gained wide acceptance in the United States. These two types of diuretics do, however, exemplify two separate routes by which one may achieve water diuresis. Decinine (Fig. 1) has properties which relate to both these routes. It is a natural product derived from various *Lythraceae.* Decinine occurs only in some genera; we usually obtain most of it by extracting and separating out the lythrine from the plant material and converting this to decinine by reduction at the site designated $\alpha - \beta$. This reduction profoundly enhances the activity of this structure. Alkaloids from this plant, other than lythrine or decinine, have little or no diuretic activity.

The failure of Addisonian patients to excrete water at a normal rate following a water load was noted by Rowntree and Snell (1931). The 'Robinson-Kepler-Power' or water-load test was introduced in 1941 as a test for adrenal insufficiency in man (Robinson, Power, and Kepler, 1941; Gaunt, Birnie, and Eversole, 1949). Numerous publications have confirmed the defect in water excretion in experimental animals and have established the ability of glucocorticoids to promptly and completely repair this defect in

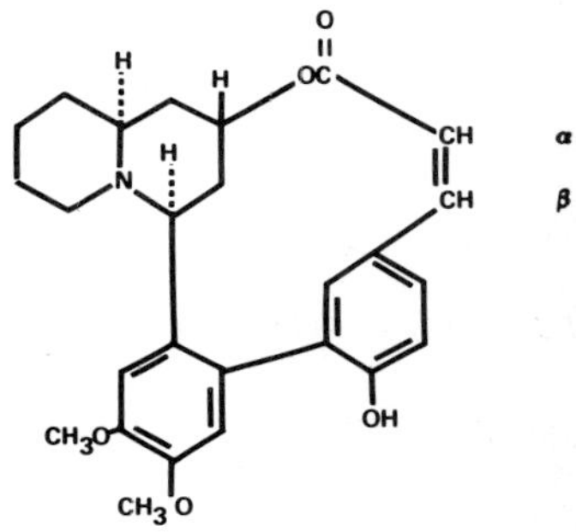

LYTHRINE DECININE (2H across α–β)

Lythraceae plant family (22 genera; ca 500 species)

Heimia	myrtifolia	Brazil
Heimia	salicifolia	Mexico
Decodon	verticillatus	New Jersey

20 known alkaloids

Fig. 1. Structure and reduction of decinine.

water excretion. While extrarenal factors are undoubtedly also involved, there is clearly a substantial influence of glucocorticoids upon the renal handling of water.

The foregoing observations imply that glucocorticoids may alter renal tubular permeability to water. Since glucocorticoids also have anti-inflammatory utility which may be based upon influences on the integrity and permeability of basement-membrane structures elsewhere, the renal tubular reduction of water permeability may also result from modification of basement-membrane constituents of the nephron. In line with these views is the influence of glucocorticoids upon glomerular losses of protein in nephrosis. These relationships have been discussed previously (Wiebelhaus, Sosnowski, and Maass, 1966).

We reasoned that any nonsteroidal structure which could repair the water-excretion defect of the adrenalectomized (ADX) rat might have useful water-diuretic activity and/or anti-inflammatory action and hopefully be devoid of some of the other pharmacologic effects which limit the use of steroids.

Over a number of years we had screened many structures for diuretic activity, and found many agents which could not clearly be classified as to mode of action and some agents which we definitely thought had some water-diuretic activities. All of these compounds, and standard saluretic agents, were run in water-loaded ADX rats. Compounds with interesting activity in this test were also examined for anti-ADH activity in both rats and dogs and for saluretic activity in rats. The method has been described in previous publications (Wiebelhaus *et al.*, 1966, Maass *et al.*, 1968).

METHODS

Adrenalectomized Water-loaded Rat

A water-load test was carried out in ADX in rats. Adrenalectomized animals have a defect in their ability to excrete a water load within a finite time interval. Since this defect in water unloading may be specifically corrected by glucocorticoids, this protocol has been utilized as a means of estimating glucocorticoid-like activity.

Adult male Charles River (C-D) rats, weighing 180–260 g, were adrenalectomized and then given food *ad lib.* along with 0.9% saline for drinking water for the next 26 hr. For the next 18 hr the rats were fasted and saline was replaced with tap water. The animals were then divided into control and test groups with a group of sham-ADX rats utilized as a positive control. All rats were given 0.2 ml of 0.9% saline/100 g body weight 1 hr prior to water loading. Nonsteroidal test compounds were dissolved or suspended in the saline administered to each group. Steroids were administered s.c. in 30% ethanol in 0.1 ml/100 g body weight. One hour after administration of the test compounds, each rat received an oral load of 5 ml of distilled water per 100 g body weight. Immediately after administration of the water load the rats were placed in metabolism cages, four rats per cage, and the excreted urine volume was recorded every 30 min for the next 3 hr. The 3-hr urine volume was calculated as a percentage of the water load administered. Sham-operated rats excreted approximately 70% of the water load within 3 hr. Adrenalectomized rats excreted approximately 40% of the water load in this time, while a significantly improved excretion of the water load was statistically defined as an excretion of 50% or more within 3 hr.

The definition of significant activity is as follows: percentage water load excreted $\geqslant$ 50%; Na^+ excretion $\geqslant$ 0.96 mEq/group of 8 rats; K^+ excretion $\geqslant$ 0.64 mEq/group of 8 rats.

Rat Anti-ADH Method

Groups of eight adult rats were fasted from food and water for 16 hr prior to testing. There was usually a one-control group to six-test group ratio among the animals being tested. Test procedure was as follows: The animals were housed, four per metabolism cage, and drug was administered orally to the test group at the zero hour; at the same time both control and test groups received 1 mU pitressin/100g body weight s.c. and a gavage containing 5% ethanol, 5% propylene glycol, and 0.21% NaCl at a dose of 5 ml/100g body weight. One hour later the same animals received a repeated dose of pitressin s.c. and a second gavage (2.5% ethanol and 0.20% NaCl at a dose of 5 ml/100 g body weight. Urine volumes were measured at 1 and 2 hr. Pooled urine samples from both control and test groups were collected at the end of 2 hr. Test values were recorded as percentage water load excreted and mEq electrolytes excreted per group as compared with controls.

The definition of significant activity is as follows. A compound is considered active if it produces an increased water-load excretion $\geqslant$ 7.4% above control values; Na^+ $\geqslant$ 0.80 mEq/group of 8 rats; N^+ $\geqslant$ 0.17 mEq/group of 8 rats.

Rat Diuretic Screening Methods

Adult male albino rats of the Wistar strain weighing 200–400 g each were fasted overnight with water allowed *ad lib.* The following morning the rats were divided into groups of four in such a way that their weights were evenly distributed throughout the series. Eight rats (two groups of four each) were used as controls for each group of animals and for each dose of test compounds. Each control rat received an oral load of 2.5 ml of 0.9% NaCl/100 g body weight administered by means of a graduated syringe fitted with a small rubber catheter. The desired mg/kg dose of test compound was added to each 25 ml of saline contained in a vessel whose contents were continuously stirred with a magnetic stirrer so that insoluble compounds would be uniformly distributed. The saline-drug solution (or suspension) was administered orally to each rat of a test group at a volume of 2.5 ml/100 g body weight. Immediately after drug administration the rats were placed in metabolism cages with each subgroup of four rats in a separate cage. Urine was collected for the next 5 hr. The total 5-hr urine volume for each group of eight rats was then measured.

The results were expressed in terms of the percentage of the volume of the saline load excreted during the 5-hr period:

$$\frac{\text{Volume of urine (8 rats)}}{\text{Volume of saline load (8 rats)} \times 100.}$$

It was found that control groups excreted an average of 60% of the volume of the saline load with a standard deviation of 10.8%. The excretion of 82% of the volume of the saline load administered can be considered a positive diuretic effect within 95% confidence limits. With a variety of standard diuretic agents reliable dose-response curves were obtained whether one determined sodium excretion or only urine volume; i.e. the latter criterion was found to be reliably related in a direct manner to natruresis. The significant Na^+ effect was 1.45 μEq above control Na^+.

Sodium-Deficient Rat Test

Normal male albino rats weighing 150–200 g each were placed on a sodium-deficient diet (Nutritional Biochemicals, Cleveland, Ohio) for a period of five days. On the evening of the fifth day, food was removed for the duration of the experiment. On day 6 the water cups were removed from the cages and each rat given 3.0 ml of 0.85% NaCl s.c. and 5 ml of water orally. This NaCl load provided 10 mg Na^+ per rat. The drug was given in the water load; in the case of insoluble agents, the drug was administered as a suspension. Eight rats were employed for each control group and each test group. The rats were placed in metabolism cages (four rats per cage) and the urines were collected for the following 6 hr. After measuring the urine volumes, the samples were analyzed for sodium and potassium.

The Definition of Significant Activity is as follows. The responses for any single dose are considered biosignificant if they differ from controls by the following amounts: Na^+ excretion $\geqslant$ 2.5 mg/rat; K^+ excretion $\geqslant$ 10.0 mg/rat; Na/K ratio $\geqslant$ 2.5.

Dog Anti-ADH Test

A fasted dog was given a water load equal to 5% body weight using a stomach tube approximately 1½ hr before the start of the experiment. Half of this load (2.5%) was again given 30 min prior to venoclysis.

The unanesthetized animal was lightly restrained on a dog board, catheterized, and given a 5% dextrose infusion at 0.5 ml/min. In order to help suppress ADH release from the posterior pituitary, a stat injection of 50 ml of 30% ethanol was administered over a 10-min period. Urine volumes collected over 10 min were recorded and graphed (urine volume *versus* pitressin dose). When the volume became sufficiently high (60 ml/10 min), control injections of pitressin (Vasopressin, Parke, Davis) were given at 0.3 or 0.35 mU/kg i.v. Following a suitable control (about a 40% drop in urine flow) drug is given i.v. or orally and the same dose of pitressin is repeated at various post-drug intervals.

During the course of the entire experiment the dog was given a 2% water load via stomach tube every 40 min, or at such a time when approximately half of the previous load had been eliminated.

Results were calculated as the percentage inhibition of the pitressin control.

RESULTS

Adrenalectomized rats were unable to form dilute urines and excreted only a small amount of the administered water load (Table 1). Administration of standard saluretic agents did not restore the ability of rats to dilute the urines and urine volumes were only slightly increased. Prednisone administration did restore the ability to dilute the urines and eliminate the water load.

The abilities of several standard saluretics plus prednisone and decinine to restore water excretion in the ADX rat are represented in Fig. 2. In confirmation of previous reports the glucocorticoid is very effective in this test and the maximal response, i.e., 90% water-load excretion, actually exceeds the values for untreated sham-operated rats which excrete about 78% of the water load. Decinine also restores water excretion to levels equal to the sham-operated controls but does level off slightly below prednisone. A variety of saluretic agents which have different sites of action were not effective in this test.

Table 1. Adrenalectomized water-loaded rat test

Percentage volume excreted		Urinary osmolality	
Shams	ADX	Shams	ADX
77.83 (61.2–94.1) 93 values	39.04 (16.0–53.4) 93 values	109.3 (72–141) 12 tests	207.1 (112–264) 12 tests

Test compounds and urinary osmolalities

Hydrochlorothiazide	283–415	Butazolidin	220–322
Triamterene	174–209	Indomethacin	438
Acetazoleamide	212–232	Diazepam	198–224
Furosemide	253–284	Cyproheptadine	245–248
	Prednisone 115–147		

The percentage volumes are calculated on the basis of the loading volumes given. Data on percentage excreted for the saluretic agents appear in Fig. 2.

When we tested other steroids with known glucocorticoid properties we found that their order of potency in the water-loaded ADX rat test paralleled their reported potency as glucocorticoids (Fig. 3). Aldosterone is not very active in this test, but the 9*a* F-hydrocortisone which, like aldosterone, has very substantial mineralocorticoid activity but also has very substantial gluco-

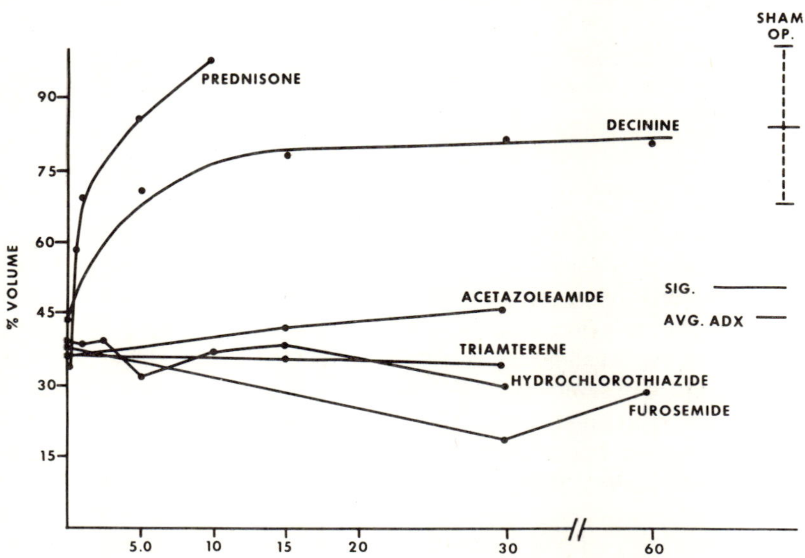

Fig. 2. Comparative responses in water-loaded ADX rat. Sham-operated rats excrete percentage volumes ranging from 61.2–94.1% with an average of 77.8%. The average percentage volume excretion for ADX rats is 39.0%. Increases for ADX rats to 50% or more are significant ($p = 0.05$).

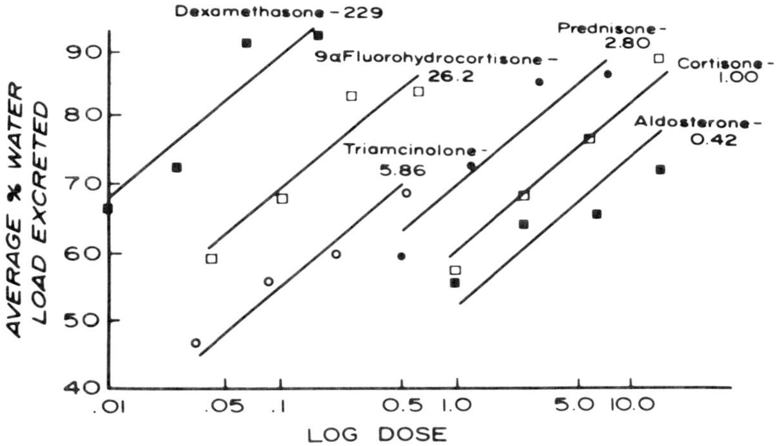

Fig. 3. Water-excretion restoration by steroids with known glucocorticoid properties in water-loaded ADX rats. The abscissa is expressed as log dose in mg/kg. (From Maass *et al.*, 1968. Reprinted by permission of the publishers of the *Journal of Pharmacology and Experimental Therapeutics.*)

corticoid activities, is much more effective than is aldosterone. Dexamethasone was easily the most potent, as was to be expected.

Table 2 shows the relative potencies of this same series of steroids in clinical use for arthritis (Boland, 1959) and potencies in the granuloma test in laboratory animals (Silber, 1959), compared with the potencies of these agents, as we have measured them, in the water-loaded ADX rat. By all three modes of measurement the orders of potencies are identical and the correlation shown by the relative potencies is also rather good.

Decinine has been shown to have good activity in a variety of laboratory anti-inflammatory tests. The minimal effective doses of decinine in a series of

Table 2. Comparison of clinical and granuloma-test potencies of steroids with potencies in water-loaded ADX rat test

Compound	Clinical potency[a]	Inhibition of granuloma formation relative potency[b]	ADX water-load test relative potency
Aldosterone	0	< 1	0.42
Cortisone	1	1	1.0
Prednisone	3	2	2.8
Triamcinolone	3–4	5.2	5.9
9αFluorohydrocortisone	10–15	12	26.2
Dexamethasone	> 30	100–200	229

[a]From Boland, 1959.
[b]From Silber, 1959.

Table 3. Decinine anti-inflammatory activity

Test	MED (mg/kg p.o.)[a]
Rat paw edema	5
Carrageenin abscess	1–5
Granuloma	5
Adjuvant arthritic rat	10–25

[a]MED, minimal effective dose.

such tests are shown in Table 3. Like the glucocorticoids, decinine was inactive in the rat erythema test.

While the efficacy of any agent in the water-loaded ADX rat would be analagous to activity in man in a truly pathological degree of adrenal dysfunction, it is quite possible that relatively low levels of adrenal secretion, which are not detected or classified as pathologic, may exist in man, and such an individual could respond to an agent of this type. States of electrolyte and water imbalance may also influence the degree of activity to be shown by glucocorticoid-like effector agents.

Since ADH is a normal common moderator of water excretion we have determined the affect of decinine in both water-loaded rats and dogs which have been given pitressin. For the anti-ADH rat test we used a method which is essentially the method published by Hofmann (1967). At pitressin doses of 1 mU (2 X's) urine volumes are usually about 10% of the volume of the 'loading' solutions (Fig. 4). The osmotic concentrations of the urines from the pitressin-treated rats ranged from 589–921 mOsm. For untreated rats the concentration was less than 211 mOsm; figures above that level were statistically significant ($p = 0.05$). At the 1-mU dosage of pitressin drug treatment increasing the volume 7.4% above the control is a significant ($p = 0.05$) change. In Fig. 4 the dose-response curve, in terms of percentage load volume excreted as urine in 2 hr, is given for doses of pitressin from 0.0625–1.0 mU per 100 g body weight of the rats.

In Fig. 5 are shown the urine volume responses and urinary dilution effects of prednisone, lythrine, and decinine when given to pitressin-treated rats. The urine volume increases with prednisone are significant but are quite limited even at high doses. The urines are more dilute but still hypertonic, indicating that prednisone cannot completely reverse the effects of pitressin. Lythrine, at high doses, increased urine volumes to levels above untreated controls and at the doses of 30, 60, or 90 mg/kg reduces urine concentration to the range of 100–200 mOsm. Decinine produces dramatic increases in urine volume and urinary dilution but at lower doses than required by lythrine. The responses in excess of untreated controls could be attributed to antagonism of residual endogenous circulating ADH. Small amounts of the hormone might still be present in spite of the water-alcohol loads. Another

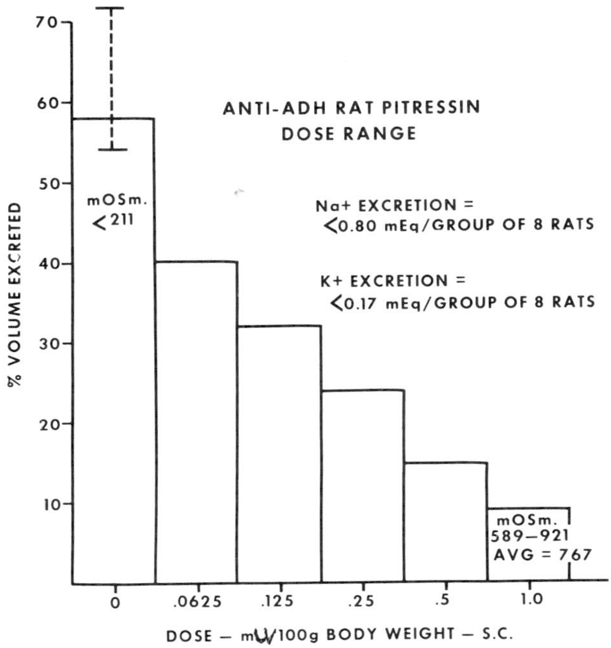

Fig. 4. Dose-response curve in terms of percentage load volume excreted as urine in 2 hr for pitressin doses from 0.0625-1.0 mU/100 g body weight of rats. Any treatment which increases percentage volume of administered toad excreted to values 7.4% or more above the values for the 1.0-mU dosage group is a significant result.

explanation is that these alkaloids are not only completely overcoming the effects of pitressin, but are causing additional water excretion by influencing some process in addition to that controlled by pitressin. This point will be discussed later.

Triamterene, hydrochlorothiazide, acetazoleamide, and furosemide at doses which are very effective in saline-loaded rats caused small very limited increases in urine volumes in the hydrated pitressin-treated rats. This data will be shown later as part of a tabulation of comparative efficacy of these agents *versus* decinine in a variety of rat diuretic tests.

In order to test activity against pitressin in dogs we gave oral water loads to hydrate the animals and in addition gave some ethanol to suppress further the output of endogenous ADH. The protocol is outlined at the top of Fig. 6[1]. At 30–40 min intervals water loads equal to 2% of body weight were given to sustain hydration and maintain a reasonably stable level of urine flow. Stat injections of 0.3 mU of pitressin/kg at the times indicated produced marked

1 We wish to acknowledge the assistance and advice of Dr. A. Gilman in developing our dog 'anti-ADH' test procedures.

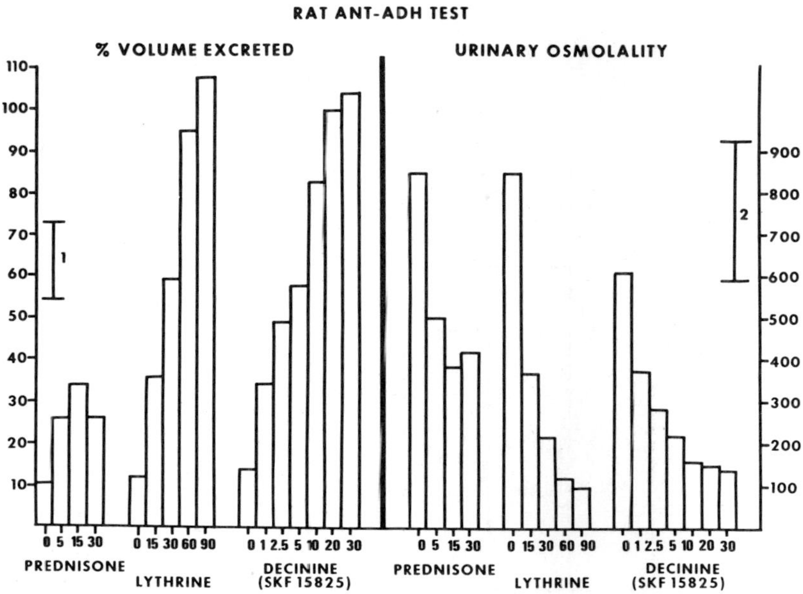

Fig. 5. Urine volume responses and urinary dilution effects of prednisone, lythrine, and decinine when given to pitressin-treated rats. Positive controls (1.0 mU doses of pitressin) are run each day. 1, Range of percentage volume with no pitressin; 2, range of urinary concentrations with 1 mU pitressin.

temporary drops in urine volume and simultaneous increases in urinary osmolality. During a 4-hr experiment each of three responses to pitressin were quite comparable, i.e., there was no 'drift' of responsiveness to the pitressin during the test. The short biological half-life of pitressin is reflected in the short duration of response and the lack of evidence of any residual effects from any of the separate intravenous doses. The concentrations of Na^+ and K^+ never fell outside the ranges indicated. Dose-response curves were obtainable with dosages of pitressin ranging from 0.3 to 0.7 mU i.v. stat doses. The high dose of pitressin reduces urine flow rates to very low levels.

The ability of decinine, at low oral doses, to reduce or block the effects of pitressin in the dog is demonstrated in several experiments, the results of which are shown in Fig. 7. After a dose of 1.25 mg/kg the effects of pitressin given 60 min later are modestly reduced, but at 160 min after decinine was given a 0.3mU dose of pitressin was essentially completely blocked. At 200 min after decinine even a 0.6 mU dose of pitressin was largely blocked. At the dose of 0.625 mg/kg of decinine the blocking of pitressin is less complete than at the higher doses and the blocking is much more pronounced at 150 min than at 60 min. Since these tests were run, we have collected metabolic data which show that after oral doses of decinine to dogs peak blood levels are reached at 2–3 hr and fall off rather slowly. The onset of anti-ADH activity relates very well with the timing observed for peak blood levels of decinine after oral dosing.

The efficacy of decinine, as compared with prednisone and various types of saluretic agents in the rat anti-ADH test and the water-loaded ADX rat test, is shown in Table 4. Decinine is very effective in both tests, whereas prednisone is fully effective only in the water-loaded ADX rat. In the ADH rat it is obvious that ADH acting at the most distal portions of the nephron is still able to exert most of its function even in the presence of prednisone. A variety of primary saluretics have only very slight activity in either test, indicating that saluretics acting at a number of different sites cannot produce any substantial degree of water excretion in either of these two water-loading

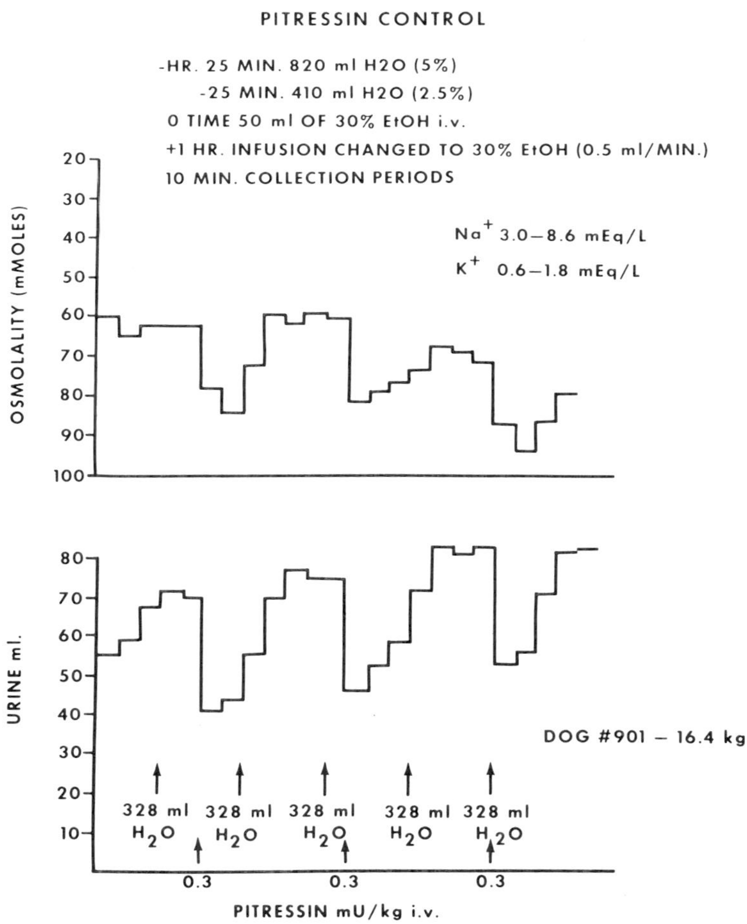

Fig. 6. Effects of pitressin on urine volume and urinary osmolality in the dog. Each value represented is based on a 10-min urine collection.

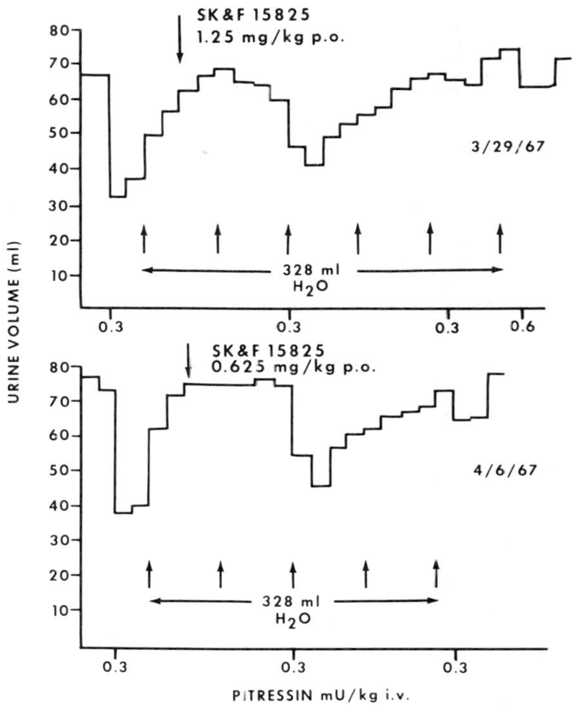

Fig. 7. Ability of decinine to reduce or block pitressin effects in the dog. Each value is based on a 10-min urine collection. The duration of the experiment of 3/29/67 was 280 min; the duration of the experiment of 4/6/67 was 240 min.

tests. A comparison of these agents in two different rat saluresis tests in which the animals receive sodium loads was made and the results appear in Table 5.

The saline-loaded rat test has been previously described (Wiebelhaus *et al.*, 1965). In brief, rats are given 0.9% NaCl at 2.5 ml/100 g body weight and urine is collected for 5 hr. Urine outputs exceeding control values by 22% or more are significant. In the sodium-deficient rat test (Wiebelhaus *et al.*, 1965) the rats are on a Na^+-deficient diet for five days before test.

Decinine has marked activity in both sodium-loaded rat tests. In the sodium-deficient rats large amounts of both sodium and potassium are excreted. Prednisone has very limited activity in both tests. Triamterene is very effective in both tests; in the sodium-deficient rat it shows its characteristic K^+-blocking activity. Hydrochlorothiazide, acetazoleamide, and furosemide are all very active in both tests and in the sodium-deficient rat show both natruretic and kaliuretic responses.

The activity of saluretics in sodium-loaded rats only and the marked natruretic effects of decinine in sodium-loaded rats, together with the prop-

Table 4. Comparative diuretic responses

					Water-loaded rats				
Compound	Oral dose (mg/kg)	ADH-treated rats (% volume)	Oral dose (mg/kg)	ADX rats (% volume)	Compound	Oral dose (mg/kg)	ADH-treated rats (% volume)	Oral dose (mg/kg)	ADX rats (% volume)
Decinine	0	14	0	44	Hydrochlorothiazide	0	10	0	40
	1	34	5	71		5	20	1	39
	2.5	49	15	78		15	18	2.5	40
	5	58	30	81				5	32
	10	83	60	80				10	37
	20	101						15	39
	30	104						30	30
Prednisone	0	12	0	34	Acetazoleamide	0	10	0	38
	5	21	0.5	59		15	36	15	43
	15	27	1.0	69		30	47	30	46
	30	27	5	86					
			10	98	Furosemide	0	10	0	39
						30	47	30	19
Triamterene	0	8	0	38		60	59	60	29
	15	31	15	36					
	30	31	30	34			7.4% > C		50%
		7.4% > C		50%					

Table 5. Comparative diuretic responses

Sodium-loaded rats											
				Sodium-deficient rats						Sodium-deficient rats	
Compound	Oral dose (mg/kg)	Saline-loaded rats (% volume)	Oral dose (mg/kg)	Na^+ (mg/rat)	K^+ (mg/rat)	Oral Compound	Oral dose (mg/kg)	Saline-loaded rats (% volume)	Oral dose (mg/kg)	Na^+ (mg/rat)	K^+ (mg/rat)
Decinine			0	2.0	5.7	Hydrochlorothiazide			0	1.2	5.5
	1	18	5	10.5	13.1		0.15	93	5	6.7	15.2
	5	76	15	18.9	18.0		0.50	95	15	10.8	13.7
	15	136	30	28.4	22.5		1.0	119			
	30	146	60	29.3	22.9		2.5	126			
	60	179					5	119			
							10	116			
Prednisone			0	0.3	3.5		15	127			
	2 s.c.	43	2	2.6	10.2						
	10 s.c.	49	10 s.c.	4.7	14.2	Acetazoleamide			0	0.2	4.0
							15	94	15	19.7	17.9
Triamterene			0	0.6	3.8		30	112	30	28.5	20.7
	2	77	5	3.9	5.7						
	5	85	15	8.7	4.5	Furosemide			0	1.0	3.5
	10	105	30	14.7	4.0		30	158	30	9.0	16.7
	15	111					60	224	60	31.6	28.1
	30	139									
	60	151						22%		2.5 > C	10 > C
		22%		2.5 > C	10 > C						

erty of causing water elimination as markedly hypotonic fluid in water-loaded rats and dogs, demonstrates an unusual set of results and requires some attempt at explanation, although there are further obvious experiments which have not yet been done. These results could be explained if one hypothesizes that decinine can reduce the permeabilities of the distal nephron to both Na^+ and water, although not necessarily to the same extent for each. In the water-loaded animal treated with decinine distal filtrate Na^+ concentrations may be lower than normal and Na^+ transport is adequate to remove most of the cation from the filtrate. In the sodium-loaded rat distal Na^+ concentrations may be comparatively high and a modest limitation of Na^+ permeation may significantly limit diffusion and/or transport of Na^+. Vasopressin may also influence a Na^+ pump so that some of the natruresis may be attributable to antagonism of this component to ADH action (Finn, 1968; Finn and Rockoff, 1971).

Figure 8 is a schematic in which approximate division of the nephron into various segments which differ somewhat from their neighbors in function are shown. The movement of water is probably restricted except for the descending limb of Henle's loop (DLH) and the cortical and medullary collecting duct. These areas may both be sites of action for decinine. Since it can completely block the effects of ADH and this effect is a terminal event in the

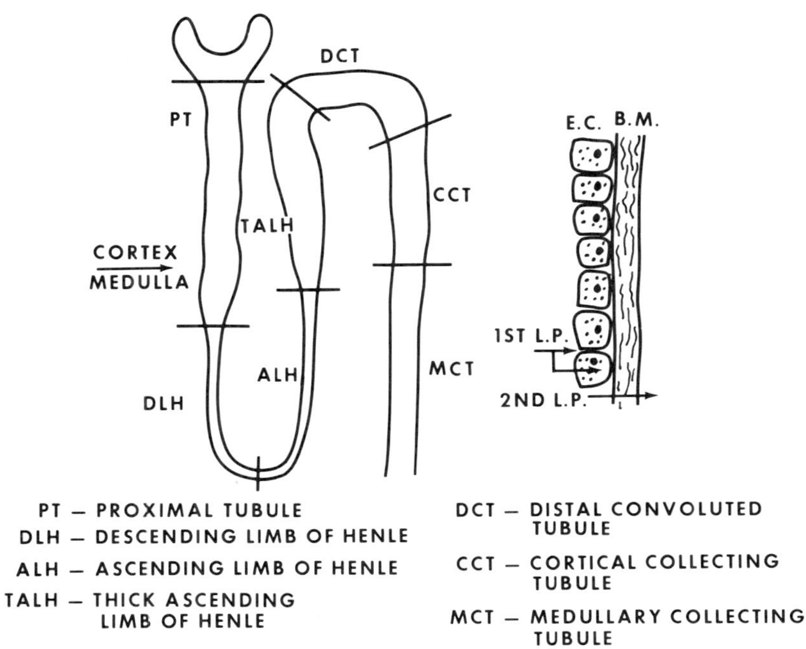

Fig. 8. Schematic division of nephron into segments differing in function from their neighbors.

nephron, decinine must influence the collecting duct, perhaps at both the medullary and cortical levels. Since decinine can also largely restore water excretion in ADX rats it must share a common point of influence with prednisone. Prednisone must act at sites proximal to ADH since it shows little antagonism to ADH in the rat. This leaves the DLH as a potential site of action for both decinine and prednisone. As far as Na^+ passage across the distal tubule is concerned, if we consider both diffusion and active transport, Na^+ may traverse the distal nephron at all levels and any interference with Na^+ permeability at any distal site is possible. In view of the very substantial Na^+ output by Na^+-deficient rats treated with decinine any effect of the alkaloid on Na^+ permeability must extend to the late distal tubule in order to prevent substantial diminution of the cation content of the filtrate before it leaves the collecting ducts. It seems unlikely that decinine owes its action to flushing of the proximal nephron followed by distal removal of Na^+, since acetazoleamide, which probably acts proximally, has very little activity in the hydrated-ADH rat or in the water-loaded ADX rat.

Since decinine produces urine volumes greater than controls which receive no pitressin in the ADH rat test, it may have diuretic effects other than that related to antagonism of ADH. Decinine also has water-diuretic effects in the ADX rat where failure to excrete water is not likely to be completely due to the action of ADH. These observations suggest that while decinine can completely block ADH effects, it is probably not a specific antagonist of ADH. It is probable that ADH affects water passage through the epithelial cells lining the collecting duct or via lateral cell processes. Decinine may also act at the site of the epithelial lining cells or could be acting at a second level of permeability, e.g., the basement membrane. If decinine is acting in a fashion related to the effects of glucocorticoids, as suggested by its activity in the water-loaded ADX rat and a common pattern of efficacy in anti-inflammatory tests, then one could conclude that decinine is acting on the basement membrane.

Finn (1968) and Finn and Rockoff (1971) have concluded that vasopressin can stimulate active Na^+ transport by toad bladders. Blocking this effect of ADH could then be contributing to natruretic effects of decinine in salt-loaded rats.

Describing the diuretic properties of a specific compound essentially answers the question: "Why discover and develop a water diuretic compound?" An agent such as decinine should be of use in any circumstances where the ADH function is at a higher level than required for a normal water balance, or where there is a relative adrenal insufficiency, or a reduced renal response to adrenal glucocorticoids. Morrison and Chalmers (1960) and Dingman *et al.* (1958) have reported on the water-diuretic effects of prednisone in man and its diuretic efficacy in combination with saluretics. Inappropriate ADH secretion or post-operative anuria are instances in which an anti-ADH compound may be of value. Intensive saluretic therapy may result in a degree of hyponatremia and relative refractoriness to further saluretic therapy. Congestive heart failure patients frequently exhibit hyponatremia. These latter clinical situations may represent attempts to maintain extracellular fluid compartments at higher than normal levels, possibly by means of elevated ADH secretion. Since decinine can repair the water-excretion defect in ADX rats it may have some utility in nephrosis. As with the saluretics a water diuretic could conceivably be of value in the treatment of hypertension.

Biochemical and micropuncture studies could provide much more basis for an accurate description of the action of decinine. We have initiated studies on water flux with toad bladder *in vitro* and some preliminary work on the renal medullary cyclic AMP system.

REFERENCES

Boland, E. W. 1959. The treatment of rheumatoid arthritis with adrenocorticosteroids and their synthetic analogues: an approach of certain developments of the past decade. Ann. N. Y. Acad. Sci. 82: 887–901.

Dingman, J. F., J. T. Finkenstaedt, J. C. Laidlaw, A. E. Renold, D. Jenkins, J. P. Merrill, and G. W. Thorn. 1958. Influence of intravenously administered adrenal steroids on sodium and water excretion in normal and Addisonian subjects. Metabolism 7: 608–623.

Finn, A. L. 1968. Separate effects of sodium and vasopressin on the sodium pump in toad bladder. Am. J. Physiol. 215: 849–856.

Finn, A. L., and M. L. Rockoff. 1971. The kinetics of sodium transport in the toad bladder. J. Gen. Physiol. 57: 326–348.

Gaunt, R., J. H. Birnie, and W. J. Eversole. 1949. Adrenal cortex and water metabolism. Physiol. Rev. 29: 281–310.

Hofmann, L. M. 1967. Azido pyrimidine diuretics (SC-16102, SC-16100): ADH antagonism assay in the rat. Arch. Int. Pharmacodyn. Ther. 169: 189–199.

Maass, A. R., G. Sosnowski, V. D. Wiebelhaus, and J. Weinstock. 1968. Acylphenothiazine antiinflammatory agents with steroid-like activity. I. 2-chloro-10-(β-dimethylaminopropionyl)-phenothiazine-5-oxide hydrochloride. J. Pharmac. Exp. Ther. 163, 239–249.

Morrison, R. S., and T. C. Chalmers. 1960. Combined diuretic and steroid therapy in cirrhosis with ascites. Ann. N. Y. Acad. Sci. 88: 907–914.

Robinson, F. J., M. H. Power, and E. J. Kepler. 1941. Two new procedures to assist in the recognition and exclusion of Addison's disease: a preliminary report. Proc. Staff Meetings, Mayo Clinic. 16: 577.

Rowntree, L. G., and A. M. Snell, 1931. A Clinical Study of Addison's Disease. W. B. Saunders Co., Philadelphia.

Silber, R. H. 1959. The biology of antiinflammatory steroids. Ann. N. Y. Acad. Sci. 82: 821–828.

Wiebelhaus, V. D., G. Sosnowski, and A. R. Maass. 1966. Glucocorticoid activity in the water-loaded ADX rat-relationship to antiinflmmatory activity. Third International Congress of Nephrology, abstr.

Wiebelhaus, V. D., J. Weinstock, A. R. Maass, F. T. Brennan, G. Sosnowski, and T. Larsen. 1965. The diuretic and natriuretic activity of triamterence and several related pteridines in the rat. J. Pharmac. Exp. Ther. 149: 397–403.

Renal Function during Intravenous Urography

Gilbert H. Mudge
Departments of Medicine and of Pharmacology and Toxicology
Dartmouth Medical School
Hanover, New Hampshire

Intravenous urography (IVU) is widely employed throughout the medical world. The test itself is of obvious interest to the radiologist and the clinician. Parenthetically, one might comment on the important role that so-called diagnostic agents have played in physiological research. Many of these are obvious. However, it is appropriate to recall the study of Richards and Walker (1930) on phenol red and indigo carmine. The latter dye had indeed been used as a test of renal function. Both dyes are quite strongly bound to plasma protein. Dr. Richards made the critical observation that the concentration in the glomerular filtrate was the same as in an ultrafiltrate across collodion membranes. This helped to establish the nature of glomerular filtration and has also been one of the few pieces of direct data on which much subsequent renal pharmacology has of necessity been based.

Within the past decade new agents have been introduced for urography and also for the rapidly expanding field of angiography. These are all tri-iodinated derivatives of benzoic acid and they differ slightly in the substitutent at the 3 or 5 position. They are all handled by the kidney in the same manner. We have studied diatrizoate, which is available commercially as Hypaque®, Renografin®, or Cardiografin®. It is prepared as either the sodium or meglumine salt, or sometimes a combination. Diatrizoate is not bound to plasma proteins, does not undergo metabolic alteration, is filtered at the glomerulus, is not secreted in man and dog, and, except under unusual circumstances, is not reabsorbed (Saxton, 1969; Lobentz *et al.*, 1972). In other words, it is handled by the kidney in the same manner as inulin.

With this as a background, one might well ask: Why study it further? If it behaves like inulin, what else is there to learn? The question is a fair one, and there are several answers. Unlike inulin, diatrizoate is administered in doses sufficiently large to produce an osmotic diuresis. What effect does this have on kidney function during the radiological procedure? X rays are conventionally taken from 1 to 30 min. To what extent does renal function change during this interval? How do these changes influence either the urinary concentration or the rate of excretion of the contrast agent? Phrasing it differently and perhaps in more general terms, what aspects of renal function specifically influence radiographic quality? There is also a most fascinating problem from the radiological literature, namely that the sodium salt becomes more concentrated in the urine than the meglumine salt (Benness, 1970a; Cattell *et al.*, 1970). This has been observed by several investigators, but the mechanism is not worked out. Finally there is the question of nephrotoxicity. Acute renal failure occurs rarely after angiography and even less frequently after IVU. From the pharmacological point of view, the important question is quite simple. Why does it occur at all?

METHODS

Our studies were conducted in dogs under pentobarbital anesthesia. Water had been restricted and vasopressin was infused continuously. This produced low urine flows at maximal osmolality. Urine was collected from ureteral catheters. Samples were usually taken at ½-min intervals during the early response, and thereafter at longer ones. Standard clearance procedures were used with inulin as a measure of glomerular filtration rate (GFR). Diatrizoate was measured with ^{125}I-labeled material. No X rays were taken.

We have mimicked two types of urography, the first with rapid injection of the contrast agent within 30 sec, the second with infusions over 10 min. For each procedure we have examined three doses. Our intermediate dose was equivalent to 1.5 ml/kg body weight of 50% Hypaque®. For the rapid or bolus injections, we compared the sodium and meglumine salts at all doses. With the slow infusion these were compared only at the high dose.

RESULTS

Let us first consider the data with rapid injections of the contrast agent (Fig. 1). Urine flow rises promptly, increasing about 50-fold within 2 min. Solute excretion also increases promptly. There is an early peak due to washout of preformed urine from the lower urinary tract. Diatrizoate excretion also increases rapidly. Urine osmolality falls as diuresis begins. At the same time there is a sudden increase in urea excretion. When expressed as the urea to inulin clearance ratio this peaks at about 3 min and then subsides rapidly.

These changes in GFR are less dramatic with infusion urography (Fig. 1). Urine flow increases far more gradually. After the washout period the GFR does not fall as far as with the bolus injection. Also, with the infusion technique, the changes in urea excretion are less dramatic. In the summary data (Fig. 2), at approximately equivalent doses the bolus type of injection

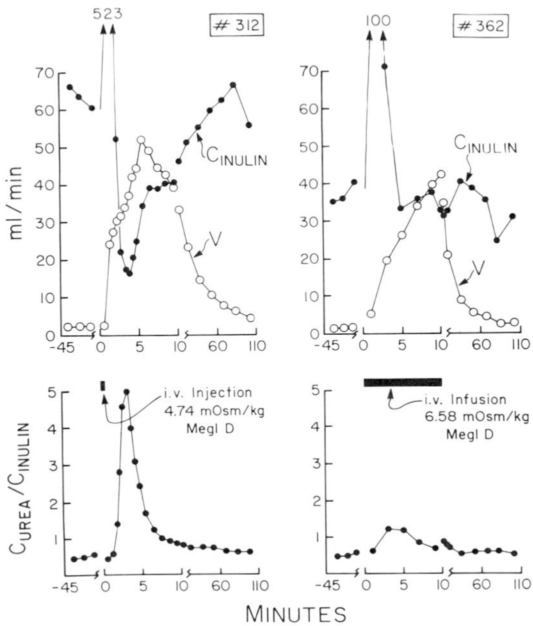

Fig. 1. Comparison of renal response to rapid (#312) and slow (#362) intravenous injection of contrast agent. V, Urine flow.

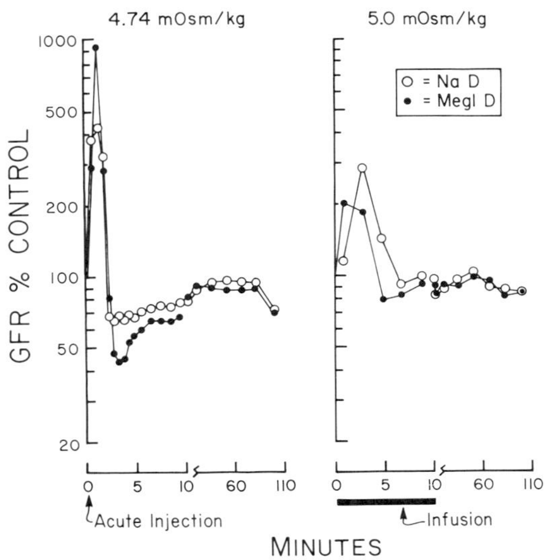

Fig. 2. Summary of changes in GFR following rapid and slow administration of diatrizoate as either sodium or meglumine salt. In this and similar figures, average values are given for 4–6 experiments per group. In the infusion experiments contrast material equivalent in osmolality to 25% sodium diatrizoate was infused at 6.7 ml/min for 10 min; the total dose of 5 mOsm/kg is the average of all animals.

clearly provokes a drop in GFR. With the slow infusion, there is almost no change.

The secretion of urea is clearly related to the washout of urea from the medulla. With the rapid onset of diuresis, the urea concentration in the tubular fluid falls to less than that of the interstitium, and urea diffuses from medulla to tubular fluid down its concentration gradient. This mechanism is supported by a number of observations, the most important of which involves the quantitative aspects of the amount of urea excreted. By the method of Aukland (1961) we have calculated the amount of urea initially present in the medulla. As shown in Fig. 3 the amount lost within the first 15 min is the same as the amount previously sequestered in the medulla. It is of interest that both bolus and infusion urography, at least in the doses employed, produce about the same amount of urea washout. The difference between the procedures (Fig. 1) is clearly related to the more acute changes with the more rapid injection and to the fact that the higher urea to inulin clearance ratio is strongly influenced by the greater drop in GFR.

Complex factors influence both the urinary concentration (U) and rate of excretion (UV) of the contrast agent. A schematic summary may be helpful (Fig. 4). This is drawn with rapid injection urography in mind. It emphasizes that UV_D is the product of the plasma concentration (P_D) and GFR. Both are changing rapidly in the period immediately after injection. It further emphasizes that concentration (U_D) is a function of several tubular processes, even though diatrizoate itself is not reabsorbed. These involve the reabsorption of chloride, the secretion of urea, the action of vasopressin, and the overall relationship between urine flow, total solute excretion, and free-water production.

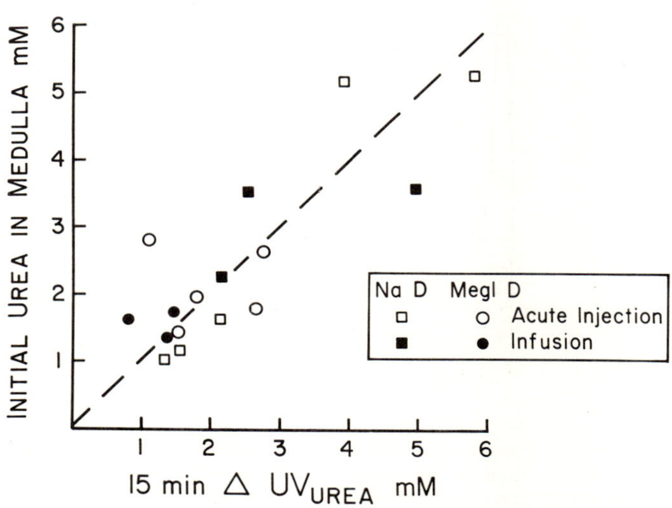

Fig. 3. Relation of increased urea excretion to initial amount of urea present in medulla. Comparison of rapid and slow administration of the two salts of diatrizoate.

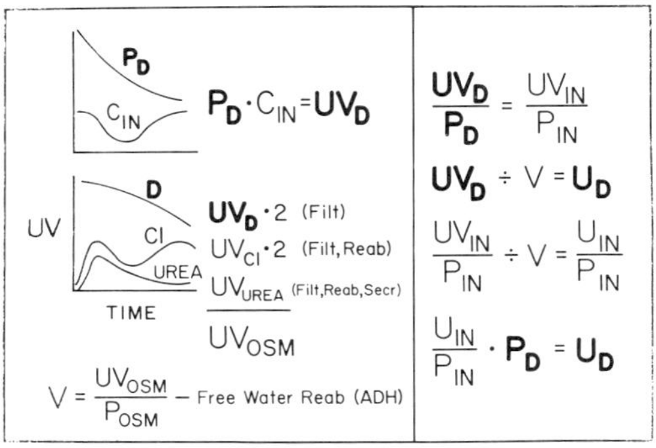

Fig. 4. Schematic summary of factors influencing urinary concentration (U) and excretion rate (UV) of diatrizoate in relation to other aspects of renal function.

Urine osmolality falls in the manner which one might predict (Fig. 5). The magnitude of the fall is clearly related to the dose of contrast agent. It is more abrupt with the bolus injection and more gradual with infusions. The patterns of recovery should be noted. With the sodium salt osmolality rises more promptly than with the meglumine. In the recovery period, the same pattern is seen with the urinary concentration of diatrizoate itself (Fig. 6).

Benness (1970a) and Cattell *et al.* (1970) have reported this in man. They attributed it to a differential effect of the two salts on the excretion of nonopaque solute, predominantly chloride and its attendant cation. However, our data do not completely support this interpretation (Fig. 7). Chloride excretion is highly unpredictable. It depends both on the control rate of

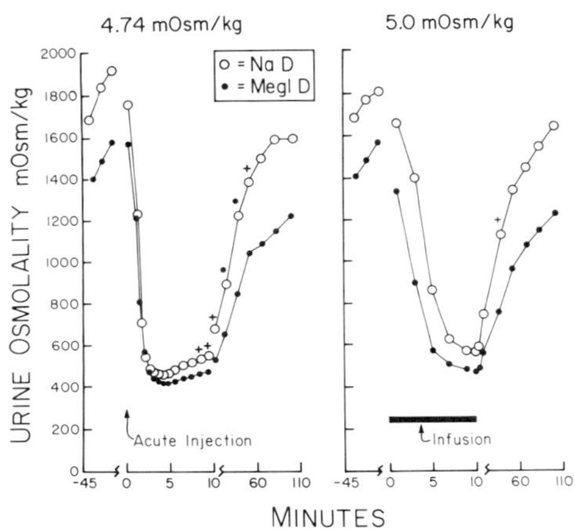

Fig. 5. Effect of intravenous urography on urine osmolality. Symbols * and + above points indicate a statistically significant difference between sodium and meglumine diatrizoate at $p < 0.05$ and $p < 0.01$, respectively.

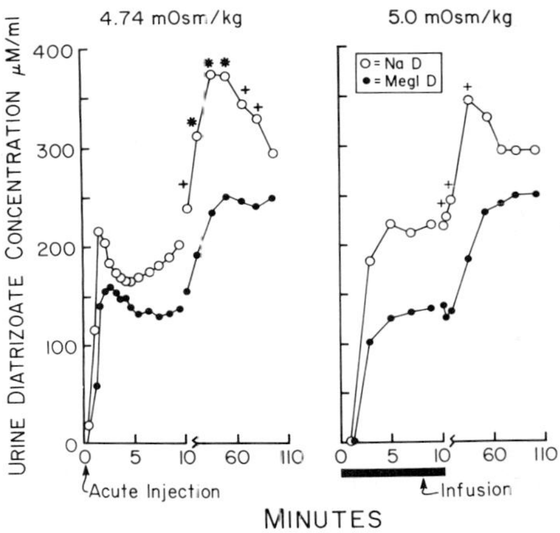

Fig. 6. Urinary concentration of diatrizoate during urography.

chloride excretion and the induced changes in GFR. Total solute excretion fails to account for the differences between the sodium and meglumine salts.

We therefore postulated that meglumine diatrizoate might preferentially inhibit the action of vasopressin on the distal nephron. Dr. John Gatzy of this laboratory has pursued this in a conclusive manner using the isolated toad bladder. The vasopressin-induced augmentation of water flow is inhibited by meglumine diatrizoate, but not by the sodium salt. Meglumine sulfate produces a partial effect. Furthermore, meglumine diatrizoate acts on the serosal and not on the mucosal side. Transferring these findings to the dog, it is our interpretation that a high plasma concentration of meglumine diatrizoate at least partially inhibits the action of vasopressin.

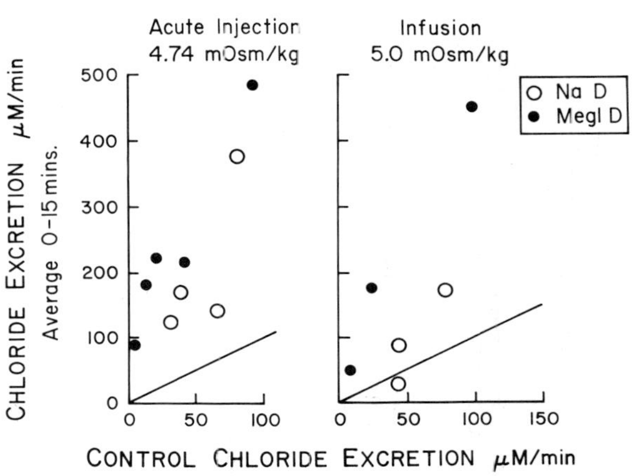

Fig. 7. Effect of urographic agents on chloride excretion.

We wish to emphasize the prediction based on the equation $U_D = P_D \times U/P$ inulin. This is well illustrated in Fig. 8. In this experiment, as in many others, P_D fell rapidly. At the same time, U/P inulin rose rapidly. Their product is given here as the calculated U_D. It is clear that calculated U_D is identical to observed U_D. With smaller doses of contrast agent, U_D fails to rise even though U/P inulin increases. The reason is clear, namely that as the urine becomes more concentrated during subsidence of diuresis, the plasma level of diatrizoate is not sufficiently high to provide maximal urinary concentrations. This late rise in urinary level has not been observed in man, a point to which we shall return.

Plasma concentration is predictable and clearly related to the method of administration. With bolus injections it is high early and then falls in curvilinear fashion. With infusions it rises gradually and then falls off once the infusion is terminated. The sodium and meglumine salts give rise to similar plasma levels. Any difference between the two is clearly not related to volume of distribution, but rather to naturally occurring differences in filtration rate.

From what has been said, excretion rate is also readily predictable (Fig. 9). In both sets of experiments, the early peak of UV_D is higher with the sodium than the meglumine salt. Two different reasons are involved. With the infusions the GFR happened to be far higher in the animals receiving the sodium salt. However, this was not the case with the bolus injections. We shall not go into detail, but the evidence is thoroughly convincing that the higher peak with sodium involves a differential effect of the two salts on renal delay time.

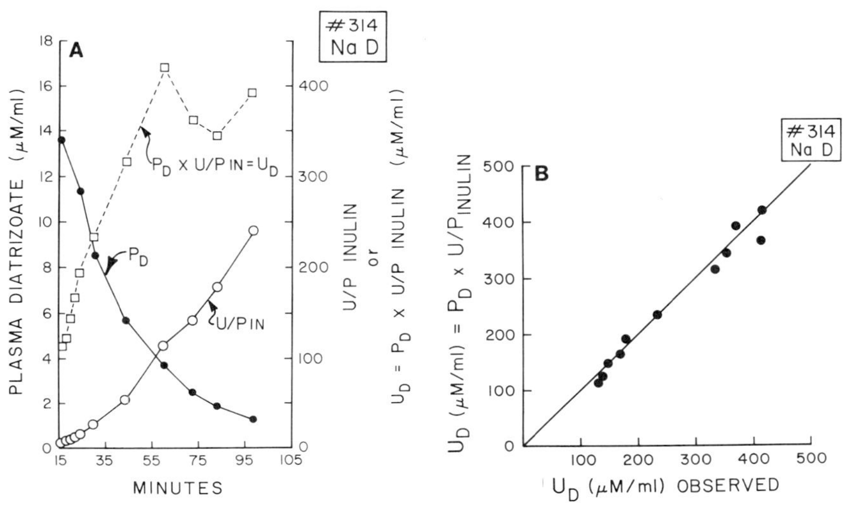

Fig. 8. Effect of simultaneous changes of plasma diatrizoate concentration and of U/P (inulin) on calculated and measured urinary concentration of diatrizoate. See text for calculations.

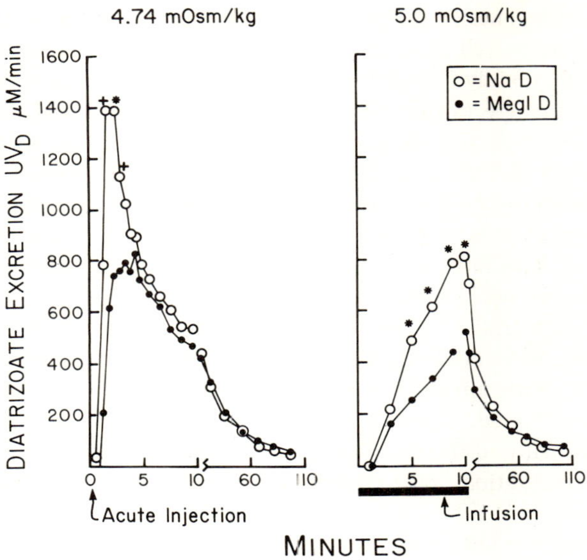

Fig. 9. Rate of diatrizoate excretion during urography.

We shall not attempt an extensive discussion of the data in relation to the many important aspects of radiology. Let us focus on a few points. The transient drop in GFR is of some interest. We believe that one of the factors is an acute increase in intratubular pressure. Gottschalk and Mylle (1957) clearly showed a rise in proximal pressure in response to osmotic diuresis. The time course from their studies is just about the same as the period of reduced GFR in ours. Although there was a slight and very brief reduction of arterial blood pressure in some experiments, particularly with the larger doses, in about half the experiments the GFR fell without any change in blood pressure. In the infusion studies diuresis began slowly and without any fall in GFR. The abruptness of diuresis is clearly an underlying factor.

The nephrogram is usually most dense shortly after the injection of the contrast agent. Previously this has been attributed to a high initial concentration of contrast agent in the tubular fluid. From our studies we are not certain that this would occur. Early after the bolus injection, even though the filtered load is at its highest, so also is the induced diuresis. Concentrations in voided urine are almost constant during the first 10 min. We suggest that the density of the early nephrogram may involve an additional factor. Our inference that intratubular pressure rises acutely is supported by the increase in kidney size noted radiologically (Arkless, 1969). If this occurs by dilatation of the tubules, which we believe to be the case, it may be calculated that the volume of tubular fluid increases almost two-fold during this period. While this is only a derived value, subject to several assumptions, it is of sufficient magnitude that it may be a real factor in determining the nature of the nephrogram.

Rare cases of nephrotoxicity occur after high-dose aortography or renal arteriography. They occur far less often after the intravenous procedure. From a pharmacological point of view, one would like somehow to correlate toxic reactions with local drug concentrations. With this as a goal, our data provide one suggestion. With high doses and in the antidiuretic animal the urinary concentration is far higher than previously reported. Actually in some experiments the urine was almost 25% diatrizoate, which is half the concentration of the injected material. The half-life of diatrizoate in the dog is 25 min, in man, 120 min. This is due to the greater GFR in the dog when expressed on a basis of body weight. From this we would predict that, with selected doses, the urinary level would rise at a later time in man, and actually later than has been studied to date. If so, these high late concentrations might have some bearing on the problem of nephrotoxicity. In support of such a notion is the clinical impression that transient renal failure is particularly apt to occur in patients who have been unduly dehydrated (Talner, 1972). Further studies in man seem warranted.

This raises the old question of the role of dehydration in urography. This has been and still is a slightly controversial subject. There is agreement that it involves the stimulation of the posterior pituitary, the release of vasopressin, its action on the water permeability of the distal nephron, a subsequent increase in U/P inulin and, by the same token, a rise in the urinary concentration of the contrast agent. However, at second glance the situation is quite complex. First, there is the dose of the contrast agent. This has not received adequate attention. Because of the nature of the renal response to osmotic diuresis, it is quite possible that the action of vasopressin might be far more important with one dose than with another. Second, there is the question of timing. The factors operating at 5 min may not be the same as those at 30 min. Third, it has been well shown in several clinical studies that water restriction *per se* is remarkably unpredictable in the extent to which the urine then becomes concentrated (Sherwood *et al.*, 1968). Fourth, the osmolality before injection is a poor guide to the renal response *during* urography. Figure 10 shows two experiments at the same dose, one with the highest control urinary osmolality (2300 mOsm/kg), the other with the lowest (600 mOsm/kg). In acute diuresis these fall to about 500 and 300, respectively. Urine concentration of diatrizoate during the first 10 min is about 440 and 250 mOsm/liter, respectively, taking into account the attendant cation. In other words, the four-fold difference in control osmolality becomes translated to less than a two-fold difference in the concentration of the contrast agent *during* urography. Fifth, there is an interesting question involving the release of vasopressin as a result of urography. The contrast agents are strongly hypertonic solutions. One study on patients in water diuresis shows clearly that vasopressin was released after the injection of the contrast agent (Ben-

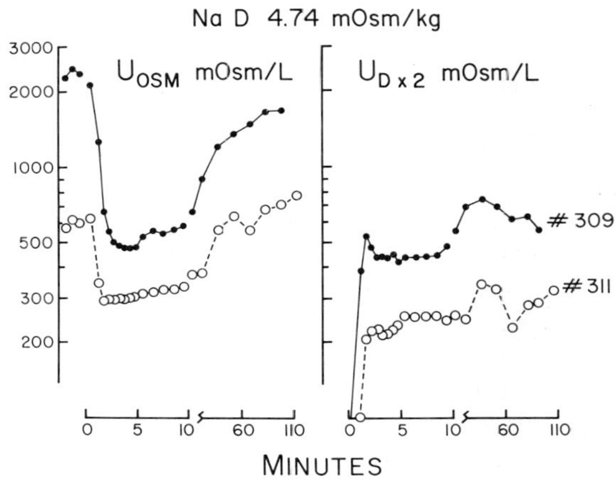

Fig. 10. Changes in urinary osmolality and diatrizoate concentration during urography. Comparison of two experiments with highest and lowest control urine osmolalities. Diatrizoate concentration has been multiplied by 2 to account for accompanying cation.

ness, 1970b). Sixth, there is our own observation that the contrast agent may partially block the action of vasopressin. Seventh, it is common radiological practice to apply abdominal pressure. This distends the ureters and pelvis. Acute obstruction may have another effect, namely to concentrate the urine (Kiil and Aukland, 1961). However, this reaction has not been evaluated under conditions of urography. Eighth, there is the dimension added by considering sodium chloride excretion. Our data are reasonably clear that the degree of chloruresis is somehow related to the control rate of chloride excretion. Cattell (1970) reported in a single patient that the urinary concentration of the contrast agent was far higher after salt depletion. In terms of final solute excretion, unreabsorbed chloride and unreabsorbable diatrizoate must compete with each other to become concentrated within the urine. Given this truism, if the urinary concentration of the contrast agent were to be of primary importance for radiography, it might logically be more proper to restrict the intake of salt rather than that of water. We suggest that this might be more logical. We do not pretend that it would be practical. Indeed, the only reason we mention it at all is to emphasize just one point, namely the complexity of the renal response to urography.

REFERENCES

Arkless, R. 1969. The normal kidney's reaction to intravenous pyelography. Am. J. Roentgen. 107: 746–749.

Aukland, K. 1961. Renal tubular permeability to urea with special reference to accumulation of urea in the renal medulla. Scand. J. Clin. Lab. Invest. 13: 646–660.

Benness, G.T. 1970a. Urographic contrast agents. A comparison of sodium and methylglucamine salts. Clin. Radiol. 21: 150–156.

Benness, G.T. 1970b. Evaluation of anti-diuretic hormone in intravenous urography. 'Sniff urography.' Clin. Radiol. 21: 157–162.

Cattell, W.R. 1970. Excretory pathways for contrast media. Invest. Radiol. 5: 473–486.

Cattell, W.R., I.K. Fry, R. Lane, and J.L. Tsay. 1970. Comparison of the renal excretion of Hypaque 45% and Urografin 60%. Brit. J. Radiol. 43: 309–313.

Gottschalk, C.W., and M. Mylle. 1957. Micropuncture study of pressures in proximal and distal tubules and peritubular capillaries of the rat kidney during osmotic diuresis. Am. J. Physiol. 189: 323–328.

Kiil, F., and K. Aukland. 1961. Effect of high ureteral pressure on urine concentration during water diuresis. Scand. J. Clin. Lab. Invest. 13: 268–275.

Lobentz, W.B., Jr., W.E. Lassiter, and C.W. Gottschalk. 1972. Renal tubular permeability during increased intrarenal pressure. J. Clin. Invest. 51: 484–492.

Richards, A.N., and A.M. Walker. 1930. Quantitative studies of the glomerular elimination of phenol red and indigo carmine in frogs. J. Biol. Chem. 87: 479–498.

Saxton, H.M. 1969. Urography. Brit. J. Radiol. 42: 321–346.

Sherwood, T., A. Breckenridge, C.T. Dollery, F.H. Doyle, and R.E. Steiner. 1968. Intravenous urography and renal function. Clin. Radiol. 19: 295–302.

Talner, L.B. 1972. Urographic contrast media in uremia. Radiol. Clinics N. Am. 10: 421–432.

Studies on Urate Handling in Man Utilizing Pyrazinamide

Thomas H. Steele
Department of Medicine
University of Wisconsin Center for the Health Sciences
Madison, Wisconsin

The elimination of uric acid in man, primarily a function of the kidney, assumes considerably greater importance for this purine metabolite than for many other metabolic end products because of the tendencies of uric acid and monosodium urate to crystallize in urine and tissues (Gutman, 1964). In addition to the involvement of hyperuricemia in uric acid nephropathy and acute gouty arthritis, chronic hyperuricemia may be related via intrarenal urate deposition to the development of hypertension and chronic renal failure (Verger *et al.*, 1967). For these reasons it seems justifiable to characterize as fully as possible the renal transport processes affecting urate excretion in man. Unfortunately, suitable animal models applicable to man have been difficult to come by. With the exception of the chimpanzee, a species with apparently analogous renal urate transport processes (Fanelli, Bohn, and Reilly, 1971), all other species studied have demonstrated significant differences, either in renal urate handling or in other aspects of urate homeostasis, as compared with man. Because of these difficulties we have chosen to study urate handling primarily in man, realizing the experimental limitations inherent in this approach.

TUBULAR SECRETION OF URATE IN MAN; THE PYRAZINAMIDE SUPPRESSION TEST

The enunciation of a 'three-component hypothesis' by Gutman and Yü (1961) laid the ground-work for many of our present concepts. According to that hypothesis, urate is filtered freely by the glomeruli and subsequently undergoes both reabsorption and secretion by the tubules. The urinary uric acid is comprised of a mixture of the filtered urate escaping reabsorption and other urate derived from tubular secretion. Although earlier workers had assumed that urate was filtered and partially reabsorbed (Berliner *et al.*,

1950), direct evidence for its tubular secretion in man was presented by Praetorius and Kirk (1950) who studied a patient with substantial net secretion of urate, probably as the result of a renal tubular reabsorptive defect. Gutman, Yü, and Berger (1959) subsequently demonstrated a modest amount of net urate secretion in patients with mild chronic renal disease by inducing an osmotic diuresis and simultaneously administering uricosuric agents.

Given the existence of tubular secretion of urate, its role and importance in regulating the rate of uric acid excretion remained a subject for conjecture. The observation that the antituberculous agent pyrazinamide (PZA) appeared to inhibit the tubular secretion of urate (Davis *et al.*, 1965) suggested that the use of PZA in man might provide a suitable pharmacologic method for assessing the importance of renal urate *secretion.* Specifically, the rate of urate excretion could be compared before and during the maximum action of PZA, the decrement in urate excretion produced by PZA being ascribed to secretory inhibition (Fig. 1). In normal persons PZA decreased urate excretion by approximately 80%, with residual excretory rates averaging less than 2% of the filtered load (Steele and Rieselbach, 1967; Gutman, Yü, and Berger, 1969). Although these results could have been explained by an accelerated rate of urate reabsorption induced pharmacologically by PZA, recent work suggests that the hypouricosuric action of PZA results from the inhibition of tubular secretion. Pyrazinamide initially is metabolized to pyrazinoic acid which, at low plasma concentrations, appears to inhibit the tubular secretion of urate (Weiner and Tinker, 1972). At high plasma concentrations pyrazinoic acid is uricosuric in the dog (Weiner and Tinker, 1972) and chimpanzee (Fanelli and Weiner, 1973), a characteristic reminiscent of

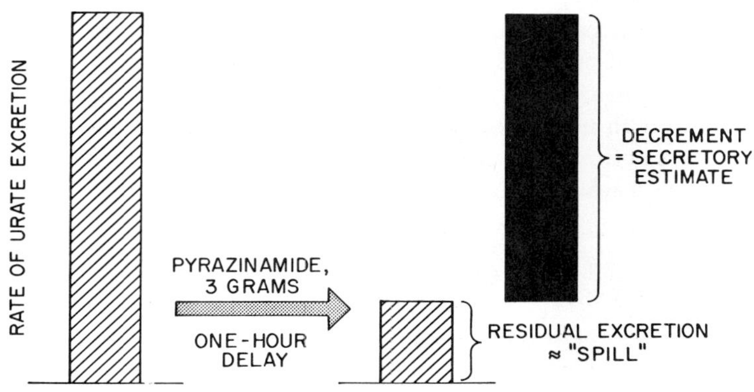

Fig. 1. Diagram of a 'pyrazinamide-suppression test.' The decrement in urate excretion produced during the maximal antiuricosuric action of PZA was taken as a minimal estimate of urate secretion in the original interpretation of the test (see text). The amount of nonsuppressible urate excretion ('spill') was assumed to represent filtered urate escaping reabsorption.

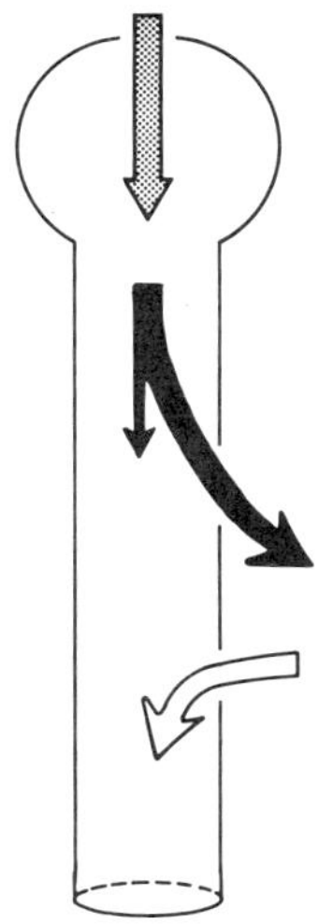

Fig. 2. Model for renal urate handling underlying the original interpretation of the PZA-suppression test. In this model extensive urate reabsorption occurs entirely prior to secretion.

several other agents affecting urate excretion (Gutman, 1966). Thus, the antiuricosuric effect of PZA most likely results from the antisecretory action of small amounts of pyrazinoic acid generated by the metabolism of PZA (Weiner and Tinker, 1972).

The original interpretation of the PZA-suppression test (Steele and Rieselbach, 1967) was based on the simplest formulation derived from the 'three-component hypothesis' (Gutman and Yü, 1961), namely that filtered urate first undergoes extensive reabsorption with 98% being abstracted from tubular fluid (Fig. 2). Subsequently, urate would be returned to tubular fluid via tubular secretion. The amount of PZA-suppressible urate excretion then could be considered an index of the tubular secretion of urate (Fig. 1), requiring only the additional assumptions that PZA almost completely inhibits the tubular secretion of urate and interferes minimally, if at all, with its reabsorption. According to that interpretation, 80% or more of the urinary uric acid in normal persons would originate from tubular secretion (Steele and Rieselbach, 1967).

SUPPRESSION OF URICOSURIC RESPONSES BY PYRAZINAMIDE

The application of the PZA-suppression test in a variety of situations, however, produced some surprising results. Several chemical and pharmacologic agents and disease states causing increased urinary urate losses were investigated with PZA. Initially, Yü, Kaung, and Gutman (1970) clearly demonstrated that the administration of glycine, an amino acid long thought to inhibit urate reabsorption, caused a uricosuric response which could be completely eliminated by PZA pretreatment. Those studies suggested that the uricosuric effect of glycine might result from the stimulation of tubular secretion of urate rather than the inhibition of its reabsorption. Similar observations were obtained (without and with PZA pretreatment) after the administration of benziodarone (Podevin *et al.*, 1967; Gougoux *et al.*, 1970), ethacrynic acid (Steele and Oppenheimer, 1969), and certain iodinated radiographic contrast media (Postlethwaite and Kelley, 1971). In addition, the uricosuric effect of hydration (Diamond *et al.*, 1972) and the hyperuricosuric states accompanying certain cases of Wilson's disease (Wilson, Mitchell, and Goldstein, 1971) and Hodgkin's disease (Bennett *et al.*, 1972) could be eliminated by PZA. Likewise, a major portion of the greatly increased urate excretion per nephron in unilaterally nephrectomized renal transplant donors was suppressible by PZA (Shelp and Rieselbach, 1968).

In all these hyperuricosuric states, the interpretation of PZA-suppressible urate excretion as an index of tubular secretion led to the conclusion that increased tubular secretion of urate (or secretory stimulation) resulted in the accelerated urinary uric acid losses. This conflicted rather strikingly with traditional interpretations of the actions of uricosuric agents, in that these compounds usually had been assumed to act as a result of their inhibiting urate reabsorption. It also seemed surprising that the renal lesions of Wilson's disease, a condition often accompanied by defects in the proximal tubular reabsorption of amino acids and other solutes, could lead to an increase in urate secretion. During previous studies in man, modulations in urate excretion had demonstrated little relationship to changes in the excretion of other partially reabsorbed solutes. For example, following volume expansion to 102% of control body weights with isotonic saline, sodium excretion increased briskly but urate excretion remained unchanged (Fig. 3). Furthermore, at any level of sodium excretion following volume expansion, increases in the excretion of inorganic phosphorus, a proximal tubular 'marker,' were not accompanied by proportional uricosuric responses (Fig. 4).

Recent studies in animal models, however, have helped to clarify these results. Although an earlier micropuncture study in the rat utilizing [^{14}C] uric acid could not be interpreted as showing evidence of proximal tubular secretion of urate (Kramp, Lassiter, and Gottschalk, 1971), more recent experiments by Greger, Lang, and Deetjen (1971) demonstrated net secretion of urate within the proximal tubule of the rat. Although the 'amount of urate remaining' in the late proximal tubule of superficial nephrons in the rat kidney was greater than the filtered load, simultaneous whole-kidney uric acid excretion values were substantially less than the amount filtered. These observations suggested that urate is secreted and then subsequently reabsorbed in the rat nephron. In addition, microperfusion studies demonstrated the existence of bidirectional fluxes for uric acid across proximal tubular epithelium, with the secretory flux predominating (Lang, Greger, and Deetjen, 1972, 1973).

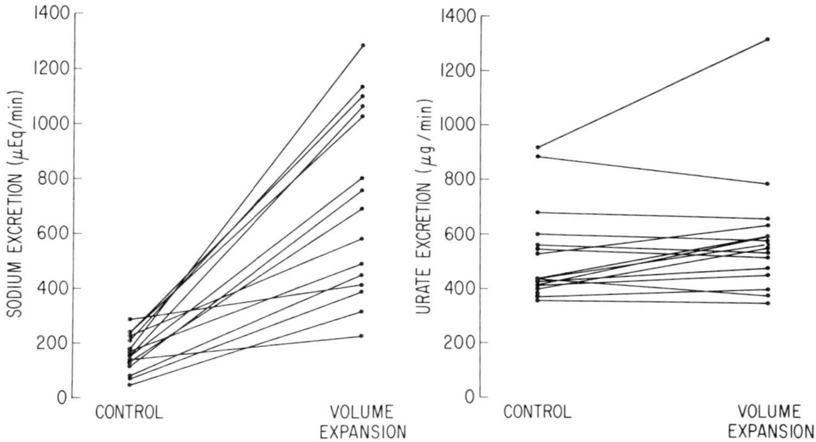

Fig. 3. Comparison of changes in sodium and urate excretion during 2% volume expansion with isotonic saline in 15 normal persons (Steele, 1969). Although sodium excretion increased briskly, urate excretion usually showed little change.

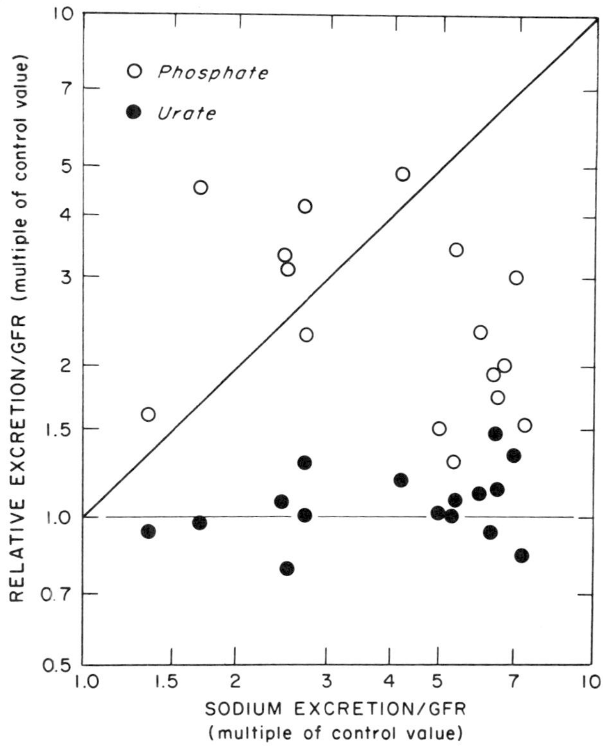

Fig. 4. Comparison of relative changes in inorganic phosphate and uric acid excretion, as functions of sodium excretion, following 2% volume expansion in normals. With increasing rates of sodium excretion, the excretion of phosphate (a proximal tubular 'marker') increased but urate did not.

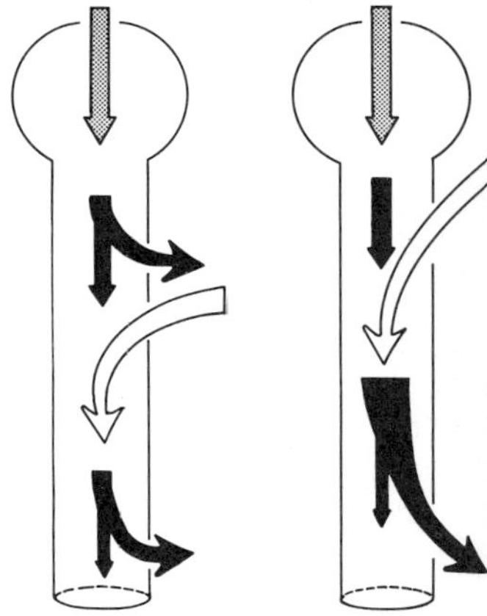

Fig. 5. Possible models for renal urate handling in man, employing post-secretory reabsorption. It should be noted that, in either case, intrarenal urate secretory and reabsorptive fluxes are larger than in the model of Fig. 2. The presence or extent of presecretory reabsorption of urate in man is currently unclear.

Clearance studies in the chimpanzee by Fanelli, Bohn, Reilly, and Weiner (1973) indicate that a similar situation may exist in that species. These investigators demonstrated that the administration of large doses of mersalyl to the chimpanzee increased uric acid excretion to rates far greater than the simultaneous filtered loads. Although the normal urate-to-inulin clearance ratio (C_{urate}/C_{inulin}) in the chimpanzee approximates that in man, this ratio approached values as high as 2 following mersalyl administration. These results suggest that, by the inhibition of urate reabsorption, mersalyl unmasked a large urate secretory flux normally present in the chimpanzee. It seems reasonable to postulate that a similar relationship between the secretion and reabsorption of urate may occur in man, namely that urate secretion occurs prior to or coextensive with its reabsorption and that the magnitudes of intrarenal urate secretion and reabsorption are far greater than had been predicted from previous experiments (Fig. 5). Perhaps prophetically, this possibility had been suggested nine years previously by Gutman (1964).

IMPORTANCE OF URATE SECRETION IN MAN

In man relationships between urate secretion and reabsorption have been more difficult to delineate. In our laboratory, working with Dr. Geoffrey Boner, uricosuric responses to intravenous probenecid were measured under standardized conditions in seven normal persons (Steele and Boner, 1973). The studies then were repeated on a subsequent day in the same participants after the subjects had been pretreated with PZA. The increase in urate excretion after probenecid averaged 1129 (± 150) μg/min, with a simultaneous change in urate clearance equivalent to 18.4 (± 2.1) % of the filtered load. After PZA pretreatment, however, the uricosuric response to probenecid in the same subjects averaged only 235 (± 58) μg/min, with C_{urate}/C_{inulin} (× 100) increasing by only 4.1 (± 0.6) %. Thus, PZA pretreatment significantly diminished the uricosuric response to probenecid. Secretory inhibition by PZA might have permitted post-secretory reabsorptive mechanisms to deal more efficiently with reduced intratubular urate loads, allowing the abstraction of a greater fraction of the urate from tubular fluid.

An alternate possibility is that PZA interfered with the uricosuric response to probenecid by inhibiting the renal binding or secretion of probenecid, thereby diminishing the amount of the uricosuric agent acting at reabsorptive sites. This possibility was examined indirectly by Dr. Boner by measuring the decrement in net p-aminohippurate (PAH) secretion (T_{PAH}) produced by probenecid in three persons, both without and with PZA pretreatment (G. Boner and T. H. Steele, unpublished). Each experiment was carried out with plasma PAH concentrations rising steadily between 5 and 10 mg/100 ml. At these plasma levels T_{PAH} varies directly with the plasma PAH, and a decrease in T_{PAH} (concomitantly with rising plasma levels) indicates an inhibition of net PAH secretion in the absence of renal hemodynamic changes. The results of these three pairs of studies are summarized in Fig. 6. In each instance PZA pretreatment did not substantially affect the magnitude of T_{PAH}; furthermore, the decrement in T_{PAH} produced by probenecid was

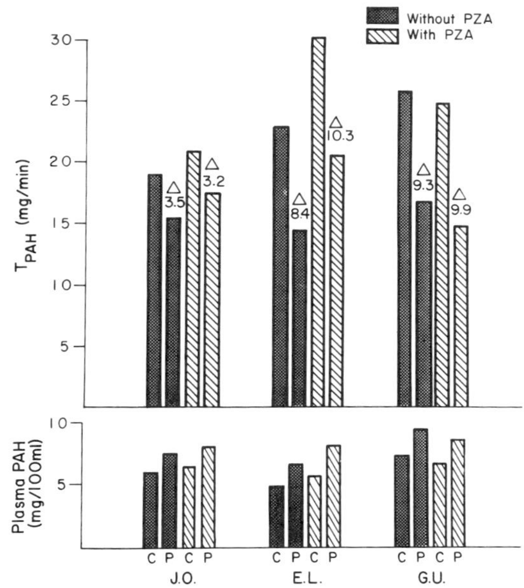

Fig. 6. Failure of PZA pretreatment to affect probenecid-induced inhibition of T_{PAH} in three persons (Boner and Steele, unpublished). C, Measurements during control periods; P, measurements after probenecid, 500 mg i.v.

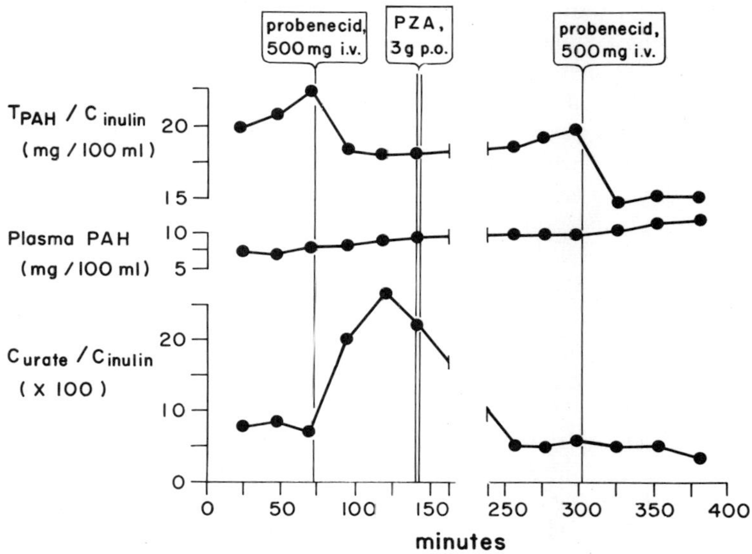

Fig. 7. Example of similar depressions of T_{PAH} by probenecid, before and after PZA (Boner and Steele, unpublished). The minimal uricosuric response to probenecid following PZA administration should be noted.

not affected by PZA. Similarly, in 'double' studies, when PZA was administered immediately after measuring the uricosuric effect of probenecid and sufficient time allowed to elapse for its action to develop, T_{PAH} decreased by a similar amount after a second dose of probenecid was administered (Fig. 7). Although these studies indicated that PZA does not alter the effect of probenecid on PAH secretion, they did not rule out the possibility that an interaction between PZA or pyrazinoate and probenecid may occur at urate transport sites. Indeed, recent studies in our laboratory indicate that the secretion of PAH and urate proceed independently of one another in man (Boner and Steele, 1973).

Pyrazinamide pretreatment also sharply ameliorates the acute uricosuric action of intravenous chlorothiazide in many persons (Steele and Boner, 1973). Although PZA interferes with the uricosuric response to chlorothiazide, the simultaneous natriuretic and phosphaturic properties of chlorothiazide persist unimpaired (Table 1). This suggests that the acute uricosuric response to intravenous chlorothiazide, like probenecid, is due in part to the enhanced excretion of secreted urate. However, as with probenecid, PZA might interfere with the renal actions of chlorothiazide at urate transport sites without simultaneously affecting sodium or inorganic phosphate reabsorption.

Recently, we have studied the effect of PZA on a uricosuric response not produced by a pharmacologic or chemical agent. Although previous studies

Table 1. Partial suppression of uricosuric responses to intravenous chlorothiazide by PZA pretreatment

	$\Delta\ C_{urate}/C_{inulin}$ (X 100)	$\Delta\ C_{Na}/C_{inulin}$ (X 100)	$\Delta\ C_{phosphate}/C_{inulin}$ (X 100)
Without PZA	9.6 (± 1.2)	5.1 (± 0.8)	13.2 (± 1.0)
PZA pretreatment	4.9 (± 0.8)	6.3 (± 0.4)	14.5 (± 0.9)
P	< 0.02	NS	NS

Mean values (± s.e.m.) in 20 paired experiments in normal persons (see text). Delta (Δ) indicates value after chlorothiazide, 500 mg i.v., minus control during water diuresis. Data are summarized from Steele and Boner (1973).

showed that the infusion of isotonic saline affects urate excretion only slightly (Steele, 1969), experiments by Cannon, Svahn, and DeMartini (1970) indicated that the infusion of 2.5% sodium chloride produces a brisk uricosuric response in many persons. In studies performed recently by Dr. Manuel in our laboratory, normal volunteers underwent volume expansion with 3% sodium chloride after control measurements were made during water diuresis (Manuel and Steele, 1974a). An example of one such study is summarized in the solid circles of Fig. 8. After volume expansion with 3% sodium chloride, urate excretion and clearance increased briskly. Likewise, sodium excretion and fractional excretion rapidly rose to very high levels. Two days later the same procedure was repeated but after PZA pretreatment. As shown by the open circles in Fig. 8, urate excretion and clearance commenced at very low levels after PZA and changed only minimally during 3% sodium chloride infusion. In sharp contrast, the absolute and fractional excretions of sodium were comparable with values obtained without PZA pretreatment. The increments in urate excretion and clearance, between water diuresis and sodium chloride periods, were far greater in the study without PZA pretreatment. Similar results were obtained in other individuals who manifested significant uricosuric responses to 3% sodium chloride infusion (Table 2). The amelioration of the uricosuric response by the suppression of tubular secretion of urate with PZA suggests that intact tubular secretion plays an important role in the uricosuric response to 3% sodium chloride. The results cannot be explained on the basis of an inhibitory action of PZA or pyrazinoate on the renal action of a second pharmacologic agent, indicating that the suppression of uricosuric responses by PZA need not involve an interaction between pharmacologic agents.

The reverse situation occurred during recent studies of prolonged hydrochlorothiazide administration in man (Manuel and Steele, 1974b). Normal subjects underwent a standard 'PZA-suppression test,' measuring urate excretion and clearances before and after PZA administration. Each person subsequently ingested hydrochlorothiazide, 100 mg daily, for two weeks. The PZA-suppression study was then repeated. After two weeks of hydrochloro-

Table 2. Pyrazinamide suppression of uricosuric responses to 3% NaCl

	Δ Urate excretion (μg/min)	Δ C_{urate}/C_{inulin} (X 100)	Δ Sodium excretion (μEq/min)	Δ C_{Na}/C_{inulin} (X 100)
Without PZA	258 (± 44)	5.7 (± 0.3)	1686 (± 194)	9.0 (± 0.6)
PZA pretreatment	122 (± 12)	1.8 (± 0.3)	1464 (± 184)	7.9 (± 1.3)
P	< 0.05	< 0.003	NS	NS

Mean values (± s.e.m.) in 10 paired experiments in normal persons (see text).
Delta (Δ) indicates value during 3% NaCl infusion, 20 ml/min, minus control during water diuresis. Data are summarized from Manuel and Steele (1974a).

thiazide, baseline C_{urate}/C_{inulin} ratios had decreased significantly (Fig. 9). On the other hand, the C_{urate}/C_{inulin} values obtained during maximal action of PZA were not affected significantly by prolonged hydrochlorothiazide treatment (Fig. 9). Previous studies had shown that C_{urate}/C_{inulin} in PZA-treated persons decreased significantly during acute ethacrynic-acid-induced

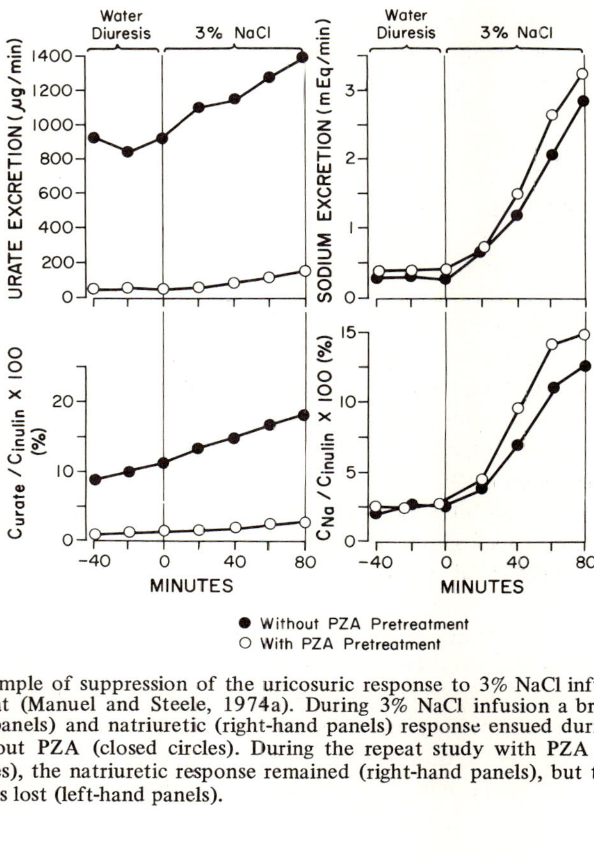

Fig. 8. Example of suppression of the uricosuric response to 3% NaCl infusion by PZA pretreatment (Manuel and Steele, 1974a). During 3% NaCl infusion a brisk uricosuric (left-hand panels) and natriuretic (right-hand panels) response ensued during the initial study without PZA (closed circles). During the repeat study with PZA pretreatment (open circles), the natriuretic response remained (right-hand panels), but the uricosuric response was lost (left-hand panels).

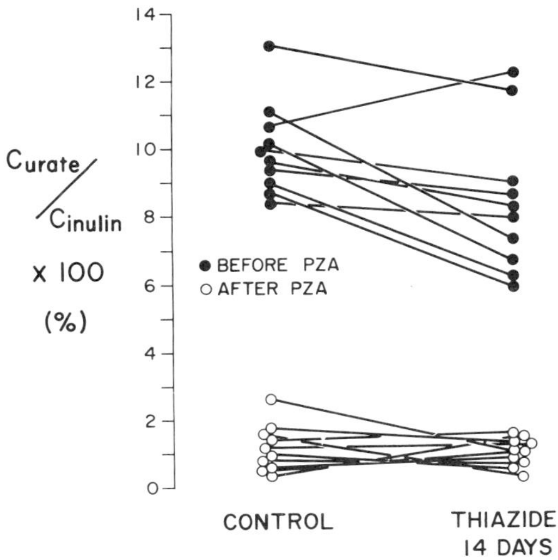

Fig. 9. Changes in Curate/Cinulin following hydrochlorothiazide, 100 mg daily for 14 days (Manuel and Steele, 1974b). Most of the change occurred in the PZA-suppressible component of C_{urate}/C_{inulin}.

volume contraction, but remained unchanged after ethacrynic acid in PZA-pretreated saline repleted controls (Steele, 1969). In contrast to the situation occurring during acute ethacrynic-acid-induced volume depletion, the changes in renal urate handling occurring during prolonged thiazide therapy probably reflect influences other than solely those generated during acute volume contraction. This view is in contrast to the proposal by Suki *et al.* (1967) that chronic thiazide diuretic treatment results in enhanced renal urate reabsorption brought about primarily through a volume contraction stimulus. Perhaps intrarenal circulatory adjustments, not occurring during acute volume contraction, are important in the pathogenesis of hyperuricemia occurring during chronic diuretic therapy. In any event, the changes in renal urate handling during prolonged thiazide administration occurred primarily in the PZA-suppressible portion of the urinary urate. This suggests either that urate secretion may have been adversely affected or, alternatively, that the reabsorption of secreted urate became more avid after hydrochlorothiazide treatment.

In summary, the functional arrangements and interrelationships between urate secretory and reabsorptive sites within nephrons in man remain a subject for considerable speculation. Results from animal models and more indirect data from studies in man are consistent with the hypothesis that large intrarenal urate secretory and reabsorptive fluxes interact with one another, a large amount of secreted urate subsequently being reabsorbed. Assuming this is the case, the inhibition of urate secretion by PZA would not estimate quantitatively either urate secretion or reabsorption. Indeed, the PZA-induced inhibition of even a relatively small fraction of a large urate secretory flux might be sufficient to diminish strikingly uric acid excretion by permitting greater reabsorptive efficiency at post-secretory sites under conditions of lessened intratubular urate loads. While currently defying precise quantitative interpretation, the data with PZA still strongly suggest a pivotal and crucial role for tubular urate secretion in maintaining the normal renal contribution to urate homeostasis in man.

ACKNOWLEDGMENTS

Supported by USPHS Grants AM15162, AM15512, and AM05630, and grants from the Wisconsin Heart Association.

REFERENCES

Bennett, J. S., J. Bond, I. Singer, and A. J. Gottlieb. 1972. Hypouricemia in Hodgkin's disease. Ann. Intern. Med. 76:751–756.

Berliner, R. W., J. G. Hilton, T. F. Yü, and T. J. Kennedy. 1950. The renal mechanism for urate excretion in man. J. Clin. Invest. 29:396–401.

Boner, G., and T. H. Steele. 1973. Relationship of urate and p-aminohippurate secretion in man. Am. J. Physiol. 225:100–104.

Cannon, P. J., D. S. Svahn, and F. E. DeMartini. 1970. The influence of hypertonic saline infusion upon the fractional reabsorption of urate and other ions in normal and hypertensive man. Circulation 41:97–108.

Davis, B. B., J. B. Field, G. P. Rodnan, and L. H. Kedes. 1965. Localization and pyrazinamide inhibition of distal transtubular movement of uric acid-C^{14} with a modified stop-flow technique. J. Clin. Invest. 44:716–721.

Diamond, H. S., R. Lazarus, D. Kaplan, and D. Halberstam. 1972. Effect of urine flow rate on uric acid excretion in man. Arthritis Rheumat. 15:338–346.

Fanelli, G. M., D. L. Bohn, and S. S. Reilly. 1971. Renal urate transport in the chimpanzee. Am. J. Physiol. 220:613–619.

Fanelli, G. M., D. L. Bohn, and S. S. Reilly. 1973. Effects of mercurial diuretics on renal transport of urate in the chimpanzee. Am. J. Physiol. 224:985–992.

Fanelli, G. M., and I. M. Weiner. 1973. Pyrazinoate excretion in the chimpanzee; relation to urate disposition and the action of uricosuric drugs. J. Clin. Invest. 52: 1946–1957.

Gougoux, A., G. Michaud, P. Vinay, and G. Lemieux. 1970. The uricosuric action of benziodarone in man and dog. Clin. Res. 18:747 (abstr.).

Greger, R., F. Lang, and P. Deetjen. 1971. Handling of uric acid by the rat kidney. I. Microanalysis of uric acid in proximal tubular fluid. Pflügers Arch. Ges. Physiol. 324:279–287.

Gutman, A. B. 1964. Significance of the renal clearance of uric acid in normal and gouty man. Am. J. Med. 37:833–838.

Gutman, A. B. 1966. Uricosuric drugs, with special reference to probenecid and sulfinpyrazone. Adv. Pharmacol. Chemother. 4:91–142.

Gutman, A. B., and T. F. Yü. 1961. A three-component system for regulation

of renal excretion of uric acid in man. Trans. Ass. Am. Physicians 74:353–365.
Gutman, A. B., T. F. Yü, and L. Berger. 1959. Tubular secretion of urate in man. J. Clin. Invest. 38:1778–1781.
Gutman, A. B., T. F. Yü, and L. Berger. 1969. Renal function in gout III. Estimation of tubular secretion and reabsorption of uric acid by use of pyrazinamide (pyrazinoic acid). Am. J. Med., 47:575–592.
Kramp, R. A., W. E. Lassiter, and C. W. Gottschalk. 1971. Urate-2-^{14}C transport in the rat nephron. J. Clin. Invest. 50:35–48.
Lang, F., R. Greger, and P. Deetjen. 1972. Handling of uric acid by the rat kidney. II. Microperfusion studies on bidirectional transport of uric acid in the proximal tubule. Pflügers Arch. Ges. Physiol. 335:257–265.
Lang, F., R. Greger, and P. Deetjen. 1973. Handling of uric acid by the rat kidney. III. Microperfusion studies on steady state concentration of uric acid in the proximal tubule. Consideration of free flow conditions. Pflügers Arch. Ges. Physiol. 338:295–302.
Manuel, M. A., and T. H. Steele. 1974a. Pyrazinamide suppression of the uricosuric response to sodium chloride infusion. J. Lab. Clin. Med. In press.
Manuel, M. A., and T. H. Steele. 1974b. Changes in renal urate handling after prolonged thiazide treatment. Amer. J. Med. In press.
Podevin, R., F. Paillard, C. Amiel, and G. Richet. 1967. Action de la benziodarone sur l'excrétion de l'acide urique. Rev. Franc. Études Clin. Biol. 12:361–367.
Postlethwaite, A. E., and W. N. Kelley. 1971. Uricosuric effect of radiocontrast agents. Ann. Intern. Med. 74:845–852.
Praetorius, E., and J. E. Kirk. 1950. Hypouricemia: with evidence for tubular elimination of uric acid. J. Lab. Clin. Med. 35:865–868.
Shelp, W. D., and R. E. Rieselbach. 1968. Increased bidirectional urate transport per nephron following unilateral nephrectomy. Abstr. Am. Soc. of Nephrol. 60 (abstr.).
Steele, T. H. 1969. Evidence for altered renal urate reabsorption during changes in volume of the extracellular fluid. J. Lab. Clin. Med. 74:288–299.
Steele, T. H., and G. Boner. 1973. Origins of the uricosuric response. J. Clin. Invest. 52:1368–1375.
Steele, T. H., and S. Oppenheimer. 1969. Factors affecting urate excretion following diuretic administration in man. Am. J. Med. 47:564–574.
Steele, T. H., and R. E. Rieselbach. 1967. The renal mechanism for urate homeostasis in normal man. Am. J. Med. 43:868–875.
Suki, W. N., A. R. Hull, F. C. Rector, and D. W. Seldin. 1967. Mechanism of the effect of thiazide diuretics on calcium and uric acid. J. Clin. Invest. 46:1121 (abstr.).
Verger, D., C. Leroux-Robert, P. Ganter, and G. Richet. 1967. Les tophus goutteux de la médullaire rénale des urémiques chroniques. Nephron 4:356–370.
Weiner, I. M., and J. P. Tinker. 1972. Pharmacology of pyrazinamide: metabolic and renal function studies related to the mechanism of drug-induced urate retention. J. Pharm. Exp. Ther. 180:411–434.
Wilson, D. M., J. S. Mitchell, and N. P. Goldstein. 1971. Renal urate excretion in patients with Wilson's disease. Abstr. Am. Soc. Nephrol. 91 (abstr.).
Yü, T. F., C. Kaung, and A. B. Gutman. 1970. Effect of glycine loading on plasma and urinary uric acid and amino acids in normal and gouty subjects. Am. J. Med. 49:352–359.

Use of Furosemide in Hyponatremic Disorders

Robert W. Schrier

Department of Medicine
University of Colorado Medical Center
Denver, Colorado

Hyponatremia due to impaired capacity to dilute the urine may be observed in patients with sodium-retaining states including congestive heart failure, cirrhosis, and nephrotic syndrome. Since these patients may be receiving diuretics for treatment of their edema, the diuretics are frequently incriminated as the cause of the hyponatremia. This possibility is not unreasonable, since diuretics such as furosemide and ethacrynic acid are known to inhibit sodium transport in the ascending limb of the Henle loop in normal man and animals and thus limit maximal renal diluting capacity (Seldin *et al.*, 1966; Earley and Friedler, 1964; Clapp and Robinson, 1968). Alternatively, however, in edematous patients with hypertonic urine it is possible that these diuretic agents might have a net effect of improving the capacity to excrete solute-free water. Such an effect could result from diuretic-induced increased tubular fluid delivery to diluting sites beyond where the diuretic acts. In this regard, patients with edema-forming states may have impaired ability to excrete dilute urine at least partially because of limited delivery of tubular fluid to the distal diluting segments of the nephron (Bell, Schredl, and Bartter, 1964).

Studies were therefore performed to examine the effect of intravenous furosemide (1 mg/kg) on renal diluting capacity in a group of patients with hyponatremia associated with congestive heart failure, cirrhosis, and nephrotic syndrome (Schrier *et al.*, 1973). The results of these studies are shown in Fig. 1. The administration of the furosemide resulted in a net increase in free-water clearance in five out of seven of the patients with hyponatremia and sodium retention. In the remaining two patients negative free-water excretion approached zero, so that these patients also demonstrated relative improvement in the ability to excrete solute-free water. The mean urinary

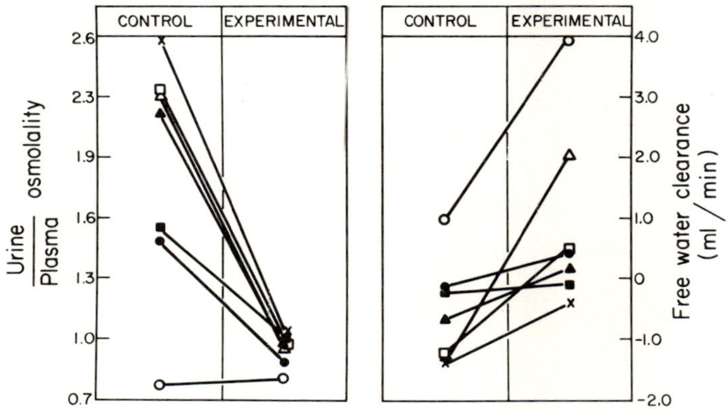

Fig. 1. Effect of intravenous furosemide on the urine to plasma osmolality ratio (left-hand side) and free-water clearance (right-hand side) in edematous patients with hyponatremia. Each pair of points represents a single patient and is the mean of 3–5 consecutive clearance periods.

osmolality was 526 mOsm/kg H_2O before and 251 mOsm/kg H_2O after the administration of furosemide. The mean free-water excretion increased from −1.3 to +.45 ml/min, and in two patients maximal values of 2 and 4 ml/min were achieved. These findings therefore indicated that the acute administration of furosemide can potentially counteract the water retention and hyponatremia associated with sodium-retaining states. It should be emphasized, however, that in certain instances secondary effects of the diuretic administration, such as reduced blood volume, could increase release of vasopressin and thereby promote water retention and intensify the hyponatremia.

In previous studies in edematous patients with hyponatremia the administration of hypertonic mannitol also has been demonstrated to dilute the urine and increase free-water excretion (Bell, Schedl, and Bartter, 1964; Schedl and Bartter, 1960). The infusion of hypertonic mannitol, however, may have increased blood volume and thereby suppressed endogenous vasopressin (ADH) independent of any alteration in fluid delivery to the distal nephron. In the present experiments furosemide-induced urinary electrolyte and water losses were not replaced; thus, suppression of ADH release by volume expansion could not have accounted for the improved diluting ability. Taken together, therefore, these results are compatible with the interpretation that the primary cause of hyponatremia in edematous states may be enhanced proximal tubular fluid reabsorption and diminished tubular fluid delivery to the diluting segment of the nephron. Such a mechanism does not, however, exclude a role of persistent secretion of ADH. Studies were thus performed to examine whether the furosemide-induced hypotonic urine could be converted to a hypertonic state by the administration of exogenous vasopressin. If the patient's hyponatremia was associated with appropriate suppression of ADH, then a response to exogenous vasopressin might be demonstrable. The results of the infusion of exogenous vasopressin during the furosemide-induced hypotonic urine production are shown in Fig. 2. In five patients in the present study in which vasopressin was administered during the furosemide diuresis neither an effect on urinary osmolality nor free-water clearance was observed. This finding indicates that the production of hypotonic urine in such patients during the administration of either furosemide or hypertonic mannitol does not exclude the role of persistent secretion of ADH as one of the pathogenetic factors in the development of the hyponatremia. The effect of furosemide to inhibit sodium reabsorption in the medullary portions of the Henle loops or to increase medullary blood flow may diminish the degree of medullary hypertonicity but would not be expected to produce a hypotonic medullary interstitium. Such effects of the diuretic might therefore diminish urinary osmolality to isotonic but not hypotonic levels, providing that osmotic equilibration between the tubular fluid and medullary interstitium occurs. Thus the most likely explanation for the vasopressin-resistant hypotonic urine which occurred during furosemide administration would seem to be a failure of complete osmotic equilibration. The cause of this incomplete equilibration was probably the increased rate of solute and fluid flow through the collecting ducts during the furosemide-induced diuresis. There are indeed several precedents for the occurrence of vasopressin-resistant hypotonic urine in association with increased solute excretion, including humans with impaired renal function (Tannen *et al.*, 1969), normal dog (Wesson *et al.*, 1950), and normal monkey (Tisher, Schrier, and McNeil, 1972).

The use of furosemide in another clinical setting also has been investigated (Hantman *et al.*, 1973). Some patients with the syndrome of inappro-

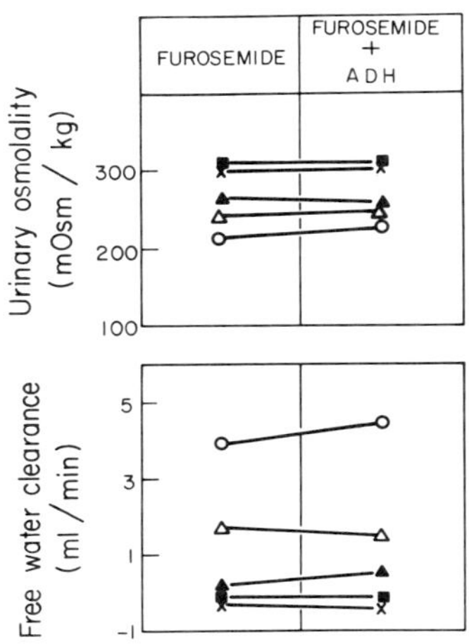

Fig. 2. Effect of exogenous vasopressin (ADH) on urinary osmolality and free-water clearance during furosemide-induced diuresis. Symbols represent the same patients shown in Fig. 1. Values are the means of 3–4 consecutive clearance periods before and after intravenous or subcutaneous administration of vasopressin.

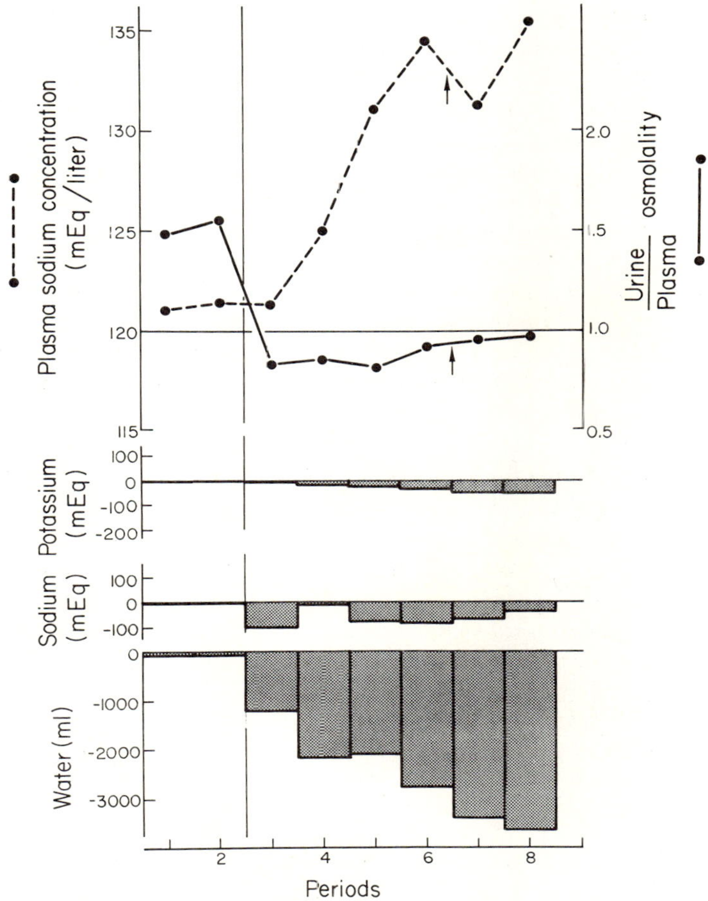

Fig. 3. Use of furosemide and hypertonic saline in the rapid correction of hyponatremia in patient (C.H.) with SIADH. The control periods in this and subsequent figures are separated from the periods collected after furosemide administration by the vertical line. The last dose of furosemide is indicated by the arrow. Each period indicates 1-hr duration of time. Furosemide administration was associated with hypotonic urine and an increase in plasma sodium concentration in the absence of either a positive sodium or potassium balance. The cumulative potassium, sodium, and water balances are shown in the bottom three panels of the figure.

priate ADH secretion (SIADH) may have life-threatening symptoms of cerebral dysfunction associated with severe hyponatremia. In such symptomatic patients with SIADH severe fluid restriction is inadequate to produce an acute negative water balance and rapidly increase serum sodium concentration. In these patients with symptoms of water intoxication, such as increased neural excitability, obtundation, coma, or convulsions, the infusion of hypertonic saline has been the most frequent treatment used. However, since patients with SIADH have retained water, and thus have an increased volume of total body fluids, further volume expansion during the infusion of hypertonic saline could be deleterious. Moreover, because of this volume-expanded state, hypertonic-saline infusions are rapidly excreted and thus may only transiently increase serum sodium concentration. The most appropriate therapy therefore would be rapidly to correct the low serum sodium concentration by producing an acute negative water balance. The results in a patient with SIADH whose plasma sodium concentration was corrected rapidly in this manner are shown in Fig. 3. An acute negative water balance was induced by administering the diuretic, furosemide, to increase urine flow and simultaneously the urinary electrolyte losses were replaced by a hypertonic infusion of sodium chloride and potassium chloride. In this patient the cumulative negative water balance necessary to raise the plasma sodium concentration from 121 to 135 mEq/liter was obtained in 6 hr and amounted to 3600 ml. Since, as shown in the middle panels of Fig. 3, the sodium and potassium balances were slightly negative, none of the rise in plasma sodium concentration could be contributed to the addition of electrolytes to the body fluid compartments. Rather, the negative water balance was the primary cause of the increase in plasma sodium concentration. The rapid rise in serum sodium concentration in five patients with SIADH who were treated by using this same therapeutic approach is shown in Fig. 4. As in the previous patient the sodium and potassium balances were not positive, and the negative water balance was, therefore, primarily responsible for the increases in plasma

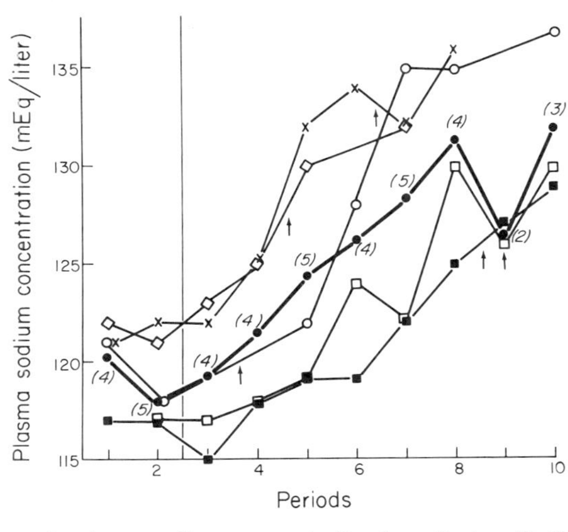

Fig. 4. Increases in plasma sodium concentration in patients with SIADH treated with furosemide and hypertonic saline. Each symbol indicates an individual patient except the symbol (-•-) which indicates the mean values for all the patients. The numbers in parentheses indicate the number of determinations made for each period. The arrows indicate the last dose of furosemide for each patient.

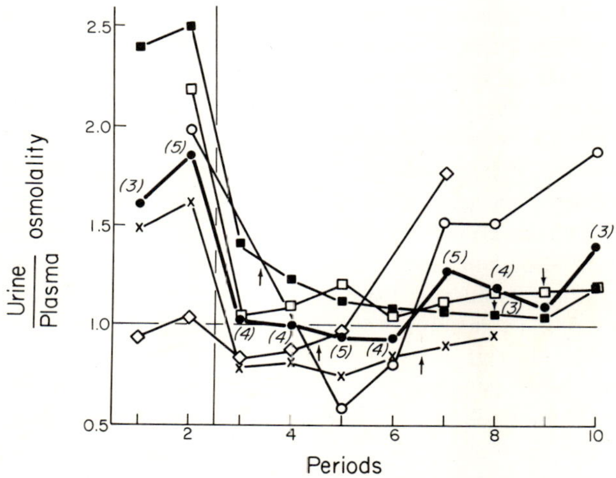

Fig. 5. The effect of furosemide on urinary dilution in patients with SIADH. Each symbol indicates an individual patient except the symbol (-•-) which indicates the mean values for all the patients. The numbers in parentheses indicate the number of determinations made for each period. The urine of three of the five patients became hypotonic after receiving intravenous furosemide and the urine-plasma osmolality ratio approached 1 in the other two patients. The arrows indicate the last dose of furosemide for each patient.

sodium concentration. In Fig. 5 are shown the urinary to plasma osmolality ratios before and after the administration of furosemide. In all circumstances the urinary to plasma osmolality ratio diminished after furosemide administration, and in three of the five patients the urine became hypotonic. It should be emphasized, however, that the urinary sodium and potassium concentrations, rather than the osmolality of the urine, are primarily involved in the effect of any diuresis on plasma sodium concentration. If urinary osmolality falls to hypotonic levels, owing primarily to a decrease in nonelectrolyte solute excretion, the plasma sodium concentration will not increase. The sodium- and potassium-free water losses are thus primarily responsible for the rise in plasma sodium concentration, and such an effect potentially could determine whether the urine is hyper-, hypo-, or isotonic during the furosemide-induced diuresis. Moreover, if urinary sodium and potassium losses are replaced in a concentrated solution, the absolute urine volume rather than the urinary osmolality or cation concentration is of primary importance in achieving the necessary negative water balance to increase the serum sodium concentration. It should, therefore, be apparent that any method which induces a brisk diuresis can be used to correct symptomatic hyponatremia rapidly in patients with SIADH. In this regard, other potent diuretics such as ethacrynic acid may be useful. The use of hypertonic mannitol or hypertonic saline may also lead to the excretion of urine in which the sum of urinary sodium and potassium concentrations is less than that of the plasma sodium concentration. Such a diuresis would therefore ultimately correct the hyponatremia by producing a negative water balance. It should, however, be re-emphasized that both the infusion of hypertonic mannitol and saline are associated with further volume expansion in patients with SIADH who are already in a volume-expanded state. Moreover, in addition to avoiding further volume expansion, the negative water balance necessary to increase plasma sodium concentration in such patients can be more rapidly obtained with potent diuretics such as furosemide.

In Fig. 6 are shown data which support the suggestion that the vasopressin-resistant hypotonic urine induced by furosemide diuresis is related to the increase in solute and water delivery to the collecting duct with incomplete osmotic equilibration of the tubular fluid with the medullary interstitium. In the patients with SIADH who were studied the occurrence of hypotonic urine was observed primarily at high rates of urine flow and solute excretion.

In summary, it has been demonstrated that the use of intravenous furosemide in patients with edematous disorders such as congestive heart failure, cirrhosis, and nephrotic syndrome may be associated with improved rather than worsening of urinary diluting capacity. In some of these patients hypotonic urine may actually occur during a furosemide diuresis despite the effect of furosemide to inhibit sodium reabsorption in the Henle loops where the initial urinary diluting process occurs. This hypotonic urine during furo-

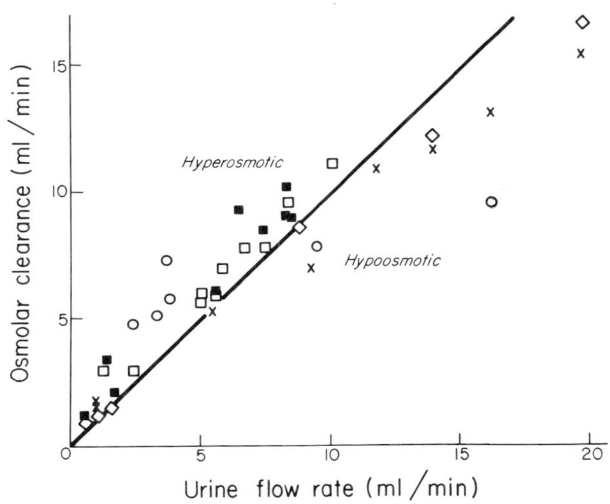

Fig. 6. Osmolar clearances and urine flow rates before and after furosemide administration in patients with SIADH. Values for individual periods are plotted and each symbol indicates an individual patient. The three patients whose urine became hypotonic did so at the highest osmolar clearances and urine flow rates.

semide is unresponsive to exogenous vasopressin administration, therefore suggesting incomplete equilibration between tubular fluid and the medullary interstitium.

Furosemide has also been demonstrated to be of value in the treatment of patients with SIADH and severe symptoms of water intoxication. In such patients with life-threatening central nervous system symptoms water restriction is too slow a treatment, and the rapid infusion of hypertonic sodium chloride infusions will further expand these patients and be rapidly excreted. The approach described herein involves inducing a rapid diuresis with furosemide while simultaneously replacing the urinary cation losses, particularly sodium and potassium. Lastly, it has been emphasized that the efficacy of this treatment in producing a negative water balance and increasing plasma sodium concentration is primarily dependent on the increase in urine volume rather than the urinary osmolality or cation concentrations, providing the urinary electrolyte losses are replaced in a more hypertonic solution than the urine.

ACKNOWLEDGMENTS

The authors are indebted to Lisbeth Streiff, Vicki Neel, and Dorothy Byrd for technical assistance and to Mrs. Linda Benson for secretarial assistance. This work was supported by grants HE 13319-01 and AM 21753 from the National Institutes of Health, and by grant NGR 05-025-007 from the National Aeronautics and Space Administration, and grants from the Bay Area Heart Association and Hoechst Pharmaceutical Company.

REFERENCES

Bell, N.H., H.P. Schedl, and F.C. Bartter. 1964. An explanation for abnormal water retention and hypoosmolality in congestive heart failure. Am. J. Med. 36:351–360.

Clapp, J.R., and R.R. Robinson. 1968. Distal sites of action of diuretic drugs in the dog nephron. Am. J. Physiol. 215:228–235.

Earley, L.E., and R.M. Friedler. 1964. Renal tubular effects of ethacrynic acid. J. Clin. Invest. 43:1495–1506.

Hantman, D., B. Rossier, R. Zohlman, and R.W. Schrier. 1973. Rapid correction of hyponatremia in the syndrome of inappropriate secretion of antidiuretic hormone. Ann. Int. Med. 78: 870–875.

Schedl, H.P., and F.C. Bartter. 1960. An explanation for and experimental correction of the abnormal water diuresis in cirrhosis. J. Clin. Invest. 29:248–261.

Schrier, R.W., D. Lehman, B. Zacherle, and L.E. Earley. 1973. Effect of furosemide on free water excretion in edematous patients with hyponatremia. Kidney Internatn. 3:30–34.

Seldin, D.W., G. Eknoyan, W.N. Suki, and F.C. Rector, Jr. 1966. Localization of diuretic action from the pattern of water and electrolyte excretion. Ann. N. Y. Acad. Sci. 139:328–343.

Tannen, R.L., E.M. Regal, M.J. Dunn, and R.W. Schrier. 1969. Vasopressin-resistant hyposthenuria in advanced chronic renal disease. New Engl. J. Med. 280:1135–1141.

Tisher, C.C., R.W. Schrier, and J.S. McNeil. 1972. Nature of the urine concentrating mechanism in the macaque monkey. Am. J. Physiol. 223:1128–1137.

Wesson, L.G., W.P. Anslow, L.G. Raisz, A.A. Bolomey, and M. Ladd. 1950. Effect of sustained expansion of extracellular fluid volume upon filtration rate, renal plasma flow and electrolyte and water excretion in the dog. Am. J. Physiol. 162:677–686.

Index